RECENT ADVANCES IN CROHN'S DISEASE

DEVELOPMENTS IN GASTROENTEROLOGY

VOLUME 1

Also in this series:

2. Motta PM, Didio LJA, eds: Basic and clinical hepatology. 1981.
ISBN 90-247-2475-9

series ISBN 90-247-2441-4

RECENT ADVANCES IN CROHN'S DISEASE

Proceedings of the 2nd International Workshop on Crohn's Disease,
Noordwijk / Leiden, 25-28 June 1980

edited by

A.S. PEÑA
Department of Gastroenterology,
State University of Leiden, Leiden,
The Netherlands

IRENE T. WETERMAN
Department of Gastroenterology,
State University of Leiden, Leiden,
The Netherlands

C.C. BOOTH
Clinical Research Centre,
Northwick Park, Harrow,
U.K.

W. STROBER
National Cancer Institute,
National Institutes of Health, Bethesda, MD,
U.S.A.

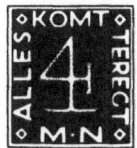

1981

MARTINUS NIJHOFF PUBLISHERS
THE HAGUE / BOSTON / LONDON

Distributors:

for the United States and Canada

Kluwer Boston, Inc.
190 Old Derby Street
Hingham, MA 02043
USA

for all other countries

Kluwer Academic Publishers Group
Distribution Center
P.O. Box 322
3300 AH Dordrecht
The Netherlands

This volume is listed in the Library of Congress Cataloging in Publication Data

ISBN-13: 978-94-009-8275-8   e-ISBN-13: 978-94-009-8273-4
DOI: 10.1007/978-94-009-8273-4

Published February 1981.

FOREWORD

The study of disease entities as complex as Crohn's disease will increasingly require comprehensive knowledge of formerly unrelated areas of the medical sciences. To promote this broad approach, a conference was organized in which geneticists, morphologists, immunologists, and virologists participated as well as clinicians whose work is focused on Crohn's disease. Ample time was given to the presentation of major new findings in each of these areas, and comments were given by the participants in the various sections. This approach yielded many new ideas, because individuals with very different backgrounds were able to address old problems from fresh angles.

This volume, published in January, 1981, contains the papers presented during the workshop held in June, 1980, in Noordwijk/Leiden, The Netherlands. In addition, we have included the extensive discussions, edited by experts in the field, which followed each presentation. Finally, each main category is followed by a summary of the topic covered as well as many valuable conclusions concerning the significance of recent work and ideas for new directions in research. In the Preface, J.B. Kirsner gives a comprehensive review of the material, and in an Afterword A.J.Ch. Haex deals with a number of other aspects.

We believe that this volume will be of value to a wide spectrum of scientists and clinicians and that it will help to establish the multidisciplinary approach to Crohn's disease as the one that should predominate in the future.

The Editors

CONTENTS

PREFACE

by Joseph B. Kirsner
The Louis Block Distinguished Service Professor of Medicine
University of Chicago, Chicago, U.S.A.

The "Coming of Age" of Crohn's disease

"Natura non facit saltus"
Nature does not proceed by leaps, but rather reveals its
secrets slowly, quitely and grudgingly. Notable advances
of today have their background in work often carried out
decades before.
Carl Linnaeus, Philosophica Botanica, (Section 77), 1751

It is perhaps difficult in 1980 to realize that not too
long ago, Crohn's disease was an unknown entity; and that for
many years after its classic description by Crohn, Ginsberg
and Oppenheimer in 1932, this entity was infrequently discussed and rarely investigated. Today, Crohn's disease is
regarded as one of the more challenging problems in medicine;
in part, because of its rising incidence in many parts of the
world; in part, because of the intriguing associated systemic
problems and in part, because Crohn's disease clinically and
investigationally involves so many scientific disciplines:
internist, psychiatrist, pharmacologist, gastroenterologist,
radiologist, surgeon, pathologist, immunologist, geneticist,
biochemist, cell biologist, among other basic sciences.

The immediately impressive feature of this book then is that it is a compilation of nearly 100 papers presented in a three-day meeting in The Netherlands in June 1980, attended by approximately 100 physicians and scientists; a constellation of topics and participants that would not have been possible a few years earlier. This workshop also is a testimony to the highly informed administrative talent of the programs' organizers: Prof.Dr. A.J.Ch. Haex and Dr. A.S. Peña of Leiden, The Netherlands, who selected the speakers and arranged the meeting. In refreshing contrast to the usual international symposium, the emphasis here is upon recent or newer observations, especially in the areas of epidemiology, histopathology, genetics, microbiology, immunology, and some aspects of therapy. As such, the book contains much valuable information on the nature of Crohn's disease; especially of interest to the investigator. The organization of the material, as shown in the contents, reflects currently attractive research areas.

Though focussed on selected research aspects of Crohn's disease, the individual presentations and the subsequent discussions reflect an awareness; perhaps an anticipation of additional knowledge yet to come. Where then are we today in our understanding of Crohn's disease?

We know more of its clinical features and its course than ever before. An enormous number of complications; local and systemic; now have been identified; in themselves intriguing pathogenetically since they implicate the diseased bowel and its internal milieu as the source of these difficulties. They also direct attention to concepts of individual vulnerability and individual resistance to both the bowel disease and the associated systemic disorders. However, the underlying cause or causes of Crohn's disease remain obscure; and this continuing deficiency provides the motivation for these proceedings.

Although several recent papers report a declining incidence (Aberdeen, Scotland and Stockholm county, Sweden), the rising incidence of Crohn's disease elsewhere in the world is intriguing; all the more so in view of the similar clinical features of Crohn's disease everywhere, despite different ethnic populations, environmental circumstances, dietary habits and socio-cultural customs. Possible explanations have included some type of virus, unusual microbial agents, dietary constituent,(i.e., excessive intakes of sugar), environmental pollutant, tobacco or contraceptive steroids; but without decisive supporting evidence. Carefully organized epidemiological studies of Crohn's disease, except in a few discrete geographic areas have been lacking; studies that could provide useful clues for further investigations. Epidemiological studies and other cooperative clinical projects would be greatly enhanced by more easily applied and more uniform criteria of diagnosis, and by generally acceptable quantified assessment of clinical activity. Despite considerable application in the United States via the National Cooperative Crohn's Disease Study [NCCDS], the Crohn's disease activity index has not proved to be an easily utilized measure of disease activity. The initial part of this workshop, directed to this particular question therefore considers an important practical problem. The challenge is especially great because of the absence of any single pathognomonic feature or laboratory test of Crohn's disease, the relatively non-specific clinical and histopathological manifestations, and because of the associated clinical problems. Despite their many similarities, the two entities: Crohn's disease and ulcerative colitis, correctly should be separated in any consideration of inflammatory bowel disease; for this object to be attained. Despite current limitations, the more uniform objective assessment of clinical activity should be an attainable goal, worthy of further effort. Once achieved, the information should accelerate future cooperative clinical studies of Crohn's disease.

More complete morphologic understanding of the Crohn's tissue reaction always has been accepted as a potentially clarifying approach to the nature of the disease. Knowledge in this area has been limited by the available methodology;

a deficiency now being remedied in part by more careful light microscopy and by the use of transmission and scanning electron microscopy, histochemical and immunohistochemical studies. These approved techniques reveal the intensity of the Crohn's inflammatory reaction, affecting every constituent of the bowel wall [epithelial cells, blood vessels, muscle layers and neural elements),multiple cellular types, including polymorphonuclear leucocytes, lymphocytes, eosinophils, basophils, mast cells, Paneth cells and macrophages; and the widely disseminated though focal distribution of the identifiable Crohn's lesion. A handicap of the present morpholocigal approach is imposed by current limitations in knowledge, as to what to look for, how to seek it and where to look. The granuloma, though easily recognized and often emphasized as diagnostic, is not specific to Crohn's disease. Granulomas are not evident in 50 percent of patients; their regional distribution varies and, apparently, once having been present, they may disappear. While some animal transmission studies have utilized the granuloma and the site of the "causative agent" of Crohn's disease, decisive supportive evidence has not appeared. Whether or not the granuloma reflects an adaptive protective response of the host to an etiological agent awaits much more knowledge of both Crohn's disease and host defenses in general.

The specificity of the histologic changes also remains in question. The focal nature of the early Crohn's lesion, its scattered distribution along the entire gastrointestinal tract, and the micro-ulcerations of the dome epithelium of the Peyer's patches on the other hand, are observations of potential etiologic significance; perhaps compatible with an unusual viral or microbial agent but also perhaps corresponding to the "focal" distribution of the lymphoid follicles in the bowel wall. Future studies of the nature of the Crohn's disease tissue reaction should evaluate not only the possible role of mast cells and Paneth cells, but also there the prostanoids, thromboxane, lysosomal enzymes of monocytic origin; and intestinal endorphins and enkephalins.

The search for pathogenic bacteria, viruses and other microbial agents has been in progress since the entity was first described. Beginning with the exclusion of the tubercle bacillus, then Shigella, E. histolytica and lymphopathia venereum virus, all hitherto known bacterial, viral and parasitic agents appeared to have been eliminated. However, the recent identification of "new" bacterial causes of enteritis and colitis i.e., Yersinia Pseudotuberculosis, Campylobacter fetus ss. jejuni, and Aeromonas hydrophila has rekindled microbiological interest in Crohn's disease. Today, the microbiological focus is upon such anaerobic organisms, as Eubacteria and Peptostreptococcus [strains C_{18}, Me_{46}, Me_{47}] cell-wall defective, Pseudomonas-like bacteria, various strains of E. coli, Mycobacteria and Mycoplasma. However, convincing data for the etiological involvement of any infectious agent in Crohn's disease has not been published.

Microbial interest has centered also upon a possible viral etiology; based upon such indirect information as the presence of lymphocytotoxic antibodies in the family household contacts of Crohn's patients; and the apparent presence of a "transmissible agent" the cytopathic constituent in Crohn's disease tissue injected into animals [mouse, rabbit]. However, while some observations are intriguing, including either the development of ulcerative colitis or Crohn's disease among married couples [five such reports], the evidence to date is inconclusive. The demonstration of similar in vitro cytopathic effects, though less often, with non-IBD intestinal tissues, the negative results of other investigators utilizing a variety of virological techniques, the inability to reproduce the disease with cultured agents obtained from resected Crohn's tissue, the inability to identify viral particles or intraepithelial microorganisms on electron microscopy and the non-fulfillment of Koch's postulates, all of these observations indicate the need for restraint in the acceptance of the viral etiology. Nevertheless, the demonstration of replicating, transmissible cytopathic agents in Crohn's disease tissue is at least worthy of further cooper-

ative examination; especially with more subtle virus-demon-
strating techniques. All that is known of Crohn's disease
clinically and histopathologically, is compatible with microbiological involvement of some type. Microbiological concepts
worthy of further study might include an "imbalance" of the
normal entero-colonic microflora, and hypersensitivity of the
gut-associated immune apparatus to constituents of the endogenous normal bacterial flora, and to bacterial products
[lipopolysscharides, endotoxins].

The possible involvement of the immunological mechanism
in inflammatory bowel disease, first proposed by Kirsner and
Palmer in 1954, continues to be a highly active research
area. The immunological studies to date have demonstrated a
central role of the gastrointestinal tract in the immunological homeostasis of the body and the importance of the gut-
associated lymphoid tissue and the locally protective role of
secretory IgA at the gastrointestinal epithelial surface.
Although immunological processes probably play some role in
Crohn's disease, an immunological basis for this disease has
not been established. The many immunological observations
[both humoral and cellular] in Crohn's disease at present are
confusing and difficult to interpret; including circulating
antibodies against bacterial, viral, food, human and rat
colon, as well as enterobacterial and various tissue antigens, defective cutaneous anergy, the variations in B and T
cell numbers and proportions, imbalances in various T cell
subsets [normal total T cell numbers and marked decreases in
proportion and absolute numbers of the cells bearing Fc receptors for IgM], IgM-type lymphocytotoxic antibodies against
B cells, the absence of a consistent correlation between
major immunoglobulin classes and the activity of the inflammatory bowel disease, the variable lymphocyte responses to
mitogens, the possible presence and the role of circulating
immune complexes, the increased monocytic lysosomal enzyme
activity, the alterations in complement [elevated C_3, C_4 and
increased metabolism of Cl_q and C_3 and the activation of the
alternate complement pathway]; all of these findings, and

others, appear to be secondary epiphenomena rather than primary etiologically significant features of the disease. Since studies of the blood do not necessarily reflect the local immunological status of the gastrointestinal tract, techniques are being developed for isolating and assessing the comparable immunobiological activities of non-epithelial cell populations obtained from the intestinal wall; especially lymphocytes and macrophages. Such studies have demonstrated increased numbers of B type lymphoid cells in the intestinal infiltrates, T cells, and variable numbers of IgA, IgM, IgG, IgD and IgE cells in the lamina propria; "killer" lymphocytes, and other lymphocyte subsets. Since the present methodology does not permit the separation of "pure" lymphocytes, the studies to date on mixed lymphocytes populations, probably have limited significance. Nevertheless, further investigation of gut mucosal immune defenses, including antigenic penetration of the bowel mucosa, and possible defect in the mucosal secretory [IgA] immune system are attractive approaches. The presence of elements of the complement system, $[Cl_q, C_3]$ and increased number of immunoglobulin-containing cells and immune complexes in Crohn's disease tissue are compatible with a local immune mediated reaction, perhaps in genetically-determined vulnerable individuals.

The concept of an individual [genetic] predisposition to IBD derives from the selective occurrences of IBD after enteric [food poisoning] and viral infections [infectious mononucleosis], the increased incidence of Ankylosing Spondylitis, a disorder with an established autosomal dominant gene mechanism, and especially from the observed multiple instances of IBD in the same family. Numerous surveys now have documented the familial occurrence of Crohn's disease in at least 20 percent and up to 35 percent of patients, exceeding the most generous estimates of IBD incidence in the general population. The familial tendency appears stronger in Crohn's disease than ulcerative colitis. Most of the familial occurrences are in one additional family member, but numerous families of three or more, up to eight affected members have been reported. First-degree relatives are more vulnerable. The intermingling of these two disorders among family members is an intriguing feature. At least 11 reports have documented the occurrence of Crohn's disease among monozygotic twins. No genetic markers have been identified in Crohn's disease; and inheritable protein, enzymatic or metabolic defects or chromosomal abnormalities have not been demonstrated. The chromosomal changes reported thus far appear to be non-specific, possibly attributable to the associated under nutrition, yet unidentified metabolic alterations or to the many potent medications prescribed. The genetic mechanism implicated in the individual vulnerability to IBD are not known. The most likely explanation appears to be the combined interaction or multiple genes, the multifactorial or polygenic type of inheritance. The genetic contribution presumably would be to facilitate a state of susceptibility, locally and systemically, with the precipitation of Crohn's disease by varied external environmental circumstances. The nature of the susceptibility is not known. No consistent association has been found thus far between specific HLA antigens [HLA-A,-B,-C, or -DR locus antigens] and Crohn's disease, except for the positive correlation with HLA-B27 in those patients with ankylosing spondilytis or acute iritis. However, the possibility of other associations, positive or negative, with other HLA antigens awaits further investigations, especially since present studies have dealt with only a small portion of the human genome. This research area is all more attractive in view of the possible relationship between elements of the human genome and immunoregulatory mechanisms.

The treatment of Crohn's disease continues to involve arbitrary approaches. We are more aware today of the limitations of the medical and surgical therapy. In view of the frequent recurrences, operations now are reserved chiefly for serious complications of the disease, and the tendency is toward limited rather than radical bowel resection. In medical management, dependence upon sulphazalasine and steroids alone [usually prednisone] alone often is insufficiently to control Crohn's disease continuously. Experience support the usefulness of a program of management, including emotional and physical rest, the restoration and maintenance of optimal nutrition as essential to an adequate response to medications; symptomatic measures to review abdominal discomfort and diarrhea ["steroids-savers"], and the judicious use of antibacterial, anti-inflammatory and "immuno-suppresive" drugs, each adapted to individual responses. For many drugs i.e., sulphazalasine and metronidazole the rationale is unclear; for "immuno-suppresive" medication, requiring up to six months for recognizable therapeutic benefit, whose allegedly immuno-suppresive effects in Crohn's disease have not been demonstrated, and for drugs such as superoxide dismutase and d-penicillamine, whose biological properties and clinical effects are poorly understood, we can only speculate on their therapeutic advantages and limitations. The "scientifically" more acceptable approach of "controlled clinical trials" thus far has failed to provide new insights into the nature of Crohn's disease as revealed by the therapeutic response. The various therapeutical measures currently recommended for Crohn's disease probably have no specific influence upon the tissue reaction per se; but rather, a dampening or inhibiting effect upon the inflammatory/immune Crohn's process; applied simultaneously with efforts to improve host defenses. Clinical improvement does seem attributable more to the individual capacity to contain the disease than to any "specific" drug effect. If this concept is valid, then future studies of Crohn's disease should emphasize fundamental investigations of systemic and local [gut] host defenses, the nature of immunocompetence and immunoregulation; the relationship of human immune response genes to the MHC chromosomal region and to the body's defense against microbial and viral agents, and how these mechanisms may influence the individual's response to endogenous and exogenous microbial agents. There already is evidence of an increased susceptibility to certain infections among individuals bearing a given B lymphocyte alloantigen; and japanese investigators have succesfully identified

HLA-linked control of immune responses to microbial antigens. The combination of microbial factors, host immune responses and genetic influences will encompass the more likely mechanisms in the pathogenesis of IBD.

This approach then is perhaps the major "message" of these proceedings. None of the concepts advanced here probably will endure additional scientific scrutiny. Nevertheless, they document the broadening scientific interest in Crohn's disease, and they examine at least preliminary, some newer ideas. The proceedings also demonstrate the involvement of more, better prepared researches in the study of Crohn's disease than in the past; a major advance. The Second International Workshop on Crohn's Disease thus constitute a "portal of entry" to research in progress, as well as to research in the future. As such, it documents the "coming of age", the blossoming of Crohn's disease as a medical disorder worthy of the most careful clinical and scientific investigation. Such developments alone are sufficient to renew the hope that the 1980 Holland Workshop, by encouraging more perceptive research by well-trained investigators, eventually will increase the basic knowledge of Crohn's disease; a necessary prelude to the more effective control and perhaps even the cure of what has emerged as one the more challenging medical disorders of our time.

SECTION A

DEFINITION AND ASSESSMENT OF ACTIVITY

Section Editor: S.C. Truelove

DEFINITION OF CROHN'S DISEASE

F.T. DE DOMBAL

A priori, it must be admitted that the task of this section - to define Crohn's disease - is at the present time
impossible. True definition of a disease must depend upon an
understanding of its fundamental nature which far exceeds our
present imperfect understanding of Crohn's disease. There is
for Crohn's disease no "philosopher's stone", no single test
or feature the presence of which is solely associated with
the disease; and hence in a very real sense, we cannot define
it.

Karl Popper, one of the great scientists of the twentieth
century, would have argued that this is not necessarily the
case. He would have argued in favour of a "nominalist" or
"right to left" definition - that is to say one in which
scientific opinion agreed upon a subset of features which
appear to characterize Crohn's disease patients, and then
agreed [like a kind of shorthand] to use "Crohn's disease" as
a term to describe the ailment from which such patients suffer.

However, until very recently, the picture was even more
gloomy for there has been no clear-cut multinational statement of what workers around the world have agreed to call
Crohn's disease, and hence even a "nominalist" definition has
not been possible. For this reason, in the last four years, a
large-scale multinational survey of patients with inflammatory bowel disease has been carried out under the auspices of
the Research Committee of the World Organisation of Gastro-
Enterology with the aim of characterising those features
[around the world], which are said to be associated with both
ulcerative colitis and Crohn's disease.

By 1978 some 1090 patients from 21 centres had been registered into this study.

Most centres were able to supply data from consecutive, prospective series of cases. Of the 1090 patients registered into the survey, 585 were diagnosed as having ulcerative colitis and no less than 471 as having Crohn's disease. Only 34 cases were rejected from the trial, 26[2.4%] because no agreed diagnosis could be made. Data collection was outstanding; of a possible 67,584 items of information, no less than 62,699 [92.8%] were collected and forwarded for analysis.

Further details of this survey are set out at some length in a recent special supplementum of the Scandinavian Journal of Gastroenterology (1). It is not proposed to reiterate these data in depth in this presentation, but it may be of interest, to re-emphasize some of the features shown by this survey to characterize patients with Crohn's disease around the world.

Table 1. Features associated with 585 patients suffering from ulcerative colitis and 471 patients suffering from Crohn's disease, after Myren (1).

| | Associated with | |
Feature	Crohn's disease	ulcerative colitis
Clinical	severe pain complications tenderness/mass wasting/distension	6+ bowel action/day bleeding per rectum 3+ mucus per rectum 3+
Radiology	segmental change stenosis dilatation fistulae skip lesions	
Endoscopy	normal findings patchy change	ulcers/bleeding continuous change
Biopsy	giant cells granuloma transmural change	ulcers mucosal change

As regards clinical features, severe diarrhoea [more than 6 bowel actions per day], and marked rectal bleeding or passage of mucus were more characteristic of ulcerative colitis than Crohn's disease. By contrast severe abdominal pain, perianal complications, abdominal tenderness, emaciation or wasting, abdominal mass or distension were all significantly [p<0.01] more frequently noted in patients ultimately diagnosed as having Crohn's disease.

Similarly, as regards radiological findings, segmental change, stenosis, dilatation, fistulae, and skip lesions were all associated with Crohn's disease. Interestingly, other features, such as ulcers or polyps were noted in roughly equal proportions of patients with Crohn's disease and ulcerative colitis.

Turning to endoscopy findings the chief distinguishing feature of Crohn's disease seems to be its "geographical" distribution. Crohn's disease patients were characterized by normal findings or patchy change, ulcerative colitis patients by contact bleeding and by continuous mucosal change throughout the field of vision. Once again, ulcers and polyps were seen with equal frequency in both diseases.

Often biopsy is possible at endoscopy, and the histopathological features of Crohn's disease [giant cells, granulomata, and transmural change] are amongst the most "characteristic" of all. Nevertheless, it needs to be added that not every feature is found in every biopsy specimen [possibly due to the limited size of each biopsy].

Two further general points are worthy of note. First, the World Organisation study is on-going. To date over 1500 cases have been surveyed, though the conclusions remain the same. Second, it cannot be too strongly emphasized that these characteristics do not [in an essentialist sense] define Crohn's disease, nor are they "the truth". They are simply the criteria by which over 20 centres around the world recognize a clinical entity which they refer to as "Crohn's disease". Inasmuch as the criteria in table 1 are rather consistent between centres however, they could be said [for good or ill] to constitute a "nominalist" definition - currently acceptable worldwide - of Crohn's disease.

Of course, all of the foregoing argument may be invalidated overnight by the advent of a single test which simultaneously explains [satisfactorily] the aetiology of Crohn's disease, and discriminates [reliably] between it and other diseases such as ulcerative colitis. All that can be said at the present time is that - despite much work - the prospects for such a test do not look very promising. Until the advent of such a test, therefore, the above characteristics set out in table 1 will have to suffice as an imperfect but perhaps acceptable present-day definition of "Crohn's disease".

ACKNOWLEDGEMENTS

It is a pleasure to acknowledge the contribution of all those associated with the Inflammatory Bowel Disease study of the World Organisation of Gastro-Enterology. Part of this work was aided by a grant from the Medical Research Council of the United Kingdom which is acknowledged with gratitude.

REFERENCE
1. Myren J, Bouchier IAD, Watkinson G, de Dombal FT. (1979) Inflammatory Bowel Disease, an O.M.G.E. Survey. In "Studies co-ordinated by the Research Committee of the Organisation Mondiale de Gastroenterologie". Scand.J.Gastroenterol. 14, Suppl. 56: 1-29

THE CROHN'S DISEASE ACTIVITY INDEX AS A CLINICAL INSTRUMENT

W.R. BEST and J.M. BECKTEL

INTRODUCTION

Attempts to quantify clinical activity of Crohn's disease [CD] are made difficult by the facts that it is a disease of unknown etiology and that its manifestations are nonspecific. In planning the National Cooperative Crohn's Disease Studies [NCCDS], it was apparent that some composite index of disease activity would be useful to classify initial states, to identify worsening sufficient to mandate removal from study, to quantify clinical response, and to regulate corticosteroid dosage.

The Crohn's Disease Activity Index [CDAI] was developed through multiple regression analysis, using physician's overall assessment of disease activity as dependent variable and various clinical independent variables(1). It utilizes observations readily available at a visit, uses only coefficients with intuitively appropriate signs, regresses through the origin, and rounds to one significant digit, thus:

$$CDAI = 2X_1 + 5X_2 + 7X_3 + 20X_4 + 30X_5 + 10X_6 + 7X_7 + X_8$$

where X_1=Number of soft/liquid stools in one week, X_2=Sum of abdominal pain ratings [0-3] for one week, X_3=Sum of wellbeing ratings [0-4] for one week, X_4=Number of types of extraintestinal findings [fistula, arthritis, uveitis, etc.], X_5= Opiates or Lomotil [0-none, 1-used], X_6=Abdominal mass [0-none, 2-questionable, 5-present], X_7=[47 – hematocrit] in males; [42 – hematocrit] in females, and X_8=100 -[Percentage of standard weight].

The CDAI was integral to two therapeutic trials of the NCCDS (2-4). The 8 coefficients of the CDAI were rederived

from these studies, and conformity was remarkably close(5).
There are over 60 references to CDAI in the literature; in
most it was part of a study design. It correlates with enteric protein clearance(6), B_{12} absorption(6), bile acid pool
size (7), erythrocyte sedimentation rate(8), β_2-microglobulin
levels(9), immune complexes(10), leucocyte endogenous mediator (11), and endotoxin levels(12). Reservations about the
CDAI include the subjective(13) and nonspecific(14) nature of
some input variables, questions as to whether it is sufficiently sensitive (10,15), concern over an early placebo
response (16), and the nuisance of computation (8,17,18).

We felt that a more comprehensive study of CDAI in clinical management of CD was needed. Harvey and Bradshaw [H/B]
modified the CDAI into a simple clinical index (18); we believed their index should be further evaluated and other
simplified indices explored.

PROCEDURE
Questionnaires were sent to the 13 principal investigators and 159 study physicians of the NCCDS. Valid addresses
were located for 84% [145/172]. Questionnaires were returned
by 50% [73] of these.
Data from 1,332 patient-visits [including 1,058 used
previously(5)] were subjected to multivariate regression
techniques in which special relationships between coefficients were forced.

RESULTS
NCCDS studies called for two physician roles: A was blinded to therapy, evaluated patient manifestations, could but
was not required to review CDAI; B was not blinded, did not
interact with patients directly, was responsible for dosage
adjustment according to protocol usings CDAI and other data.
Of respondents only 66% [48] had actually worked with CDAI,
and of these 77% acted only as A, 10% only as B and 13% as A
for some patients B for others. 54% participated in NCCDS as

a GI Fellow, 33% as a GI Attending physician, and 13% in some other capacity. Specific questions, number of pertinent responses [N], and percentage distribution among options follow. "The CDAI corresponds with my clinical impression of severity of illness "[41];"remarkably well"--22%,"fairly well"--71%, "so-so" --7% "poorly" --0%, and "not at all"--0%. "Relative to clinical practice, I now consider the CDAI to be" [34]; invaluable" --0% "very useful" --18%, "helpful"--29%, "of slight value"--50%, and "worthless"-- 3%. "I have used the CDAI... [in subsequent management of CD]..."[47]; "almost all the time"--6%, "frequently"--4%,"sometimes"--32%, and "never--57%. "I have done subsequent research involving the clinical course of patients with CD" [48]; "no"--77%, "yes, using CDAI"--17%, and "yes, not using CDAI"--6%. "I have personally calculated the CDAI..[and it was].."[28]: "easy to calculate" --18%, "not too hard to calculate"--61%, and "a real pain to calculate"--21%. No respondents had utilized a programmed calculator to compute CDAI(5). Other questions relating to the experience of these physicians with CD and CDAI indicated number [N] and rounded estimates of 10, 50, and 90 percentile values to be: patients monitored as physician A [if any], [31] 2, 5, and 40; as B [if any], [11] 2, 20, and 70; number of subsequent CD's managed, [45] 2, 20, and 65 [7%=none]; number of subsequent CD's on which consulted, [44] 0, 15, and 80 [23%=none]; total visits with CDAI review, [36] 4, 35, and 100; and total occasions CDAI personally computed [if ever], [24] 2, 10, and 55.

Free-form comment was invited. The most frequent concepts volunteered were that the CDAI is valuable in research but not needed in practice [19%], that familiarity with the CDAI had provided perspective in evaluating patient status [17%], that the nuisance of data collection and computation are principal reasons for routine clinical non-use [13%], and that there are some reservations as to the accuracy and pertinence of patient diary responses [4%].

Subsequent computations adopt the H/B conventions of 1-day rather than 7-day values for X_1, X_2 and X_3; deletion of

X_5, X_7 and X_8; and defining new X_5 as 1/2 of CDAI's X_6.

Regression through the origin produced the following equations for estimation of CDAI:

$$\hat{C}_A = 20.7X_1 + 36.1X_2 + 52.2X_3 + 33.5X_4 + 30.7X_5$$
$$\hat{C}_B = 20\ \ X_1 + 35\ \ X_2 + 50\ \ X_3 + 35\ \ X_4 + 30\ \ X_5$$
$$\hat{C}_C = [0.5X_1 + \ \ X_2 + \ \ X_3 + \ \ X_4 + \ \ X_5]\ x\ 40$$
$$\hat{C}_D = [\ \ X_1 + \ \ X_2 + \ \ X_3 + \ \ X_4 + \ \ X_5]\ x\ 30$$

A is the least squares regression through the origin. B rounds to the nearest 5 units. C was chosen after examining B; all coefficients are equal except that b_1 is 1/2 the others; the multiplier is 40.82, rounded to 40. D is the H/B approach, all coefficients equal; the multiplier is 29.83, rounded to 30. The standard deviations from regression are 39.1, 39.4, 40.4, and 46.2 respectively. Equations with similar constraints were developed for prediction of physicians' global estimates of disease activity [scaled 1, 3, 5, and 7]. Standard deviations from regression were 1.25 for CDAI, 1.36 for approach A, 1.36 for approach C, and 1.41 for approach D.

DISCUSSION

CDAI is not widely used in practice, but a simpler index might be. It is worth converting any index into CDAI equivalence to facilitate interpretation. The standard deviation in predicting global estimates is increased by 9% over that of CDAI in going to the optimal or our simplified five-variable indices, and by 13% in going to H/B's index. We recommend C for routine use.

CONCLUSIONS
1. Those who have used CDAI believe it corroborates clinical impressions well.
2. Few, however, believe it is particularly useful in routine management of CD.
3. A principal reason for non-use is the nuisance of comptation.

4. We developed a simple clinical index which appears superior to the index of Harvey and Bradshaw and is recommended.

ACKNOWLEDGEMENTS

From the Abraham Lincoln School of Medicine and the University of Illinois Hospital, Chicago [Dr. Best] and the V.A. Cooperative Studies Program Coordinating Center, Hines, Illinois [Mr. Becktel, now retired]. NCCDS investigators kindly permitted new computations on their data, collected under NIAMDD contract No1-AM2-2210.

REFERENCES
1. Best WR, Becktel JM, Singleton JW, Kern F.Jr.(1976) Development of a Crohn's Disease Activity Index. Gastroenterology 70:439-444
2. Winship DH, Summers RW, Singleton JW, Best WR, Becktel JM, Lenk LF, Kern F.Jr.(1979) National Cooperative Crohn's Disease Study: Study Design and Conduct of Study. Gastroenterology 77:829-842
3. Summers RW, Switz DM, Sessions JT.Jr. Becktel JM, Best WR, Kern F.Jr., Singleton JW.(1979) National Cooperative Crohn's Disease Study: Results of Drug Treatment. Gastroenterology 77:847-869
4. Singleton JW, Summers RW, Kern F.Jr., Becktel JM, Best WR, Hansen RN, Winship DH.(1979) A trial of Sulfasalazine as Adjunctive Therapy in Crohn's Disease. Gastroenterology 77:887-897
5. Best WR, Becktel JM, Singleton JW. (1979) Rederived Values of the Eight Coefficients of the Crohn's Disease Activity Index (CDAI). Gastroenterology 77:843-846
6. Kaufman S, Chalmer B, Heilman R, Beeken W.(1979) A prospective study of the course of Crohn's Disease. Am.J. Digest.Dis. 24:269-276
7. Vantrappen G, Ghoos Y, Rutgeerts P, Janssens J. (1977) Bile acid studies in uncomplicated Crohn's disease. Gut 18:730-735
8. Mee AS, Brown DJ, Jewell DP. (1978) Crohn's Disease activity index--is it useful? Gut 19:A990
9. Descos L, Andre C, Beorchia S, Vincent C, Revillard JP. (1979) Serum levels of 2-microglobulin--a new marker of activity in Crohn's disease. New.Engl.J.Med. 301:441-442
10. Fiasse R, Lurhama AZ, Cambiaso CL, Masson PL, Dive C. (1978) Circulating immune complexes and disease activity in Crohn's disease. Gut 19:611-617
11. Solomons NW, Elson CO, Pekarek RS, Jacob RA, Sandstead HH, Rosenberg IH. (1978) Leukocytic endogenous mediator in Crohn's disease. Infect.Immun. 22:637-639

12. Colin R, Grancher T, Lemeland JF, Hecketsweiler P, Galmiche JP, LeGrix A, Geffroy Y. (1979) Recherche d'une endotoxinemie dans les entero-colitis inflammatoires cryptogenetiques. Gastroenterol.Clin.Biol. 3:15-19
13. Smith RC, Rhodes J, Heatley RV, Hughes LE, Crosby DL, Rees BI, Jones H, Evans KT, Lawrie BW. (1978) Low dose steroids and clinical relapse in Crohn's disease; a controlled trial. Gut 19:606-610
14. Keighley MRB, Arabi Y, Dimock F, Burdon DW, Allan RN, Alexander-Williams J. (1978) Influence of inflammatory bowel disease on intestinal microflora. Gut 19:1099-1104
15. Present DH, Korelitz BI, Wisch N, Glass JL, Sachar DB, Pasternack BS. (1980) Treatment of Crohn's Disease with 6-mercaptopurine. New Engl.J.Med. 302:981-987
16. Vicary FR, Chambers JD, Dhillon P. (1979) Double-blind trial of the use of transfer factor in the treatment of Crohn's Disease. Gut 20:408-413
17. Hecketsweiler P, Bernier JJ, Geffroy Y.(1979) Les Essais therapeutiques au cours de la Maladie de Crohn et de la Rectocolite Hemorragique; Ethique, objectifs, methodologie. Une etude cooperative du G.R.E.C. Gastroenterol. Clin.Biol. 3:67-72
18. Harvey RF, Bradshaw JM. (1980) A simple index of Crohn's Disease activity. Lancet 1:514

ACTIVITY AND ITS ASSESSMENT IN CROHN'S DISEASE

J.F. FIELDING

INTRODUCTION

Assessment of activity in Crohn's disease is notoriously difficult (1). Yet, unless one can assess such activity the quality of patient care cannot be accurately judged and the efficacy of treatment cannot be determined. Moreover, an agreed method of assessment allows multicentre studies to be undertaken on a more uniform basis. As an initial step one must define Crohn's disease and state what is meant by activity. Thereafter, the various methods of assessing such activity can be studied. Activity may be indirectly assessed, either singly or in combination, on the basis of symptoms, signs, haematological, biochemical, immunological and/or radiological investigations. However, activity can only be truly assessed by macroscopic appearances and/or histology. It is well to remember that static histology cannot always determine the presence or absence of activity.

In this paper Crohn's disease is defined as is the meaning of activity. Indirect methods of assessing activity are discussed and a Crohn's disease activity index suggested.

RESULTS AND DISCUSSION

Crohn's disease has been defined (2) as "an inflammatory disease of unknown aetiology, almost invariably chronic, with periods of quiescence interrupted by exacerbations of varying acuteness, severity and duration. It usually involves the ileum, but may involve, either concurrently or consecutively, any part of the gastrointestinal tract.... There are associated radiological and macroscopic and histological appearances which in any given case may be either typical of, or compatible with, the diagnosis".

Activity may be defined most simply and probably most

found weight to be an accurate indicator of the presence or absence of disease activity (4); others have also found weight a useful indicator (11,12). As we are present at this meeting to indirectly honour Boerhaave and his disciples Van Swieten and de Haen we must not forget temperature as an indicator of disease activity; nor should we forget resting pulse. The value of these two parameters should be tested on a prospective basis.

A low haemoglobin, a low serum iron, low serum folate and elevated E.S.R. have all been associated with disease activity (4), with low serum iron and low folate as the better indicators. It has been my experience (4) and that of others (11), but by no means everybody's (1,12) that the E.S.R. is a relatively insensitive indicator of disease activity. Total vitamin B_{12} - binding capacity (TBBC) and serum lysozyme are other indices occasionally used (13).

It has been known for over twenty years and more recently substantiated that serum seromucoids and serum albumin are good indicators of the presence or absence of activity (11,4,12). It is my view that they are still the best indicators we have. C-reactive protein has also been shown to be an indicator of disease activity (1).

I now wish to propose a Crohn's disease activity index for your consideration. I have taken the following guidelines into consideration in its construction. It must have high indices of specificity and sensitivity. It must have a balance between symptoms, signs and laboratory investigations. These laboratory investigations must be capable of being performed in all laboratories. It must be sufficiently simple to be acceptable and capable of accurate compilation on a wide basis.

The symptoms are: overall state of health, good [0], moderate [1], poor [2]; appetite, good [0], poor [1]. The signs are: weight, steady or increased [0], diminished [1]; resting pulse, less than 85 [0], 85 to 99 [1], 100 or over [2]; temperature, less than 99°F [0], 99 to 99.9°F [1], 100°F or more [2]; clubbing, absent [0], present [1]; perianal

accurately as the presence of Crohn's disease-related biologically active inflammation. Thus the presence of a perianal
abscess is not of itself indicative of active Crohn's disease. Moreover pain from ankylosing spondylitis, or from
gallstones or a duodenal ulcer in a patient with significant
small bowel resection, is not regarded as symptomatic evidence of active Crohn's disease.

Symptomatic evidence of activity is difficult to evaluate. It must not be ignored, but it is subjective and varies
from day to day, too much reliance on it makes for inaccurate
assessment. In this context one must remember that patients
with Crohn's disease are not immune from gastroenteritis,
irritable bowel syndrome symptoms, and fibrotic stenotic
disease can be associated with severe symptoms(3). Inaccuracy
applies particularly to stool frequency (4), especially in
those who have had previous intestinal resection (5). Assessment of general well being may give sufficient information (4,6) although I have found appetite a helpful additive
discriminant (4). Unless pain is associated with and lessen-
ed by defaecation it may not be related to Crohn's disease
activity since bolus colic is not an uncommon cause of pain
in patients with Crohn's disease.

With regard to signs, finger clubbing has been shown to
be a good indicator of disease activity (7,8). The presence
of an abdominal mass has also been shown to be associated
with disease activity (6). I believe one has to define mass
more carefully before drawing such conclusions; palpation of
"thickened" bowel wall does not of itself indicate disease
activity. The presence of a squelch sign has recently been
shown to be associated with active Crohn's disease(9). The
squelch sign is present when a feeling analogous to surgical
emphysema is noted on palpation of the bowel wall and this
sensation is accompanied by a squelching sound. This finding
requires confirmation by studies of larger numbers of patients. Perianal tags are the only perianal disease which I
found to be associated with disease activity (10). I have

tags, absent [0], present [1]; abdominal mass, absent [0], present [1]; squelch sign, absent [0], present [1]. The investigative parameters are: serum albumin, normal [0], low [2]; serum seromucoids, normal [0], elevated [2].

These parameters, I believe, fulfil the above guidelines and would form a useful framework for the follow up and treatment of patients with Crohn's disease.

REFERENCES
1. Mee AS, Brown DJ, Jewell DP. (1978) Crohn's disease activity index - is it useful? Gut 19:A990
2. Fielding JF. (1971) Crohn's disease. Oxford Med.School Gaz. 24:22-27
3. Allan RN, Cooke WT. (1980) Inflammatory bowel disease. In: Recent Advances in Gastroenterology. Ed. Bouchier IAD, Churchill Livingstone Edinburgh,London and New York Vol 4: pp 124
4. Fielding JF. (1971) Clinical Assessment in the follow up of patients with Regional Enteritis; its Correlation with Haematological and Biochemical Parameters. J.Irish Med. Assoc. 64:221-224
5. Brooke BN. (1980) Index of Crohn's disease Activity. Lancet 1:711(c)
6. Harvey RF, Bradshaw JM. (1980) A simple Index of Crohn's disease activity. Lancet 1:514
7. Fielding JF, Cooke WT. (1971) Finger clubbing and regional enteritis. Gut 12:442-444
8. Kitis G, Thompson H, Allan RN. (1979) Finger clubbing in inflammatory bowel disease: its prevalence and pathogenesis. Brit.Med.J. 2:825-828
9. Fielding JF. (1980) The right iliac fossa squelch sign; a further marker of the irritable bowel syndrome. Clin.Gastroenterol. In press.
10. Fielding JF. (1972) Perianal lesions in Crohn's disease. J.R.Coll.Surg.Edinb. 17:32-37
11. Cooke WT, Fowler DJ, Cox EV, Gaddie R, Meywell MJ. (1958) The Clinical significance of seromucoids in Regional Ileitis and Ulcerative Colitis. Gastroenterology 34:910-919
12. Hees van P, Velde ten G, Hogezand van R, Driessen W, Bakker J, Lier van H, Elteren van Ph, Tongeren van J. (1980) Effect of sulfasalazine in patients with active Crohn's disease. Hepatogastroenterol. Supplement International Congress of Gastroenterol. - A.S.N.E.M.G.E. - Abstract E 38.5:311
13. Kane SP, Hoffbrand AV, Neale G. (1974) Indices of granulocyte activity in inflammatory bowel disease. Gut 15:953-959

AN INDEX OF INFLAMMATORY ACTIVITY IN PATIENTS WITH CROHN'S DISEASE

P.A.M. VAN HEES, Ph. VAN ELTEREN, H.J.J. VAN LIER and J.H.M. VAN TONGEREN

INTRODUCTION

Crohn's disease [CD] is a condition which encompasses a wide variety of complaints and symptoms. These may be related to the inflammatory activity, but even when there is little activity there may be considerable subjective complaints - for example, of abdominal pain as a result of the presence of an inactive fibrous stricture. This diversity of the causes of the complaints and the lesions found greatly impedes exact evaluation of the effect of various types of therapeutic medication on the inflammatory activity. During the preparations for a prospective study which was to establish the effects of various types of therapeutic medication on the inflammatory activity in CD, the need arose for an optimally objective and quantifiable standard of inflammatory activity. The Crohn's Disease Activity Index [CDAI] described by Best et al. (1) has, we believe, several disadvantages. With the aid of data from a retrospective study, we therefore attempted to develop a more suitable activity index - that is, an optimally objective and reproducible quantitative standard of inflammatory activity - for patients with CD.

METHODS

The retrospective study covered the data on 63 patients with CD who, during the period 1963-75, had been submitted to a total of 85 clinical examinations.

The study considered only those hospital periods in which the 18 variables listed in table 1 had all been collected. The Quetelet-index relates body weight to body height. Fisures, fistulae, and perianal abscesses were taken into account as anal and perianal lesions. Arthritis, stomatitis [aphthae], erythema nodosum, episcleritis, iritis, and irido-cyclitis were taken into account as extraintestinal lesions related to CD.

Table 1. Independent variables used in development of Activity Index.

Variable		Unit/code
x_1	rate of defaecation	number of defaecations per day
x_2	stool consistency	1= well-formed;2=soft,variable; 3=watery
x_3	blood in faeces	1=no;2=moderate;3=much
x_4	mucus in faeces	1=no;2=yes
x_5	temperature	centigrade
x_6	abdominal mass	1=no;2=dubious;3=diameter<6cm; 4=diameter 6-12cm;5=diameter >12cm
x_7	[sub]ileus symptoms	1=no;2=slight;3=moderate; 4=severe
x_8	anal/perianal lesions	1=no;2=yes
x_9	extraintestinal lesions	1=no;2=yes
x_{10}	bowel resection for Crohn's disease	1=no;2=yes
x_{11}	Quetelet index [W/H^2]	W=10xbody weight in kg;H=height in m
x_{12}	ESR	mm after 1 h
x_{13}	haemoglobin concentration	mmol/l
x_{14}	total serum protein level	g/l
x_{15}	serum albumin level	g/l
x_{16}	serum γ-globulin level	g/l
x_{17}	sex	1=male;2=female
x_{18}	stool weight	g/24 h [mean of 5 consecutive days]

Three gastroenterologists were asked, independently and without knowledge of the patient's identity, to rate the activity of the inflammation on the basis of the variables listed in table 1 for each patient.

Stepwise multiple regression analysis was used to investigate which combination of variables contributed most to the subjective ratings of the gastroenterologists.

RESULTS

It proved to be possible to develop, on the basis of nine variables, an activity index [AI] which attained a correlation coefficient of 95% with the corresponding physician's rating. Table 2 lists these variables and the constants [b_i] required for calculation of the AI.

Table 2. Variables included in the Activity Index

Variable x_i	Unit/code	Regression coefficient b_i
Constant [b_o]		-209[c]
1 albumin	g/l	- 5.48[c]
2 ESR	mm after 1 h	0.29
3 Quetelet index	W/H^2	- 0.22
4 abdominal mass	1-5[a]	7.83
5 sex	1=male;2=female	- 12.3
6 temperature	centigrade[b]	16.4
7 stool consistency	1-3[a]	8.46
8 resection	1=no;2=yes	- 9.17
9 extraintestinal lesions	1=no;2=yes	10.7

a] code given in table 1

b] 37.0°C is recorded when the patient has no fever; for febrile patients the seven-day mean evening reading is recorded.

c] when the normal values for serum albumin differ markedly from the reference values used in this study [45-55 g/l], the constant b_o and the regression coefficient of albumin [b_1] change.

The AI in a particular patient can be calculated by multiplication of the values of the 9 variables, expressed in the units or code as indicated, with the coefficient derived from regression analysis [b_i]. Addition of these results and a constant [b_o] gives the AI.

Index values below 100 points are associated with inactive disease, values between 100 and 150 indicates slight activity, between 150 and 210 moderate and more than 210 points severe inflammatory activity.

DISCUSSION

Best et al. (1) were the first to evolve a method of quantifying the inflammatory activity in CD in a less arbitrary manner than was usually done in the past. The fact that this activity index [CDAI] is now being used in a number of prospective studies, demonstrates the urgent need for such an index. Nevertheless, the CDAI has a number of disadvantages. It was evolved with the cooperation of 18 physicians in 13 hospitals. At outpatient follow-up, these physicians formulated an overall evaluation of "how the patient was doing". At the same time, a large number of subjective and objective variables were registered. The number of patients thus studied totalled 112 [three to 20 patients from each centre]. Multiple regression analysis was applied in an effort to determine which combination of variables correlated most closely with the subjective evaluation by the physician.

Best et al. (1) do not indicate whether the physician based his rating on an overall subjective impression or in part also on data from the history, results of physical examination, or laboratory findings. The interrater agreement of the subjective ratings was not studied. In the development of the CDAI several variables were arbitrarily omitted [abdominal tenderness, serum albumin level] or added [body weight]. The ultimate CDAI is made up of eight variables [stool consistency, abdominal pain, general well-being, extraintestinal symptoms of CD, use of Lomotil or opiates for diarrhoea, abdominal mass, haematocrit, and body weight].

An important objection to the CDAI is that it is largely determined by subjective variables [abdominal pain, general well-being]. The contribution of these variables to the sum of the standardised regression coefficients amounts to 39%. To register these subjective variables, the patient must be asked to keep a diary card updated for at least a week. In the development of the CDAI, the fact that the medication often given in CD may influence the subjective complaints [euphoria effect of prednisone, side-effects of salicyla-zosulphapyridine] was disregarded. Subjective complaints such as general malaise and abdominal pain are generally not reliable indications of inflammatory activity. Not infre-quently, they result from complications or residual effect of the disease such as fistulae or stenosis. The same applies to the frequency of defaecation and stool consistency [their contribution to the CDAI amounts to 19%]. Patients with CD who have undergone a bowel resection [specifically ileocaecal resection] not infrequently have a high defaecation rate and produce soft stools, even though their disease may be inac-tive. On the other hand, important objective parameters of inflammatory activity such as serum albumin level and ESR, have not been included in the CDAI. The validity of the CDAI is further reduced by the marked overlaps in CDAI score be-tween the various activity classes established on the basis of subjective rating.

The AI proposed in this paper has recently been described in full (2). It was developed by analogy to the regression analysis applied by Best et al.(1), but is made up almost en-tirely of objective variables [Table 2], of which the serum albumin level contributes most to the AI. This AI proved to be very useful in the assessment of the disease activity and of the effect of therapy during a double-blind trial of drug therapy of CD.

REFERENCES
1. Best WR, Becktel JM, Singleton JW, Kern F.Jr. (1976) Development of a Crohn's disease activity index (National Cooperative Crohn's Disease Study). Gastroenterology 70:439-444
2. Hees PAM, Elteren van PH, Lier van HJJ, Tongeren van JHM.(1980) An index of inflammatory activity in patients with Crohn's disease. Gut 21:279-286

A5   Summary of discussions relating to topics A1 to A4

Riis: A definition of activity in Crohn's disease
            would be of great value in at least three circum-
            stances. First, if the definition were simple enough
            for use in routine clinical work, it would enable
            physicians and surgeons all over the world to com-
            pare their practical experience with the disease.
            Secondly, precise definitions are essential for
            controlled therapeutic trials. Thirdly, laboratory
            studies into aetiology and pathogenesis need to be
            related to the activity of the disease.

de Dombal: The question is whether three separate defini-
            tions are required for these purposes. The "Organi-
            sation Mondiale de Gastroenterologie"[OMGE] classi-
            fication is suitable for ordinary clinical work and
            therapeutic trials. As far as scientists working on
            pathogenesis are concerned, indices are totally
            inadequate.

Booth: Any scientist working on a clinical problem must
            make his own definitions and publish them with any
            results.
            Crohn's disease and ulcerative colitis are often
            lumped together as "inflammatory bowel disease".
            This is dangerous approach as it may blur the re-
            sults of investigation, and the two diseases should
            be kept separate for scientific study. Even with
            Crohn's disease itself, it may be essential to dis-
            tinguish between those patients with the disease
            confined to the small intestine, those with both
            small and large intestine involved, and those with
            disease confined to the large bowel.

Farmer: I agree. Analysis of our clinical material at
              the Cleveland clinic has shown statistically signi-
              ficant differences in the symptomatology of patients
              with these three main anatomical locations of dis-
              ease. The existing definitions of activity take no
              note of this.

Riis: It is often stated that a high level of concor-
              dance between the CDAI index and the overall clini-
              cal assessment points to the validity of the index.
              To be provocative I would suggest that, as this
              index is based on clinical assessment, such a close
              agreement is inevitable and does not mean that the
              index measures the activity of the inflammatory
              process. In addition, this index is too complicated
              for everyday clinical use.

Jeejeebhoy: The main problem is that the index is based on
              individual symptoms whereas there are different
              patterns of disease depending on the anatomical
              location and on whether the process is mainly in-
              flammatory or obstructive due to fibrosis.

Asquith: The histological findings deserve attention. We
              saw in coeliac disease that the development of small
              intestinal biopsy enabled us to study the disease
              with an objective yardstick.

Yardley: The pathological problem is that coeliac disease
              is a diffuse process of the jejunum so that a biopsy
              is a representative sample, whereas the lesions of
              Crohn's disease are focal and biopsy specimens may
              not be representative.

Best: When we set out to devise the CDAI, we had three
              objectives. The first was to classify the state of
              the disease at the beginning of a controlled thera-

peutic trial so that we could separate patients with quiescent disease from those with highly active disease. The second was to use this classification to estimate changes in the activity of the disease in the course of a therapeutic trial. It was hoped, for example, that changes in the index value would be suitable for controlling the dose of prednisone or for deciding that a patient was deteriorating so much that he should be removed from the study for ethical reasons. The third objective was to use the difference between the initial and final scores as a measure of the success or failure of any particular form of therapy.

A CLINICAL SCORING SYSTEM FOR CHRONIC INFLAMMATORY BOWEL DISEASE IN CHILDREN

J.D. LLOYD-STILL and H.U. WESSEL

INTRODUCTION

Schachter and Kirsner (1) have attempted a definition of inflammatory bowel disease [IBD] of unknown origin in adults. None of the presently available methods of assessment of disease activity (2-4) satisfactorily encompass the wide variety of clinical manifestations of IBD in the pediatric population. In 1979 we reported (5) a new clinical score modified from the Shwachman clinical score for cystic fibrosis (6) specifically designed for use in the pediatric population that could be used for both Crohn's disease and ulcerative colitis. This report extends our observations to a present total of 92 patients seen between 1975-80.

METHODS

Table 1 shows the clinical scoring system we have devised (5). The patients were scored on five parameters shown in parentheses: general activity [10], physical examination and clinical complications [30], nutrition [20], X-rays [15], and laboratory [25]. All of the evaluations included in the score are easily elicited by any physician. The clinical score was correlated with patient age and serum albumin by linear regression analysis. Multiple stepwise linear regression analysis was used to determine the joint predictors in the clinical score for 12 clinical variables: age, score, sex, disease [ulcerative colitis and Crohn's disease], albumin, surgery, corticosteroids, family history, perianal complications, arthritis, growth failure, and site of involvement in Crohn's disease. Previous studies (5) have demonstrated reproducibility by different observers and a good correlation with other classifications of severity of disease (2-4).

Table 1. Clinical score [normal score 100 points]

General activity [10]

10	Normal school attendance; BM < 3 per day
5	Lacks endurance; BM 3-5 per day; misses < 4 weeks school per year
1	Fever; home tutor; BM > 5 per day; severely restricted activity

Physical examination and complications [30]

Abdomen	10	normal
	5	mass
	1	distention; tenderness

Proctoscopy	10	normal; no fissures
Perianal	5	friability; 1 fissure
	1	ulcers; pseudopolyps; bleeding; multiple fissures; fistulas

Arthritis	5	nil
	3	one joint/arthralgia
	1	multiple joints

Skin, Stoma-	5	normal
titis,eyes	3	mild stomatitis
	1	erythema nodosum; pyoderma; severe stomatitis; uveitis

Nutrition [20]

height	10	> 5 cm/year
	5	< optimal
	1	no growth

weight	10	normal
	5	no gain
	1	weight loss

Radiology [15]

15	normal
10	ileitis; colitis to splenic flexure
5	total colon or ileocolic involvement
1	toxic megacolon; obstruction

Table 1 continued

Laboratory [25]

Hct   5 > 40 %
            3 25-35 %
            1 < 25 %

ESR   5 normal
            3 20-40 mm
            1 > 40 mm

WBC   5 normal
            3 <20,000 cells/mm^3
            1 >20,000 cells/mm^3

Albumin   10 normal
            5   3.0 g/dl
            1 <2.5 g/dl

RESULTS

   Figure 1 shows the correlation between clinical score and
age for ulcerative colitis [N=47, mean age 9.1 ± 4.2 years]
and Crohn's disease [N=45, mean age 12.6 ± 2.5 years]. There
were 38 females and 54 males. A family history of IBD was
found in 25.5% [22/92]. The clinical score was unrelated to
patient age, but there was a significant linear correlation
with the serum albumin level [r=0.64] shown in Figure 2.

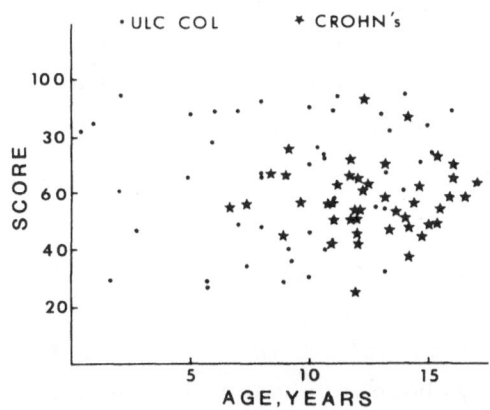

Figure 1. Correlation between
          clinical score and
          age in UC and CD

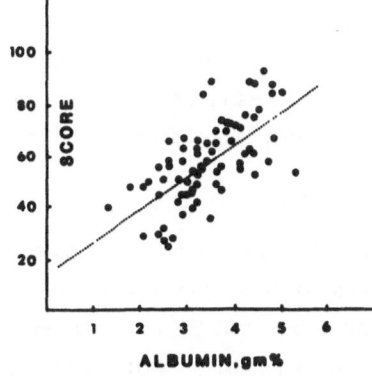

Figure 2. Correlation between
          clinical score and
          albumin

Fifteen patients who underwent surgery had a significantly lower mean score [48.9 + 15.3] than 77 patients without surgery [63.3 + 17.9], p<0.01.

Table 2 shows that the five patients undergoing surgery for ulcerative colitis had lower scores than the 10 corresponding patients with Crohn's disease; in addition, the former group had lower albumin levels and were significantly younger than the latter group.

Table 2. Patients who underwent surgery

	N	Age[yrs]	Score	Albumin g/dl
UC	5	8.22 + 1.8	36.4 + 8.7	2.66 + 0.94
CD	10	13.02 + 3.4	55.9 + 13.7	3.84 + 0.96
p		<0.05	<0.02	<0.05

Patients with ileitis had higher scores [60.3 + 11.1] than those with ileocolitis [48.7 + 11.2], p<0.01, confirming well recognized clinical observations. Sixteen patients with growth failure scored lower [51.3 + 13.2] than 76 patients without growth failure [62.8 + 18.2], p<0.01. Crohn's disease accounted for 87% of patients with growth failure.

Multiple stepwise regression analysis identified five of the examined variables as significant [F>5.0] joint predictors of the clinical score: serum albumin, positive family history, treatment with corticosteroids, surgery, and site of involvement in Crohn's disease.

DISCUSSION

This extended analysis of our pediatric patients has confirmed our previous report (5). Our data base has increased from 54 to 92 children. The limitations of the available scoring systems for inflammatory bowel disease in children have been discussed (5). We are presently using this scoring system for a variety of prospective studies in these disorders.

CONCLUSIONS

1. The clinical score is simple to perform, reproducible by different observers, and sensitive to changes in the clinical status of the patients.

2. A high incidence [25.5%] of a positive family history of IBD is documented.

3. There is a significant correlation between the level of serum albumin and the clinical score.

4. Patients, undergoing surgery, had significantly lower scores than patients without surgical treatment. [In UC lower scores than in CD $p < 0.02$]

5. Other significant observations include the lower scores for ileocolitis compared to ileitis, and for patients with growth failure.

6. Multiple stepwise regression analysis has identified five clinical variables as significant joint predictors of the clinical score: serum albumin, positive family history, treatment with corticosteroids, surgery, and site of involvement in Crohn's disease. The standard error of the estimate was $\pm 10.5\%$.

REFERENCES

1. Schachter H, Kirsner JB.(1975) Definitions of inflammatory bowel disease of unknown etiology. Gastroenterology 68:591-600

2. Truelove SC, Witts LJ. (1955) Cortisone in ulcerative colitis: final report on therapeutical trial. Brit.Med.J. 2:1041-1048

3. Best WR, Becktel JM, Singleton JW, Kern F Jr.(1976) Development of a Crohn's disease activity index. Gastroenterology 70:439-444

4. Whittington PF, Barnes HV, Bayless TM.(1977) Medical management of Crohn's disease in adolescence. Gastroenterology 72:1338-1344

5. Lloyd-Still JD, Green OC.(1979) A clinical scoring system for chronic inflammatory bowel disease in children. Dig. Dis.Sci. 24:620-624

6. Shwachman H, Kulczycki LL.(1958) Long-term study of 105 patients with cystic fibrosis. Am.J.Dis.Child. 96:6-15

CROHN'S DISEASE IN CHILDREN: DIAGNOSTIC PROBLEMS AND
PROCEDURES

A.C. DOUWES, J. FERNANDES, and M. VAN CAILLIE

INTRODUCTION

Crohn's disease [CD] is a rare condition for the pediatrician to meet and CD in childhood is likely to be mis-
diagnosed as ulcerative colitis [UC]. Management and prognosis are different in CD and in UC and early diagnosis may
enhance the results of initial medical treatment. The aim of
the present study is to evaluate which clinical symptoms and
laboratory data contribute to early suspicion and diagnosis.

PROCEDURE

The patient material consists of 36 children who have
been treated because of chronic inflammatory bowel disease
[IBD] between 1975-1980 in the Sophia Children's Hospital,
Rotterdam and the Children's Department of the Free University Amsterdam [Table 1].

Table 1. Final diagnosis in 36 children with IBD

	M	F
Crohn's disease	10	5
Ulcerative colitis	12	8
Unclassified IBD	1	

Specific examinations included radiology of upper and
lower gastrointestinal tract, colonoscopy using pediatric
sized endoscopes, agglutination-test for Eubacterium and
Peptostreptococcus species according to Wensinck (1), $CrCl_3$
test for protein-losing enteropathy and, in patients suspected to have concomitant lactose malabsorption, the hydrogen breath test by the method of Fernandes and Douwes (2,3).
Age at diagnosis and delay between initial symptoms and diagnosis is shown in table 2.

Table 2. Mean and range of age at diagnosis and diagnostic delay in years

	CD[n=15]	UC[n=20]
Age	12.6 [8.7-15.4]	10.8 [4.7-14.1]
Delay	1.2 [0.1- 2.7]	1.9 [0.1- 5.7]

RESULTS

Frequency of single initial symptoms in CD and in UC are listed in table 3, prominent laboratory findings in table 4.

Table 3. Frequency of initial clinical symptoms in children with CD and UC

Crohn's disease	%	ulcerative colitis	%
loose stools	80	blood stained stools	60
abdominal pain	60	loose stools	45
anorexia	53	mucus in stools	40
weight loss	53	abdominal pain	25
fatigue	27	salmonella enteritis	15
perianal fistulas	14	weight loss	5
blood stained stools	7	arthritis	5
stomatitis	7	anorexia	0
mucus in stools	0		

Table 4. Frequency of laboratory abnormalities in children with CD and UC

	CD[n=15]	UC[n=20]
increased ESR	100 %	40 %
increased gamma-globulin	79 %	67 %
agglutination test positive	50 %	6 %
$CrCl_3$ test abnormal	5/7	-
lactose breath test abnormal	3/9	1/2
Schilling test abnormal	1/7	-

Though no single symptom or laboratory finding is confirmative for the diagnosis of CD or UC, clusters of symptoms -if present- may be helpful in the initial diagnostic work-up. Of the 15 children with CD, 11 presented with 3 or more symptoms; another 3 patients with less than 3 symptoms had a positive agglutination test. Hence, 14 out of 15 patients with CD initially had clinical symptoms and laboratory findings which could have led to early diagnosis. The more specific examinations, i.e. radiology, endoscopy and histopathology of biopsy specimens confirmed the diagnosis of CD in

most cases. Early radiology however, did not always demonstrate recognizable changes and in some instances, subtle
lesions were only recognized on second look by an experienced
pediatric radiologist.

Localization of CD in our patients, together with the
procedures which contributed most to the diagnosis, are shown
in table 5.

Table 5.Diagnostic procedures in different localization of CD

Localization	N	Radiology	Histology Endoscopy	Miscellaneous*
colon	8	1	5	3
ileum and colon	3	3	1	0
ileum	4	3	0	1

* = angiography, perianal fistulas and/or surgical specimens

As expected, radiology was superior in demonstrating
ileal disease. Barium enemas, however, were not of great
help in assessing the diagnosis of Crohn's colitis and the
latter was diagnosed in most cases by colonoscopy. In addition, endoscopy and histopathology of biopsy specimens in 3
of the 4 patients with ileal localization and normal colonic
X-ray, revealed the presence of a low grade chronic inflammation of the colon. This finding is in agreement with observations in adults (4).

DISCUSSION
Pediatricians are becoming aware of the increasing incidence of CD in childhood. The mean delay in diagnosis in our
series is the same as reported (5) and favourably contrasts
with the delay of almost 3 years mentioned by other authors
(6). Nevertheless, a mean delay of 14 months is too long an
interval, especially in childhood. A factor complicating
early diagnosis is the high frequency of CD [8/15 in the
present material]. The condition may easily be diagnosed as
UC, partly because X-ray examination is often inconclusive.
Hence, colonic disease requires endoscopy and reliable histopathology and these studies are seldom available for the
general pediatrician.

We therefore emphasize the use of clusters of easily available clinical and laboratory data. When these lead to suspicion of disease, referral for more specific examinations is indicated.

CONCLUSIONS

1. Clusters of clinical symptoms and laboratory data should lead to early suspicion and diagnosis of CD.
2. CD in childhood is as frequent as UC.
3. CD of the ileum and colon show similar frequency.
4. Colonoscopy is necessary in all cases of CD, regardless of its localization.
5. Low grade inflammation of the colon is often present in ileal disease.

ACKNOWLEDGEMENTS
The authors are much indebted to Dr. J.L.J. Gaillard, pathologist and Dr. M. Meradji, paediatric radiologist.

REFERENCES
1. Wensinck F. (1976) Faecal flora of Crohn's patients. Serological differentiation between Crohn's disease and ulcerative colitis. In: The management of Crohn's disease. Eds: Weterman IT, Pena AS, Booth CC. Excerpta Medica, Amsterdam-Oxford pp 103-105
2. Fernandes J, Vos CE, Douwes AC, Slotema E, Degenhart HJ. (1978) Respiratory hydrogen excretion as a parameter for lactose malabsorption in children. Am.J.Clin.Nutr. 31: 597-602
3. Douwes AC, Fernandes J, Rietveld W. (1978) Hydrogen breath test in infants and children: sampling and storing expired air. Clin.Chem.Acta 82:293-296
4. Korelitz BI, Sommers SC. (1976) Rectal biopsy studies in Crohn's disease (histopathology and cell counts). In: The management of Crohn's disease. Eds: Weterman IT, Pena AS, Booth CC. Excerpta Medica, Amsterdam-Oxford pp 13-17
5. Burbige EJ, Huang S, Bayless TM. (1975) Clinical manifestations of Crohn's disease in children and adolescents. Paediatrics 55:866-871
6. O'Donoghue DP, Dawson AM. (1977) Crohn's disease in childhood. Arch.Dis.Child. 52:627-632

DESIGN, EARLY RESULTS AND OUTLOOK OF A PROSPECTIVE PAEDIATRIC CROHN'S DISEASE STUDY

D.H. SHMERLING

INTRODUCTION

An initial group of 155 children with Crohn's disease [CD] from F.R. Germany, Switzerland and Austria was submitted in 1977 to the Paediatric Crohn's Disease Working Group from 24 paediatric centers[*].

Criteria for admission to the study were:

1. Radiological criteria, established by the collaborative Crohn's disease study in F.R. Germany, Denmark and Switzerland (1) in adults and summarised in table 1 (2); every set of radiographs was reviewed without knowledge of clinical or other data of the patient by three reference radiologists (2) and accepted only upon full agreement.

Table 1. Radiological criteria [Paediatric Crohn's disease Working Group - Schlangenbad 1977]

Lesions		Localization	
M	stenosis, rigid wall, fistula, pseudo-diverticulum, intermediate segment	L	terminal ileum, ileum+ colon (contin., discont.), ileum w.skip lesion (>2), colon w.skip lesion (>2)
m	cobble-stones,spiculae, ulcers, excentric lesion, mesenteric thickening	l	proximal ileum, jejunum, ileum + colon (total), ascending colon
o	length, thickened folds, pseudo-polyps	o	oesophagus, duodenum, stomach, rectum, sigmoid, total colon

Minimal criteria: MM, Mmm, Lmmm, LMm

[*]Aachen, Berlin [FRG], Bern [Switzerland], Bonn, Dusseldorf, Erlangen, Essen, Frankfurt [FRG], Geneva [Switzerland], Giessen, Hamburg, Hannover, Heidelberg, Heilbronn, Homburg/Saar, Koln, Krefeld, Mainz, Munich, Pforzheim, Stuttgart, Tubingen, Ulm [FRG], Vienna [Austria] and Zurich [Switzerland]

2. Histological criteria: available histological material was evaluated by a reference pathologist (3), again without knowledge of any other patient data.

MATERIALS AND METHODS

105 patients [58 m., 47 f.] were accepted after thorough evaluation of retrospective data, 95 fulfilling hitherto established radiological criteria, including 21 with histological evidence, 10 additional cases were accepted on histological criteria alone. Age at diagnosis was 6-10 years in 15, 10-15 years in 84 and 15-20 years in 6 cases. 23 out of 92 patients [25%] and 19 out of 34 patients aged 13-15 years [56%] were severely growth retarded [height < 3 percentiles for age] with a mean delay in bone age of 3-4 years.

The distribution of lesions was: isolated small bowel CD in 11 [15%], isolated Crohn's colitis in 4 [6%], limited ileocolitis [ileum + right sided colon] in 38 [54%] and extensive ileocolitis in 17 [25%] of the 70 radiologically fully documented cases. In 4 patients radiological evidence for stomach involvement and in 39 cases [37%] anal/perianal lesions were present.

Symptoms and signs prior and/or at diagnosis were: abdominal pain in 90% [40% constant, 50% intermittant], anorexia in 84%, diarrhoea in 73% [in 53% intermittantly], rectal bleeding in 33% [macroscopic melaena in 6%]; arthralgia, stomatitis, erythema nodosum, liver involvement and uveitis in 17, 13, 10, 6 and 3% respectively. Anorexia was slightly more prevalent in patients with ileitis, diarrhoea and rectal bleeding significantly more frequent in extensive colonic Crohn's disease.

RESULTS AND DISCUSSION

It has rapidly become obvious that some of the 50 initially rejected patients and some of those 10 admitted according to histological criteria alone did not fulfil the chosen radiological criteria because they were submitted to the study "too early" in the course of their disease, presenting with only mild radiological alterations. Some of these patients have in the meantime developed more "diagnostic" features and will now be introduced into the study. Yet, this implies that the established radiological criteria used were those of an advanced Crohn's disease and indeed [Table 1] stenosis, fistulae and cobble-stone patterns are certainly not features of an early involvement in this disease. With increasing experience and more extensive availability of endoscopy in paediatric clinics the evidence accumulated until now shows that endoscopic findings will probably be an important candidate for an additional diagnostic criterion for early diagnosis in future cases.

A second important consequence of the evaluation of the first group of patients admitted was the decision to continue the study on a purely prospective base. New evaluation sheets for the case history, clinical findings, radiology, endoscopy, histology, laboratory data and surgery at the time of diagnosis were elaborated and should serve as a diagnostic check-list for new patients to be entered into the study. The input of these new cases is scheduled for the next months.

The third task of the study group was an evaluation study of a paediatric Crohn's disease activity index. With one exception (4) no index hitherto published (5,6) is suitable for use in children, as specific paediatric aspects of the disease, e.g., growth and development, are not included in them. The study group therefore set out a prospective programme for the establishment of a suitable index. In a first step, 3 blocks of information will be prospectively gathered at each patient-visit, with at least two observations per patient: case history [patient diary, two weeks prior to the evaluation], clinical findings and laboratory data [36 single observations per patient]. Each block will be evaluated by the examining physician according to his own "impression" as independently from the data gathered as possible. Furthermore the course of the disease since the last evaluation [improved, steady, deteriorated], the localization of the diseased bowel, the prescence or absence of prior bowel resection , the treatment at the time of the evaluation, as well as age and sex will be registered. A stepwise multiple regression analysis and correlation study will allow the establishment of a suitable and workable activity index for paediatric patients.

These three tasks are now in progress, the first entry of data for the activity index being scheduled for November 1980. Therapeutic trials will be considered when the tools described above will become operative.

REFERENCES

1. Malchow H. (1979) Report on Crohn's disease studies. Z. Gastroenterol. 27: Suppl. 51-57
2. Hauke H, Lassrich MA, Ball F. (1978) Ergebnisse einer radiologischen Studie bei Morbus Crohn im Kindesalter. Radiologie 18: 199-207
3. Schmitz-Moormann P. (1980) Histopathologie des Mb. Crohn. Round Table on Crohn's disease in Childhood, Ann. Meeting German Paediatric Assoc., Karlsruhe, 1979. Zschr. Kinderheilk., in press
4. Lloyd-Still JD, Green OC. (1979) A clinical scoring system for chronic inflammatory bowel disease in children. Dig.Dis.Sci. 24:620-624
5. Best WR, Becktel JM, Singleton JW. (1979) Rederived values of the eight coefficients of the Crohn's disease activity index (CDAI). Gastroenterology 77:843-846
6. Hees van PAM, Elteren van Ph, Lier van HJJ, Tongeren van JHM. (1980) An index of inflammatory activity in patients with Crohn's disease. Gut 21:279-286

A9   Summary of Discussions relating to topics A6 to A8

Truelove: It seems that physicians who are dealing with
children suffering from Crohn's disease consider
that they have to adopt rather different criteria to
assess activity than those of us who deal mainly
with grown-up patients.

Farmer: My opinion, based on our own studies, is that
there is certainly a difference in disease criteria
if one is dealing with the pre-pubertal child, in
contrast to the late adolescence child. The latter
are very similar to patients who are twenty-five or
thirty years old.

Riis: Our experience is that it is more a question of
pediatricians knowing that these diseases actually
exist in children. In children with Crohn's disease
who present with chronic dyspepsia, intolerance of
cow's milk, or psychological problems, the diagnosis
is often delayed until eventually a gastroenterologist sees them.

Shmerling: I completely agree that the situation in the
pre-pubertal child is a special one. Puberty should
be defined according to established criteria and
these include bone age. You are completely right
that one of the main tasks in pediatrics is to raise
the level of awareness in pediatricians that Crohn's
disease is becoming relatively common in children.

Douwes: In the Netherlands, we are not yet ready to make
an activity index for Crohn's disease in children
because our greatest problem is that at present
these children are referred to us too late.

A10 General Discussion and Conclusions
Reported by S.C. Truelove

DEFINITION AND ASSESSMENT OF ACTIVITY

The group of scientists and clinicians with particular interest in assessment of disease activity had a useful discussion from which the following points emerged:

1.   It is essential to have an index [or possibly several
indices] of disease activity, not only for use in controlled
therapeutic trials but also in scientific investigations of
the aetiology and pathogenesis of Crohn's disease.

2.   Existing indices of activity, such as the CDAI, have
already proved useful but the question is whether better
indices can be evolved.   The group considered that debating
the comparative virtues and shortcoming of existing indices
was likely to be a sterile exercise.   There was general
agreement that existing indices relied heavily on subjective
measures of assessment and that there was a need for development of indices based on objective measurements.

3.   A working party of interested members of the group
was set up for this purpose, with Dr. F.T. de Dombal as its
secretary. The working party considered that it would be best
for its members to have a special meeting to consider the
best ways to study the problem.   It is planned to have such a
meeting in about three months time.

SECTION B

MORPHOLOGICAL ASPECTS

Section Editor: J.H. Yardley

42

SIGNIFICANCE OF LIP BIOPSIES IN THE DIAGNOSIS OF CROHN'S DISEASE [ROUTINE HISTOLOGY AND IMMUNOFLUORESCENCE]

M.K. BASU, I.M. CHESNER, R.A. THOMPSON and P. ASQUITH

INTRODUCTION

Macroscopic oral lesions have been described in 4-9% of patients with Crohn's disease and ulcerative colitis (1). More recently apparently disease specific immunofluorescent changes have been found in biopsies of macroscopically normal mouths in Crohn's patients (2). The present study was carried out to compare the histology of macroscopically uninvolved oral mucosa and minor salivary glands from Crohn's patients, with that from patients with ulcerative colitis and also normal controls. We have also tried to determine the disease specificity of the immunofluorescence staining.

PATIENTS AND METHODS

Following informed consent, lower lip biopsies [including if possible minor labial salivary glands] were obtained under local anaesthesia from 14 Crohn's patients [of which 12 were suitable for routine histology], 13 ulcerative colitis patients and 10 normal controls [laboratory and clinical staff]. The diagnosis in each case was based on accepted clinical, laboratory, X-ray and histological criteria (3). Ten of the fourteen Crohn's patients had ileo-colitis, the remaining four Crohn's colitis. Of the thirteen UC patients, eight had total UC, one had sub-total UC, two had left sided disease, two had recto-sigmoiditis.

Disease activity at the time of the lip biopsy was assessed from symptoms and from levels of haemoglobin and serum albumin, orosomucoid and complement components C3 and C4. Based on these parameters, nine of the Crohn's patients and six of the UC patients were in remission; the rest had active disease.

One part of the oral biopsy specimen was fixed in 10% neutral buffered formalin, processed and stained with haematoxylin and eosin, Weigert's elastic stain and PAS technique. The incidence of abnormal biopsies in each study group was then determined without knowledge of the source of the biopsy; an abnormal biopsy was defined as showing either an epithelioid granuloma, or focal lymphocytic adenitis [Fig. 1] with acinar atrophy, tubular hyperplasia and non-specific inflammation in the lamina propria and submucosa. The sialadenitis was classified from grades 0-4, depending on the degree and distribution of inflammatory cells (4).

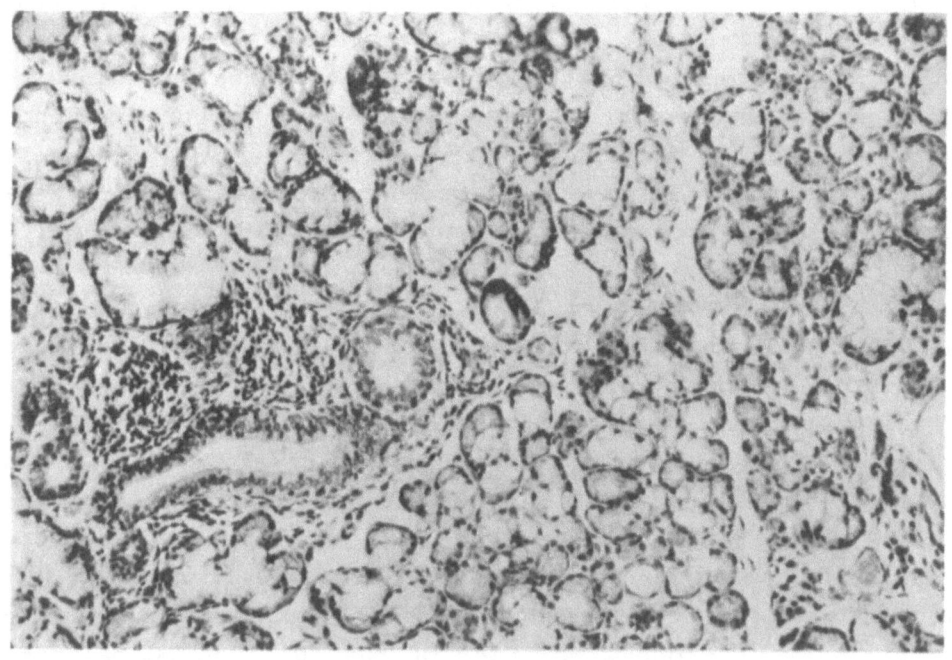

Figure 1. Focal lymphocytic infiltration in mouth biopsy from
         Crohn's patient.

Another part of the oral biopsy was processed for immuno-fluorescence studies. This piece was cryostat sectioned, washed in buffered saline and incubated with neat and then a 1/10 dilution of either autologous or heterologous serum for

30 minutes at room temperature. The slides were again washed and stained with a 1/20 dilution of fluorescein conjugated anti-human IgG [Wellcome reagents]. Following a final washing, the sections were mounted in glycerol and examined using a Vickers M40 microscope with epi-illumination and appropriate filters.

RESULTS

Routine Histology

Abnormal biopsies were found in 67% of Crohn's patients and 23% of UC patients, but were not found in any of the control subjects. However, no biopsy showed non-caseating epithelioid cell granulomata. The most frequent signs of non-specific inflammation in both CD and UC were grade 2 or 3 sialadenitis. No biopsy showed evidence of vasculitis. Neither the presence nor the degree of histological abnormality correlated with disease activity or in CD with the site of disease.

Immunofluorescence

Using autologous sera of the 14 Crohn's patients, 8 showed positive staining [2 strong]; in contrast, only 2 of 13 UC patients [1 strong] and 2 of 10 healthy controls [1 strong] showed positive staining. Moreover, using heterologous sera, most positive sera produced positive immunofluorescence with heterologous mucosa but the degree of staining was not so marked.

DISCUSSION AND CONCLUSIONS

Small focal aggregates of chronic inflammatory cells and minor parenchymatous changes occur in labial salivary glands with age but these changes are restricted to grade 1 or grade 2 changes without acinar replacement, periacinar fibrosis or tubular changes. In this study the majority of patients were aged less than 40 years and the biopsies from 9 [80%] showed grade 3 changes. Additionally, all biopsies demonstrated other histological changes, suggesting that the occurrence of abnormal biopsies in these patients was not related to age but was associated with the presence of bowel disease.

The relationship of labial sialadenitis to Crohn's disease and ulcerative colitis is not clear. Circulating anti-tissue antibodies are commonly found in certain collagen diseases (1) and it may be relevant that such antibodies are also found in Crohn's disease and ulcerative colitis. Whatever their pathogenesis, it would appear that routine histology of lip biopsies in a patient suspected of having inflammatory bowel disease, could help in confirming the diagnosis and help in distinguishing Crohn's disease from ulcerative colitis.

The immunofluorescence staining is localized to a different anatomical site than the histological changes already described and cannot therefore clearly be related to the latter. It is possible that circulating anti-mucosal antibodies formed in the intestines of patients with inflammatory bowel disease could cross-react with any mucosal membrane including that in the mouth. More likely is that an inflamed oral mucosa, occurring in inflammatory bowel disease, could allow local mouth antigens [for example bacterial antigens] to cross the mucosal barrier to stimulate local antibody production. These antibodies could then cross-react with oral epithelium. Although a positive test is not confined to Crohn's patients, in certain cases where the distinction between CD and UC is uncertain, the test could help in the differential diagnosis, especially if combined with routine histology.

REFERENCES
1. Basu MK, Asquith P. (1980) Oral manifestations of inflammatory bowel disease. In: Clinics in Gastroenterology. Inflammatory Bowel Disease. Ed. Farmer RG. Saunders London. Vol 9. pp. 307-321
2. Walker JEG. (1978) Possible diagnostic test for Crohn's disease by use of buccal mucosa. Lancet 2:759-760
3. Schachter H, Kirsner JB. (1975) Definition of inflammatory bowel disease of unknown aetiology. Gastroenterology 68:591-602
4. Chisholm DM, Mason DK. (1968) Labial salivary gland biopsy in Sjögren's disease. J. Clin. Pathol. 21:656-660

DUODENAL BIOPSY CELL COUNTS AND HISTOPATHOLOGY IN CROHN'S DISEASE

S.C. SOMMERS and B.I. KORELITZ

INTRODUCTION

Endoscopic biopsy specimens were obtained from the eso-
phagus, body of stomach, gastric antrum and duodenal bulb of
45 patients with Crohn's disease. The diagnosis was based on
appropriate clinical and radiologic criteria. The ileum, the
colon, or both were involved radiologically. No case involved the upper gastrointestinal tract.

MATERIALS AND METHODS

Endoscopic appearances were recorded, and independent
histopathologic analyses were made of serial sections of the
45 biopsies from Crohn's disease patients. Specimens were
fixed in Bouin's solution and paraffin sections were stained
with hematoxylin-phloxin-safranin. Also cell counts of 500
connective tissue cells of the duodenal lamina propria were
made, using a manual cell counter. Fibroblasts, macrophages,
mast cells, lymphocytes, plasma cells, neutrophils and eosinophils were counted (1). The microscopic fields containing
500 such cells were recorded, so that the cell population per
unit area could be determined. Not enough lamina propria
connective tissue cells were present in the gastric or eso-
phageal biopsies to permit counting 500 cells in each.

Control biopsies for histopathologic study and comparable
cell counts of duodenal lamina propria were made available by
the courtesy of Joke Kreuning, C.J.L.M. Meijer and J. Lindeman, Departments of Gastroenterology and Pathology, Acade-
misch Ziekenhuis, Leiden. The control specimens had been
fixed in formol-sublimate and stained with hematoxylin-eosin.
Numerous special stains and immunoperoxidase reacted slides
were also available. Fifty specimens had been obtained from

volunteers (2).

Means and standard deviations were computed for each connective tissue cell type, and these figures were compared with the duodenal biopsy cell counts of the 45 Crohn's disease cases and the 50 volunteer cases. The Student t-test was employed for statistical analysis, with technical assistance provided by courtesy of P.H.J. Kurver, SSDZ, Delft.

RESULTS

Histopathologic abnormalities were found in one or more duodenal biopsies in 19 of 45 Crohn's disease cases. In eight patients endoscopy had shown a mucosal reddening or erosion, while in 11 with histologic alterations the mucosa had appeared grossly normal. Twelve lesions in the gastric antrum or duodenal bulb were considered suggestive of Crohn's disease, including 3 granulomas, 2 in the gastric antrum and 1 in the duodenum. The other 9 lesions comprised 5 biopsies showing lymphedema or lymphangiectasia and 3 showing chronic inflammation and fibrosis, and one showing a crypt abscess. Most frequently lesions were present in the gastric antrum, and next in the duodenum.

There was no correlation found between endoscopically observed mucosal alterations and the presence or type of histopathologic changes. In addition, no correlation between the presence or type of lesion and clinical activity of Crohn's disease was evident. Among the 50 control biopsies, one example of duodenal inflammation and lymphangiectasia was seen.

Duodenal lamina propria cell counts gave the following values, means and standard deviations, of cells:

	Fibro-blast	Macro-phages	Mast cells	Lympho-cytes	Plasma cells	Neutro-phils	Eosino-phils
Crohn's disease [N=45]	83.9 $\pm$16.2	48.5 $\pm$12.8	1.2 $\pm$1.1	198.4 $\pm$45.1	174.7 $\pm$58.3	5.7 $\pm$15.5	0.02 $\pm$0.16
Controls [N=50]	121.3 $\pm$22.9	24.9 $\pm$12.0	4.3 $\pm$2.0	162.4 $\pm$35.6	181.3 $\pm$41.7	1.6 $\pm$2.0	6.4 $\pm$7.7

There were significant greater numbers of lamina propria macrophages and significant smaller numbers of fibroblasts and mast cells in Crohn's disease cases than in the control cases [all p<0.001]. Numbers of other cell types were not significantly different from normal.

Replicate cell counts of 13 control duodenal biopsies, using different serial sections, showed a variation of 2 to 6 percent between counts of the major cell types, and of 10 percent between counts of mast cells, neutrophils and eosinophils.

DISCUSSION

Previous studies of rectal and sigmoid biopsies from Crohn's disease patients, both whether the endoscopic appearance of the rectosigmoid was abnormal or normal, have showed increased lamina propria macrophages when cell counts are performed (3,4). Likewise duodenal biopsies now demonstrate significantly increased lamina propria macrophages, compared to appropriate controls. It is believed that mobilization of mucosal macrophages is a cytologic characteristic of Crohn's disease, both in clinically and grossly uninvolved and involved portions of the gastrointestinal tract.

Significantly reduced fibroblasts in the duodenal mucosa of Crohn's disease patients, compared to controls, have not previously been found. This is believed to reflect the increased cross-sectional area of the lamina propria due to increased numbers of leukocytes, as described by Rosekrans et al. (5) in allergic gastrointestinal disease. In the original study of this case material, with only 20 control duodenal biopsies, mast cells were found to be very significantly increased in Crohn's disease [p<0.001], while in the present report with 50 controls, mast cells are significantly less than normal in Crohn's disease [p<0.001] (6). These paradoxical results may reflect differences in fixation and staining in the Crohn's and control cases that affected the identification of some mast cells. In addition, the original 20 controls may not actually have been appropriate, which is one reason why the assistance of the Leiden group was so helpful in this project.

Histopathologic evidence of clinically and endoscopically inapparent Crohn's disease was present in the form of granuloma or microgranuloma (7) in 3 of the 45 cases [7%]. Suggestive but not conclusive abnormalities were found in an additional 9 cases, and 7 others had non-specific pathologic changes.

The pathogenesis of Crohn's disease has long been considered by one of us [SCS] to involve the absorption from the gastrointestinal lumen of a macromolecule that was part protein and part phospholipid or glycolipid (8). This material would attract macrophages into the intestinal mucosa and set up the characteristic inflammatory lesions of Crohn's disease, comprising lymphatic blockage by leukocytes, persistent lymphangiectasia, sometimes granuloma formation, and ensuing fibrosis.

Reports that the intestinal mucosa contains an increased population of IgM containing plasma cells by Meijer et al. (9), Rosekrans et al. (10) and others support the belief that individuals with Crohn's disease produce and secrete increased amounts of intestinal IgM. This immunoglobulin type forms macromolecular polymers, attracting macrophages locally to ingest and digest them. If secreted into the bowel along its length and resorbed lower down where the proteolysis is less, with or without phospholipids or glycolipids of diverse origin, the inflammatory process peculiar to Crohn's disease could thus be initiated and maintained. In mice this speculation can be tested as an experimental model, since IgM from mouse myeloma is available.

CONCLUSIONS

Biopsies of four sites of gastrointestinal mucosa from 45 patients with ileal or colonic Crohn's disease were examined histopathologically. Gastric antral or duodenal granulomas were found in 3 [7%], and in 9 additional cases there were abnormalities suggestive of Crohn's disease. No correlation

was evident with endoscopic appearances or the clinical activity of the ileocolic disease.

Cell counts of duodenal lamina propria were made and
compared statistically with 50 control biopsies. Significantly increased mucosal macrophages and significantly decreased fibroblasts and mast cells were present in Crohn's
disease cases, compared to the controls. These findings,
along with similar observations in rectosigmoid biopsies
reported previously support the concept that Crohn's disease
involves the entire alimentary canal.

REFERENCES
 1. Sommers SC, Korelitz BI. (1975) Mucosal cell counts in
    ulcerative and granulomatous colitis. Am.J.Clin.Pathol.
    63:359-365
 2. Kreuning J. (1978) Chronic non-specific duodenitis, M.D.
    Thesis Leiden
 3. Korelitz BI, Sommers SC. (1974) Differential diagnosis of
    ulcerative and granulomatous colitis by sigmoidoscopy,
    rectal biopsy and cell counts of rectal mucosa. Am.J.
    Gastroenterol. 61:460-469
 4. Korelitz BI, Sommers SC. (1977) Rectal biopsy in patients
    with Crohn's disease. Normal mucosa on sigmoidoscopic
    examination. JAMA 237:2742-2744
 5. Rosekrans PCM, Meijer CJLM, Cornelisse CJ, van der Wal
    AM, Lindeman J. (1980) Use of morphometry and immunohis-
    tochemistry of small intestinal biopsy specimens in the
    diagnosis of food allergy. J.Clin.Pathol. 33:125-130
 6. Korelitz BI, Waye JD, Feim HD, et al. Unpublished data
 7. Rotterdam H, Korelitz BI, Sommers SC. (1977) Microgranu-
    lomas in grossly normal rectal mucosa in Crohn's disease.
    Am.J.Clin.Pathol. 67:550-554
 8. Warren S, Sommers SC. (1954) Pathology of regional ilei-
    tis and ulcerative colitis. JAMA 154:189
 9. Meijer CJLM, Bosman FT, Lindeman J. (1979) Evidence for
    predominant involvement of the B-cell system in the in-
    flammatory process in Crohn's disease. Scand.J.Gastro-
    enterol. 14:21-32
10. Rosekrans PCM, Meijer CJLM, van der Wal AM, Cornelisse
    CJ, Lindeman J. Immunoglobulin-containing cells in in-
    flammatory bowel disease of the colon. Gut, in press

DOES THERE EXIST ANY CORRELATION BETWEEN CLINICAL FINDINGS
AND THE HISTOPATHOLOGY OF RECTAL BIOPSY IN CROHN'S DISEASE? A
MORPHOMETRICAL STUDY

P. SCHMITZ-MOORMANN, U. WERKMEISTER, G.W. HIMMELMANN, J.W.
BRANDES and H. EHMS

The National Cooperative Crohn's Disease Study of the
United States did not find any correlation between the grade
of inflammation of the rectal mucosa and the Crohn's disease
activity index. We recently developed a morphometrical analysis of biopsy specimens in which 80 different histologic
parameters can be measured. This kind of analysis has allowed
us to re-examine the question of the correlation between
disease activity and rectal mucosa histology.

METHODS AND RESULTS

Rectal biopsy specimens from eighty-seven patients and 81
healthy controls formed the basis of the study. All biopsies
were taken from the back wall of the rectum at a height of
5-10 cm. In each patient the extent and localization of disease was known as was the Crohn's disease activity index.

As shown in tables 1 - 5 histologic parameters relating
to total mucosa, epithelium, mucosal stroma, lymphatic tissue
and submucosa were measured; the units of measurements are
given in each table. For all of the 87 patients, each parameter was statistically correlated with the disease activity
index and a correlation coefficient [CCAI] computed.

The morphometrical data for the various histologic categories are shown in tables 1 - 5:

Table 1. Parameters of the total mucosa

	Normal	CD	CCAI
Thickness of the mucosa	429.0μ	520.8 μ	+ 0.28
Length of the crypt	253.0μ	414.0 μ	+ 0.22
Distance of the crypt	15.2μ	58.5 μ	+ 0.11
Branching of the crypt	1.0*	1.07*	- 0.05
Deformation of crypts	1.0*	1.68*	- 0.05
Ratio crypts/total mucosa			
superficial	51.3%	47.4%	
basal	52.8%	51.2%	
Ratio lymphatic tissue/mucosa	11.9%	9.4%	

* Estimated values. Grading from 1= absent to 9= maximal
CCAI = Correlation coefficient with the activity index

Table 2. Parameters of the epithelium

	Normal	CD	CCAI
Height of the epithelial cell			
superficial	24.6 μ	33.8 μ	+0.01
upper part of the mucosa	22.9 μ	31.0 μ	+0.13
lower part of the mucosa	22.6 μ	29.0 μ	+0.11
Relative content of goblet cells			
upper part of the mucosa	43.9 %	57.3 %	
lower part of the mucosa	63.5 %	55.9 %	
Reduced production of mucus			
superficial	2.08*	1.77*	-0.07
upper part of the mucosa	2.27*	2.18*	-0.14
lower part of the mucosa	2.63*	1.72*	+0.01
Leucocytic migration			
upper part of the mucosa	1.0 *	1.34*	-0.36
lower part of the mucosa	1.0 *	1.46*	+0.02
Crypt abscess			
upper part of the mucosa	1.0 *	1.23*	-0.20
lower part of the mucosa	1.0 *	1.46*	+0.10
Ulcers			
upper part of the mucosa	1.0 *	1.32*	-0.22
lower part of the mucosa	1.0 *	1.14*	+0.10

* Estimated values. Grading from 1= absent to 9= maximal
CCAI = Correlation coefficient with the activity index

Table 3. Parameters of the mucosal stroma

	Normal	CD	CCAI
Edema			
Superficial	1.0*	1.45*	+0.28
basal	1.0*	1.32*	+0.31
Fibrosis			
superficial	1.0*	1.33*	-0.12
basal	1.0*	1.41*	-0.05
Epithelioid cell granuloma			
superficial	1.0*	1.87*	+0.05
basal	1.0*	2.35*	+0.10
Content of cells**			
superficial	21.6	21.8	+0.18
basal	19.2	19.8	+0.19
Content of plasma cells**			
superficial	10.5	7.9	+0.10
basal	8.6	6.5	+0.10
Content of lymphocytes**			
superficial	3.3	5.7	+0.15
basal	2.9	5.6	+0.05
Content of histiocytes**			
superficial	2.5	3.6	-0.02
basal	2.4	3.4	+0.06

** counted in a field of 0.08 mm^2
* Estimated values. Grading from 1= absent to 9= maximal
CCAI = Correlation coefficient with the activity index

Table 4. Parameters of the lymphatic tissue

	Normal	CD	CCAI
Ratio lymphatic tissue/mucosa	11.9 %	9.4 %	
Ratio germinal centre /mucosa	9.4 %	13.8 %	
Content of cells/0.01 mm^2	88	77	-0.03
lymphocytes	69	63	-0.08
histiocytes	1.3	1.2	+0.14
plasma cells	3.0	2.1	+0.18
immunocytes	3.1	10.4	+0.01

CCAI = Correlation coefficient with the activity index

Table 5. Parameters of the submucosa

	Normal	CD	CCAI
Destruction of M. mucosae	1.0*	21.0*	+0.10
Fibrosis	1.0*	1.4*	+0.10
Epithelioid cell granuloma	1.0*	1.5*	+0.04
Content of cells/0.01 mm^2	10.5	21.5	+0.13
plasma cells	3.4	4.8	+0.10
lymphocytes	2.5	5.5	+0.13
histiocytes	2.0	3.7	-0.02

* Estimated values. Grading from 1= absent, to 9= maximal
  CCAI= Correlation coefficient with the activity index

Using this data, the following comparisons were evaluated statistically:

1. Comparison of the morphometrical data of healthy persons and those of patients suffering from CD.
2. Comparison of the localization and extent of CD with the morphology of the rectal mucosa.
3. Comparison between the activity index with its coefficients and the morphometrical data of CD.

The morphometry of healthy and affected mucosa showed an overlapping of most of the parameters. Many of these parameters show only little differences between normal and affected mucosa [Tables 1-5]. Therefore, we did not at first believe, that a discrimination between normal and affected mucosa would be possible. However, after performing a multiple stepwise discrimination analysis, using 20 selected morphometrical parameters we obtained a sharp discrimination between normal and affected mucosa without any overlapping [Fig.1].

Only incomplete evaluation of the relation between localization, extent and morphometry was possible. By making this evaluation we formed four categories to express the localization and the extent.

category 1: Only the small bowel is affected.
category 2: Only the large bowel is affected
category 3: The large bowel and the rectum are affected.
category 4: The small and large bowel as well as the rectum are affected.

56

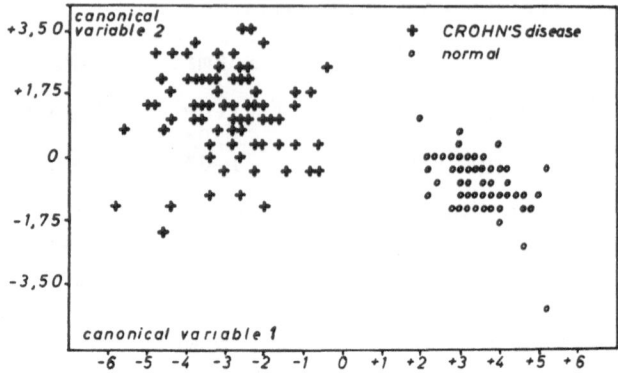

Figure 1. Computer plot of the multiple stepwise discrimination analysis of morphometrical values of the rectal mucosa.

As shown in table 6, several morphometrical parameters
showed a good correlation with this grading. Presently, we
are trying to get a sharper discrimination by a multivariate
analysis.

Our last question was whether there is a relation between
the activity index and the morphometry. We found that only a
few morphometrical parameters show a statistically significant correlation with activity index, such as the thickness
of the mucosa, the length of the crypt and cryptal abscesses
[tables 1-5].

Table 6. Comparison of localization and extent versus morphometry

Morphometrical parameters with significant correlation	Correlation coefficient
Distance of the crypt	+ 0.254
Length of the crypt	+ 0.241
Height of the mucosae	+ 0.248
Edema of lower mucosa	+ 0.328
Granuloma of lower mucosa	+ 0.229
Destruction of M. mucosa	+ 0.280
Cell content of upper mucosa	+ 0.381
Cell content of basal mucosa	+ 0.319
Cell content of submucosa	+ 0.323

In a multivariate regression analysis of the correlation
of 18 morphometrical parameters, with the activity index, the
computer plotted an excellent linear regression. This means

that there is a very good correlation between selected aspects of the morphology of the rectal mucosa and the activity index.

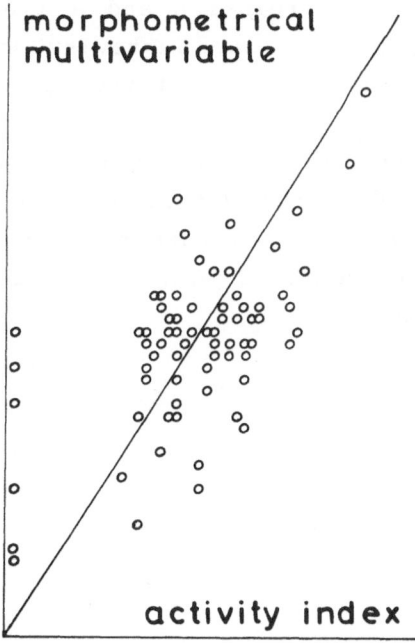

Figure 2. Computer plot of the regression analysis of 18 morphometrical parameters against the activity index.

CONCLUSIONS

Our investigation so far can be summarized as follows:

1. Rectal mucosa of Crohn's disease is definitely discerni-
    ble from normal mucosa by morphometrical investigation.
2. The morphology of the rectal mucosa in Crohn's disease
    seems to be correlated with the localization and the ex-
    tent of the disease.
3. There is a good correlation and a linear regression be-
    tween the Crohn's disease activity index and selective
    features of the morphology of the rectal biopsy.

However, it should be added that the present findings do
not bring any help to the pathologist in his daily routine
work unless we are able, to turn over these statistical results in simple diagnostical microscopy. This is under investigation at present.

B4 Summary of Discussions relating to topics B1 to B3

Mayberry: We conducted a study that was similar to that of
              Asquith. However, we concluded that the immuno-
              fluorescent test is non-specific since both colitis
              and controls can be positive. It should be noted
              also, that it is difficult to observe the fluores-
              cence, and lip biopsy is a painful procedure.

Asquith: I agree that lip biopsy is painful; that is why
              we only had ten healthy controls. Even though 20
              percent of UC patients may be positive and healthy
              controls are occasionally positive, the test is
              useful because it adds information. We have studied
              300 mouth biopsies in different situations, mainly
              in patients with aphthous ulcers. The changes noted
              in lip biopsies obtained from CD and ulcerative
              colitis patients were not found in these control
              biopsies.

Meuwissen: In addition to the lip biopsies, has Asquith
              taken biopsy specimens from aphthous lesions in the
              mouth in Crohn's disease?

Asquith: Yes, but we find it very difficult to distin-
              guish aphthous ulcers in Crohn's disease from those
              that are idiopathic or associated with coeliac
              disease.

O'Morain: Was the abnormality Sommers presented specific
              to Crohn's disease, and has he looked at UC? Also,
              has he studied lysozyme?

Sommers: We have not had duodenal biopsies to examine
               from patients with UC. The material obtained from
               Leiden contained biopsy specimens with immunopero-
               xidase stains for lysozyme. We have used them as a
               check on the number of macrophages present in the
               lamina propria, and they seemed to agree with the
               findings obtained with hematoxylin and eosine
               stained tissue.

Tijtgat: What treatment was given to Asquith's and Som-
               mer's patients?

Asquith: The UC patients were on salazopyrine except for
               two who received steroids. Approximately half the
               Crohn's group were on salazopyrine, some were on
               steroids as well, and others on steroids alone.

Sommers: Patients that had been on sulphasalazine or
               6-MP were off therapy for thirty days, and for at
               least ten days if they were on ACTH or adrenal
               steroids.

Yardley: I agree that morphometric methods may indicate
               histological changes one might otherwise not appre-
               ciate.   However, can one translate morphometric
               studies into a more practical approach for dealing
               with patients?

Schmitz-Moormann: To use morphometric techniques one must
               have an appropriate normal control, and this is
               often not feasible. Further work on morphometry is
               needed.

Sommers: A definite diagnosis of CD is possible only if a
               granuloma or microgranuloma is present.   Yet, it
               only takes about ten minutes to count five-hundred
               connective tissue-cells.   I think we are on the

61

verge of doing differential counts on tissue biopsies to identify the differences between UC and CD.
Furthermore, there is a request by the U.S. inven-
tor of the automated leucocyte counter to redesign
his machine and use it for tissue analysis.

Truelove: The most important point is that CD may be a
disorder that is generalized throughout the gastrointestinal tract, even though the obvious lesions
are focal. Some years ago Skinner, showed by morphometry that there was a marked excess of immunocytes in rectal biopsies from CD which had been
reported as histologically normal. At the same
time, Goodman showed that rectal biopsies, taken
from the apparently normal rectum in patients with
CD commonly had enhanced levels of glucosamine
synthetase.

FOCAL NON-SPECIFIC INFLAMMATION [FNI] IN CROHN'S DISEASE

J.H. YARDLEY and S.R. HAMILTON

INTRODUCTION

Greatest diagnostic reliability in Crohn's disease [CD] is attached to presence of granulomas when assessing mucosal biopsies (1,2). However, most investigators find that granulomas are detectable in less than 25% of biopsy specimens from patients with CD. Other more commonly seen forms of inflammation in CD are: a] Non-specific acute and chronic inflammation with a prominent admixture of macrophages, termed by us "granulomatous features", that at times forms indistinct collections of cells suggesting early granuloma formation; b] Conventional non-specific and acute and chronic inflammation without prominence of macrophages.

We have noted that when the distributional pattern of non-specific inflammation is considered whether or not accompanied by granulomatous features, its value as a diagnostic finding is enhanced. For this purpose we distinguish between the following distributional patterns in inflammatory bowel disease [IBD]: a] Diffuse, in which intensity of inflammation is similar everywhere. b] Patchy, in which inflammation is widespread, but with noticeable variation in intensity in different parts of the mucosa. c] Focal, in which highly localized areas of inflammation are surrounded by mucosa showing little or no active inflammation (1). This report summarizes evidence obtained by us that focal non-specific inflammation [FNI] is a regularly seen finding in CD which is useful in detecting the disorder and in differentiating between Crohn's disease and ulcerative colitits [UC].

PROCEDURES

Blinded rectal biopsy study: The distribution of non-specific inflammation was studied in rectal biopsies from

patients who had active UC, ulcerative proctitis, or indeterminate IBD (1). Clinical, radiologic, and pathologic information was used to classify the patients. Patient selection was
random except that those with UC were included only when
histologically active disease was present. There were 54
biopsies which were coded and examined by two observers.
Histologic criteria were those for focal, patchy, or diffuse
distribution described above, but without reference to granulomatous features.

Colo-rectal biopsies in CD: Information on 237 separate
colo-rectal biopsy studies classified and indexed under the
scheme described above was reviewed and summarized. Included
were all biopsies from proven or suspected Crohn's disease
and showing active inflammation which were seen at John Hopkins from 1974-78.

"En face" study of colon mucosa: In order to increase the
sensitivity and efficiency of microscopic survey, mucosa in
formalin-fixed right hemicolectomy specimens was "filleted"
from the muscularis propria, and sheets of mucosa measuring 2
by 1-1/2 cm were pressed flat with warm glass during paraffin
imbedding (3). They were then sectioned parallel to the luminal surface according to the method used to study adenomato-
sis coli (4). Ninety square centimeters of colonic mucosa in
28 tissue blocks from 3 patients with Crohn's disease were
studied histologically (3).

RESULTS

Findings in the blinded study of colo-rectal biopsy material strongly favoured association of FNI [with or without
granulomatous features] with CD [Table 1]. While FNI was not
seen in any of the 14 biopsy specimens from patients with
active UC, it occurred in 10 of 23 showing active CD. At the
same time, patchy and diffuse inflammation were also noted in
CD, emphasizing that those distributions do not exclude CD.
The results with ulcerative proctitis and indeterminate colitis [Table 1] additionally stresses the non-specific character of the distribution.

Table 1. Rectal biopsies in Crohn's disease and ulcerative
colitis[a]. Distribution of non-specific acute and
chronic inflammation

Disease	Focal	Patchy	Diffuse	Absent
Crohn's disease	10[b]	4	9	9
Ulcerative colitis	0	2	12	N/A
Ulcerative proctitis	0	1	1	0
Indeterminate colitis	2	0	4	4

a Data modified from ref. 1.
b No. of biopsies

The value of noting FNI was also borne out in the review
of routinely indexed colo-rectal biopsy studies. Among the
237 indexed studies in proven or suspected Crohn's disease
with demonstrated disease activity, granulomas were discovered in 25%, 28% showed non-specific inflammation with granulomatous features [no notation being made about distribu-
tion], and 48% revealed only non-specific inflammation without describing granulomatous features. However, in 31% of
those with non-specific inflammation without granulomatous
features, the lesion was also described as focal. During the
same period [1974-1978] this was never observed in patients
with active UC.The results give additional support to FNI as
an aid in recognizing CD and distinguishing it from UC.

Study of en face sections of colonic mucosa from CD (3)
clearly showed that the large areas surveyed from all three
patients revealed active inflammatory lesions, including
occasional granulomas, but most often as FNI either with or
without granulomatous features [Fig. 1]. Inflammatory lesions
were seen in conventional sections from only one of the same
patients, and none were found in en face sections from 3
control patients. The findings gave further emphasis to the
regular and wide spread occurrence of FNI in CD even in
grossly normal mucosa.

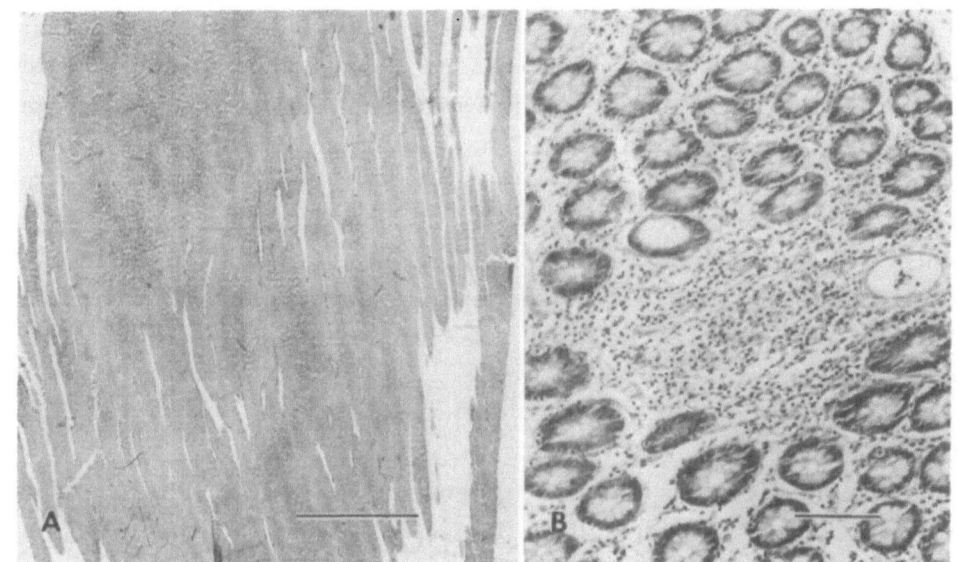

Figure 1. A. Low power view of a large sheet of grossly normal colonic mucosa from CD sectioned en face [bar=4
mm].
B. Detail of focal non-specific inflammation [FNI]
as revealed by en face section [bar=100μ m].

DISCUSSION AND CONCLUSIONS

In actual fact, non-specific, acute and chronic inflammation is the major form taken by the inflammatory process in
both CD and UC. The regular occurrence of focal inflammation
in CD has also been described previously. In an elegant computerized study, focal non-specific inflammatory lesions were
observed preferentially in CD over UC at a highly significant
level (5). Others have emphasized the related focal or irregular reduction in goblet cell mucin in CD (6, 7, 8). The
localized "aphthoid ulcers" which occur in otherwise grossly
normal mucosa in CD (9) are in all likelihood a particular
aspect of widespread FNI lesions occurring in the disease.

From the standpoint of the usefulness of rectal biopsy in
CD, it should be stressed that inflammation, including FNI
and granulomas, are sometimes detected in rectal biopsies in
CD even when the disorder seems clinically limited to the
small intestine or to the small intestine and right colon.
This was true in the blind biopsy study summarized above (1),
and was observed by others (10, 11).

Finally, it should be stressed that non-specific inflammation [with or without granulomatous features], and granulomas can be found in the same specimen, sometimes even in the same area as merging lesions. And as others at the conference has noted, FNI lesions in CD could have special relevance for pathogenic and etiologic studies in CD. This follows logically from their widespread occurrence and the fact that FNI lesions may well be the earliest recognizable histologic finding to appear in CD.

ACKNOWLEDGEMENT

Dr. Hamilton is the recipient of a Senior Fellow Award from the National Foundation for Ileitis and Colitis.

REFERENCES

1. Yardley JH, Donowitz M. (1977) In: The gastrointestinal tract. Eds. Yardley JH, Morson BC. Williams and Wilkins, Baltimore p 50.
2. Rotterdam H, Korelitz BI, Sommers SC. (1977) Microgranulomas in grossly normal rectal mucosa in Crohn's disease. Am.J.Clin.Pathol. 67:550-554.
3. Hamilton SR, Bussey HJR, Morson BC. (1980) En face histologic technique to demonstrate mucosal inflammatory lesions in macroscopically uninvolved colon of Crohn's disease resection specimens. Lab.Invest. 42:121.
4. Bussey HJR. (1975) In: Familial Polyposis coli. The John Hopkins University Press, Baltimore. p 38
5. Jones JH, Lennard-Jones JE, Morson BC, Chapman M, Sackin MJ, Sneath PHA, Spicer CC, Card WI.(1973) Numerical taxonomy and discriminant analysis applied to non-specific colitis. Quart.J.Med. 42:715-732
6. Dawson IMP. (1972) The value for diagnosis and research of special investigation on rectal biopsies in Crohn's disease. Brit.J.Surg. 59:806-809
7. Hellstrom HR, Fischer ER. (1968) Am.J.Clin.Pathol. 48:259-268.
8. Price AB, Morson BC. (1975) Inflammatory bowel disease: the surgical pathology of Crohn's disease and ulcerative colitis. Hum.Pathol. 6:7-29
9. Rickert RR, Carter HW.(1980)J.Clin.Gastroenterol.2:11-19
10. Dyer NH, Stansfeld AG, Dawson, AM. (1970) The value of rectal biopsy in the diagnosis of Crohn's disease. Scand. J.Gastroenterol. 5:491-496.
11. Geboes K, Vantrappen G. (1975) The value of colonoscopy in the diagnosis of CD. Gastrointest.Endosc. 22:18-23

B6 Summary of Discussions relating to topic B5

Sommers: The terms microgranuloma, granulomatous features
              and epithelioid cell collection are essentially
              synonyms. The lesions are very focal, and multiple
              sections are therefore important.

de Dombal: Yardley's experience regarding incidence of
              various histologic lesions agrees with those in the
              various centres that I described. I think we have
              arrived at a statement of general experience in the
              U.S.A. and elsewhere.

Strober: What is the most essential and characteristic
              lesion in CD, and what is the earliest important
              lesion? Is it the non-specific infiltrate or the
              granuloma? Also, are there limitations to ordinary
              histopathological studies?

Yardley: There are no definable limits to morphology. The
              essential point is knowing how to look at and what
              to look for. I think the nonspecific lesion is more
              likely to be the earliest lesion than either the
              granuloma or the granulomatous features. My main
              evidence for this is experimental. If you place
              tubercle bacilli into tissue and follow the reac-
              tion, the first thing that occurs is conventional
              acute and chronic inflammation followed by the gra-
              nulomatous response. I must assume, therefore, that
              the same thing happens in CD.

Sommers: Macrophages proliferate in response to the mac-
              romolecules which they ingest and digest. Rosekrans
              et al. found increased IgM-containing plasma cells

in CD. IgM is the immunoglobulin that naturally formes complexes, and this may occur without immunologic or allergic reaction.

Schmitz-
Moormann: My paper [see below] on the sequence between inflammation and granuloma touches on just this point. However, there is also focal inflammation in Yersiniosis, sometimes even with macrophages which form granuloma-like structures. I have also seen focal lesions in typical UC in the non-inflamed areas. There are many other causes, such as milk allergy and unidentified infections.

Yardley: Perhaps I haven't emphasized sufficiently the word non-specific. There was no intention to imply that the focal lesion is absolutely specific for CD and excludes other causes of inflammatory disease in the intestine.

Jewell: Since the whole of the gastrointestinal tract may be involved in CD, theories about the earliest lesion must apply to the whole of the gastrointestinal tract, including the mouth. Possibly there is a biochemical defect of permeability allowing more ready access of antigens into the lamina propria. We know that HLA antigens, and more recently possibly immune response antigens, are located in the epithelium of the gut. Such factors could enable to the whole of the gut to be mildly abnormal, and then for certain focal areas to be picked out for maximum disease because of local conditions, such as concentration of antigen.

Tijtgat: Can the histological characteristics change with treatment? It can become difficult to make the differential diagnosis by sigmoidoscopy in patients receiving steroids. Does the pathologist have the same problem?

Yardley: In patients on large doses of systemic steroids or with heavy use of steroid enemas there can be suppression of the lymphoid tissue in a rectal biopsy, but if there is active disease the basic character of the lesion is still there. I don't know what percentage of biopsies from our patients were taken during treatment, but I would guess at least 50 percent.

THE HISTOPATHOLOGICAL EVOLUTION OF CROHN'S DISEASE

T.J. CHAMBERS and B.C. MORSON

INTRODUCTION

The histopathological diagnosis of Crohn's disease rests upon the recognition of a combination of tissue changes each of which is relatively non-specific, but which together produce a characteristic histological pattern (1). Some features are always present: transmural lymphoid aggregates, mural thickening, and fissuring ulceration. In addition about 70% of cases show granulomas. Although the finding of granulomas superimposed on the above histological changes is strong supportive evidence, their presence is not essential for a diagnosis of Crohn's disease to be made. This raises fundamental questions about the significance of the granuloma in Crohn's disease, and indeed about the nature of Crohn's disease itself. There are several possible explanations for the inconstant presence of granulomas in Crohn's disease:

1] Crohn's disease may be caused by several different agents, only some of which cause granuloma formation.

2] Granulomas may appear in Crohn's disease in some patients following mucosal ulceration and consequent access to the diseased bowel wall by granuloma-inducing luminal agents. This theoretical possibility is rendered less likely by the observation that other diseases in which mucosal ulceration occurs are not associated with the presence of granulomas.

3] A single aetiological agent of Crohn's disease may only cause granuloma formation in some patients [cf tuberculoid and lepromatous leprosy].

4] Granulomas may be present only in certain phases of the disease [cf sarcoid, lymphogranuloma venereum].

We attempted to clarify the significance of the granuloma in Crohn's disease by quantitating granulomas in tissue sections and correlating the number of granulomas observed with the site of disease, length of previous history and subsequent disease course.

METHODS

The 79 patients we studied were all the patients who had undergone primary surgery for Crohn's disease at St Mark's Hospital between 1955 and 1968 in whom a ten-year follow-up was available. For each patient four random sections from areas of resected bowel involved by Crohn's disease were inspected. The number of granulomas in each section was noted, together with the origin of the section [small intestine, colon, rectum or anus]. The patients' notes were then inspected for the relevant clinical details. All patients with less than a ten-year follow-up were excluded, except from studies on the regional distribution of granulomas.

RESULTS AND DISCUSSION

Of the 79 patients in the study, 47 showed no clinical, radiological or biopsy evidence of persistence or recurrence in the 10 years after the primary operation, and the average number of granulomas in sections of involved bowel was 13. In the remaining patients who did show evidence of recurrence, there were 5 granulomas per section. Thus patients with a poor subsequent clinical course showed significantly [p<0.01] less granulomas in the primary surgical specimen than those patients who have remained clinically disease-free for 10 years. Rather unexpectedly, we noticed that there was a wide regional variation in the number of granulomas in involved bowel. Taking all the slides from involved small intestine as a group, the average number of granulomas per section was 1.1, compared with 6.1 in the colon, 18.3 in the rectum and 36.1 in the anus. This large difference in granulomas in different parts of the bowel could have accounted for the decreased number of granulomas in patients with a poor prognosis if this group had a higher loading of sections taken from proximal bowel. However, we found that in each region of the bowel [except the ileum] the number of granulomas was lower in the poor-prognosis group [see Fig. 1].

How do we account for the striking regional variation in numbers of granulomas? We felt two factors may be responsible. First, Crohn's disease is a granulomatous disorder, and as in other granulomatous disorders, granulomas may be present early and regress over a period of time. Second, that distal Crohn's disease seemed more likely to result in excision earlier than proximal disease – the more fluid bowel contents proximally may delay clinical symptoms [cf caecal vs rectal carcinoma], and proximal mucosal inflammation is less likely to lead to diarrhoea than distal inflammation [cf coeliac disease and ulcerative colitis]. The regional varia-

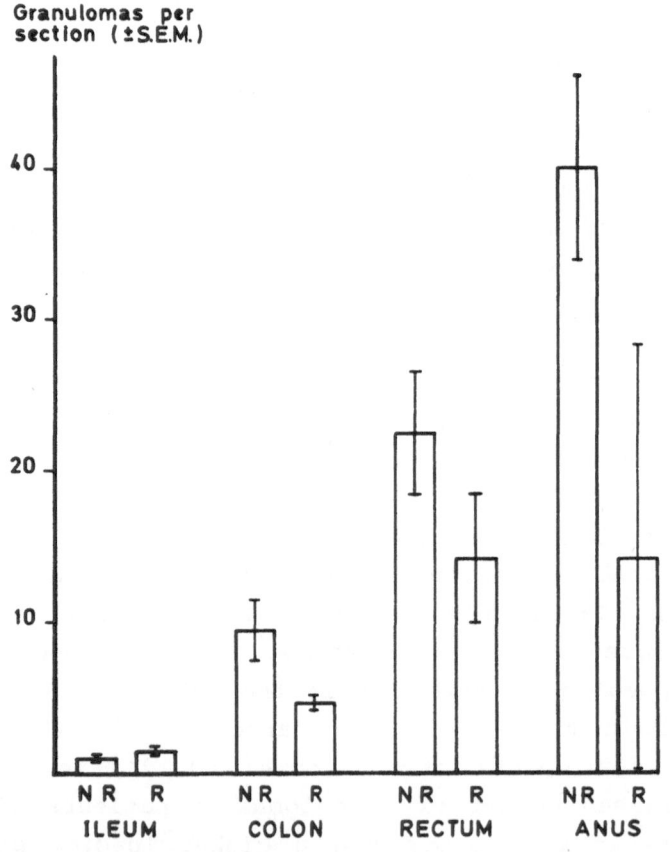

Figure 1. The number of granulomas in different regions of bowel involved by Crohn's disease, related to subsequent disease course. NR=no recurrence, R=sum of persistent and recurrent cases.

tion may thus be accounted for by postulating that early disease has more granulomas than late disease, and bowel is resected earlier in the disease course in distal Crohn's disease.

We found three lines of evidence to support this suggestion. We divided the surgical specimens into three groups: those from patients with symptoms for four years or less prior to surgery, those with symptoms for 5-8 years, and those with symptoms for more than 8 years. As shown in Fig. 2, the patients with the longest history had least granulomas.

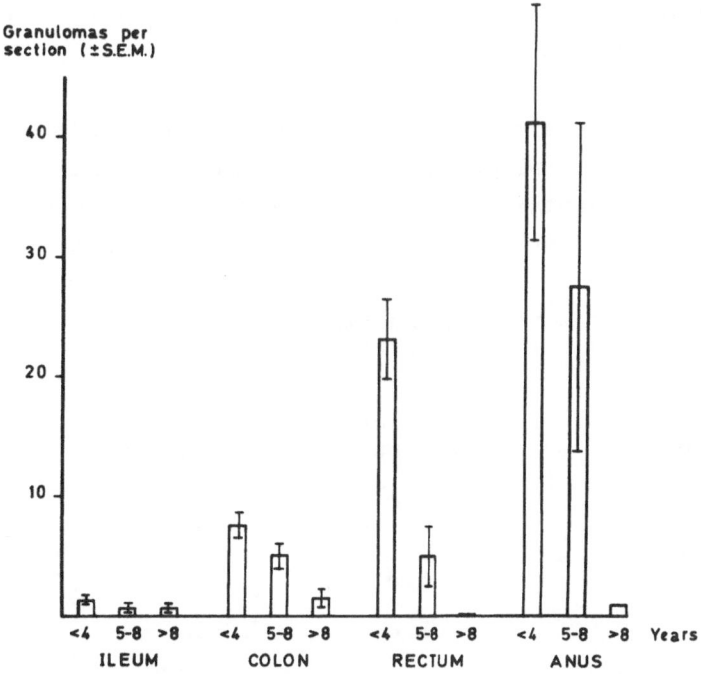

Figure 2. The relationship between duration of previous symptoms and the number of granulomas in bowel excised for Crohn's disease.

The second line of evidence resulted from a comparison between the number of granulomas in the primary resection specimen and the number in specimens removed for subsequent recurrence. The later specimens showed a highly significant reduction in granuloma content [Table 1]. The third line of evidence derives from comparing the number of granulomas in the ileum in specimens of ileal disease with the number in ileocolonic Crohn's disease. If later excision accounts for the reduced number of granulomas in ileal specimens, then those cases of ileal disease in which the colon was also involved should present earlier than usual for ileal disease and therefore contain more granulomas. We found that in Crohn's disease confined to the ileum there was a mean of 0.6 granulomas per section, while in ileocolitis, sections of the ileum contained an average of 3.7 granulomas per section. Presumably the colonic disease had led to an earlier-than-usual excision of ileum, with a consequently higher-than-usual granuloma content.

Two findings emerge from these results. The first is that the presence of granulomas in operative specimens confers an improved prognosis. Granuloma formation thus appears to be an adaptive host response for the improved elimination of the aetiological agent of Crohn's disease.

Table 1. Number of granulomas per section in surgical specimens of recurrent Crohn's disease

Origin of section	Granulomas [mean]	Standard deviation	No. of sections
Ileum	0.8	2	43
Colon	5	8.7	15
Rectum	0	–	5
Anus	4.3	4	3
Total	1.8	4.8	68

The second finding is that the number of granulomas seen in bowel involved by Crohn's disease decreases with the passage of time. In this respect Crohn's disease is therefore like other granulomatous diseases, such as sarcoid, lymphogranuloma venereum and tuberculosis, in which the usual evolution of the disease is granuloma formation in response to the aetiological agent, followed by elimination of the agent and the disappearance of granulomas. In these diseases the accompanying tissue fibrosis can lead to disordered tissue function long after the granulomas have disappeared. One reason then why granulomas are not always seen in Crohn's disease is that in many cases, by the time bowel is excised the original aetiological agent is no longer present. The fibrosis and tissue damage in the bowel wall and lymphatic drainage system persist, however, and may be the cause of the continuing fissuring ulceration and chronic inflammation. Similar chronic ulceration is seen following lymphogranuloma venereum infection, and mural thickening with fissuring ulceration can be induced in the bowel of pigs by damaging the lymphatic system (2).

If this concept of the evolution of the disease is accepted, it has implications for our approach to the clinical assessment of disease activity, the effects of treatment, and the search for the aetiological agent of Crohn's disease. Many patients with clinically active disease show on surgical histology of excised specimens only fibrosed, strictured segments of intestine with chronic inflammation and no granulomas. This suggests that many or all of the clinical symptoms and signs of Crohn's disease may be caused by tissue scarring rather than by a current interaction between host and aetiological agent. The clinical waxing and waning of disease may result from episodes of attempted healing and re-ulceration of irreversibly damaged bowel, and obstructive symptoms may be the result of disordered bowel function persisting long after the elimination of the aetiological agent. Further, since granulomas rather than clinically active disease are a sign of the presence of the aetiological agent, it would seem necessary to search for the agent in cases in which granulomas are still present.

REFERENCES
1. Morson BC. (1968) Histopathology of Crohn's disease. Proc. Roy. Soc. Med. 61:79-81
2. Kalima TV, Saloniemi H, Rahko T. (1976) Experimental regional enteritis in pigs. Scand.J.Gastroenterol. 11:353-362

HISTOLOGICAL STUDIES ON THE FORMAL PATHOGENESIS OF THE EPITHELIOID CELL GRANULOMA IN CROHN'S DISEASE

P. SCHMITZ-MOORMANN   and   H. BECKER

INTRODUCTION

The epithelioid cell granuloma is a well known lesion in Crohn's disease. It is found mostly adjacent to lymphatic tissue of the submucosa and subserosa. By the present study we have analyzed the various histologic abnormalities found in Crohn's disease and have constructed a likely sequence of events for the development of the full-blown granuloma.

METHODS AND RESULTS

Four hundred and fifty three rectal biopsies and 152 colonic biopsies form the basis of this study. Using this histologic material we correlated the frequency of epithelioid granulomas with the presence of non ulcerative diffuse colitis, local colitis, crypt abscess and ulcer or erosion. Table 1 shows that granulomas are more frequently found when crypt abcesses, erosions or ulcers are present in the rectal mucosa and in table 2 in the colonic mucosa.

Table 1. Number of granulomas in percent found in different inflammatory lesions of the rectum in Crohn's disease [453 biopsies, 156 patients]

Histologic lesion	Frequency F	Combination with epithelioid cell granuloma E	Ratio E/F
Normal	39 %	1 %	2.5 %
Colitis simplex	26 %	2 %	8 %
Local colitis	12 %	1 %	8 %
Crypt abscess	8 %	2 %	25 %
Erosion or ulcer	15 %	6 %	40 %

Table 2. Number of granulomas in percent found in different inflammatory lesions of the colonic mucosa in Crohn's disease [152 biopsies, 79 patients]

Histologic lesion	Frequency	Combination with epithelioid cell granuloma	Ratio
	F	E	E/F
Normal	12 %	2 %	17 %
Colitis simplex	19 %	1 %	5 %
Local colitis	18 %	1 %	6 %
Crypt abscess	5 %	2 %	40 %
Erosion or ulcer	46 %	7 %	15 %

In contrast, we did not find any correlation in the number or in the size of epithelioid cell granulomas within these categories [Table 3]. The mean value of the number of granulomas was about 0.9 per mm^3 of tissue, and the size of the granulomas was about 130 μ , regardless of the type of histologic lesions present. In addition no correlation between these two parameters and the site of biopsy was found. In patients with a longer history of Crohn's disease the granulomata were larger than in those with a short history.

Table 3. Number and size of epithelioid cell granulomas compared with the type of histologic lesion

Histologic lesion	Number of biopsies	Number of granulomas per cubic mm tissue	Size of granulomas in microns
Stroma infiltration			
none	10	0.64+0.44	132+37
grade 1	20	1.20+1.14	129+28
grade 2	20	0.79+0.78	138+67
grade 3	25	0.96+1.14	128+41
Local colitis			
absent	50	0.91+1.09	128+38
present	25	0.98+0.77	138+59
Crypt abscess			
absent	38	1.00+1.12	130+54
present	37	0.86+0.84	133+35
Erosion			
absent	55	0.93+0.96	126+32
present	20	0.95+1.10	148+69
Ulcer			
absent	39	0.94+1.04	133+53
present	36	0.93+0.95	130+38

DISCUSSION

Serial sections of our material reveal many intermediate stages of granuloma formation. We propose the following hypothesis concerning the sequence of events occurring during the development of the granuloma based on these different stages of the histologic lesions with which they are associated [Fig. 1].

The inflammatory process starts with a spotty non ulcerative inflammation. At this point it is characterized by a pericryptal accumulation of plasma cells and leucocytes. Next, the leucocytes migrate into the crypts, forming crypt-

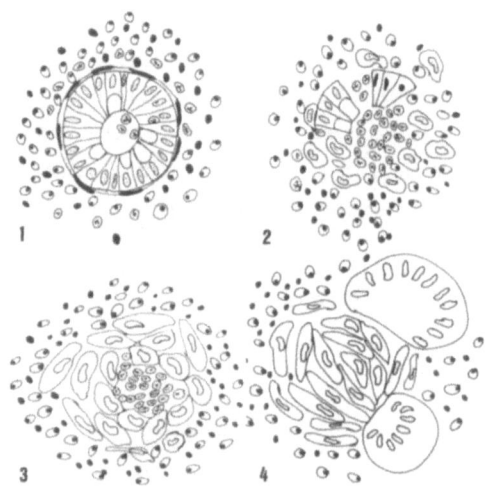

Figure 1. Development of the mucosal epithelioid cell granuloma.

1. Pericryptal inflammation with some migrating leucocytes.
2. Destruction of the crypt epithelium and development of a crypt abscess; formation of some large histiocytes.
3. Transformation of histiocytes into epithelioid cells; in the centre of the lesion some leucocytes of the crypt abscess are still visible.
4. Complete epithelioid cell granuloma in the place of the destroyed crypt area.

abscesses and simultaneously, the epithelial cells of the crypts are destroyed. During this stage large histiocytes appear in area surrounding the destroyed crypt; these histiocytes are subsequently transformed into epithelioid cells while the leucocytes in the crypt lumen are still visible. In the last stage only a epithelioid cell granuloma remains in what was once the crypt area. The stages are diagrammed.

The mucosal damage apparently depends on the extent of cryptal alterations. If the crypt damage extends only to the bottom of the crypt, a crypt abscess and, later, an epithelioid cell granuloma are produced. If the damage is localized to the upper part of the crypt, tiny superficial erosions are produced. Damage to the whole crypt produces a microscopical fissure-like ulcer. Whereas if the damage involves several neighbouring crypts, an aphthous ulcer is produced.

CONCLUSIONS

Our investigations lead to the following conclusions:

1. The development of a mucosal epithelioid cell granuloma seems to have the following sequence: local colitis-crypt abscess- destruction of the crypt with proliferation of enlarged histiocytes - transformation of histiocytes to epithelioid cells and Langhans cells - epithelioid cell granuloma.

2. According to the extent of the crypt destruction, crypt abscesses or epithelioid cell granulomas in the deeper layer of the mucosa, tiny erosions at the cryptal mouth, small fissure-like erosions or aphthous ulcers arise.

GRANULOMA, ARTERITIS AND INFLAMMATORY CELL COUNTS IN CROHN'S DISEASE

H. THOMPSON and R.S. BONSER

INTRODUCTION

This study assesses the significance of granuloma, arteritis and inflammatory cell population counts in the diagnosis of Crohn's disease.

MATERIAL AND METHODS

306 resected specimen from Leeds [128] and Birmingham [178] Crohn's series were studied for the incidence of granuloma and arteritis. The incidence of granulomata was also assessed in a series of 194 rectal biopsies studied during the last 5 years.

Cell counts were performed on rectal biopsies from 25 patients with Crohn's disease [CD], 25 patients with ulcerative colitis [UC] and 10 normal controls (1). Clinical progress of the patients was assessed independently.

A minimum of 10 blocks were examined from each resected specimen. Multiple step sections were studied from each rectal biopsy. Taylor's blue metachromatic staining technique (2) was used for identification of mast cells. Cell counts were carried out under high power with a graticule and registered on a laboratory calculator. Point counting technique was applied at lower magnification. Mathematical conversions were carried out with a stage micrometer and a calculator.

RESULTS

Granulomata

Epithelioid cell follicles with Langhan's giant cells were identified in 62.6% of all resected specimens. They occurred in all layers of the bowel wall and were distributed along the lines of lymphatic channels and blood vessels. Granulomata were found in adjacent lymph nodes in 29.5% of cases.

The incidence of granulomata in a series of 194 rectal biopsies from patients with CD during the last 5 years has been 27.3%. Granulomata have also been encountered in perianal biopsies, gastric biopsies, jejunal biopsies, appendices and rarely liver and abdominal skin.

Aphthous ulceration can be an early feature of CD and biopsy of these small ulcers frequently shows granulomata in their base. Aphthous ulceration is reversible and has been described in other disorders.

No relationship has so far been discovered between the presence of granulomata and the clinical course of the disease in this series.

Granulomata can occur occasionally in diverticular disease, as a sarcoid response to colorectal cancer and as a poorly developed reaction in UC representing a foreign body reaction.

Arteritis

The indicence of arteritis in the combined Leeds-Birmingham series of 306 patients was 9.5%. The incidence in the Birmingham series of 178 cases, which was more intensively studied was, 11.8%. The incidence of arteritis in the series of 194 rectal biopsies was only 1.5%. Vascular inflammation associated with CD can be of necrotising type with fibrinoid necrosis, as well as the granulomatous, eosinophilic or non specific inflammatory type. It can involve vessels of all sizes ranging from muscular arteries to arterioles and it can also involve veins. Mesenteric vessels occasionally show arteritis. Ischaemic necrosis secondary to arteritis is uncommon.

Rectal biopsy cell counts

The results of rectal biopsy cell counts are shown in tables 1 and 2; as expected these cell counts show an increased cell population in inflammatory bowel disease. The differential counts have no obvious diagnostic value although the presence of neutrophils and eosinophils confirms that an inflammatory response is present.

Table 1. Total cell counts in rectal biopsies[*]

	Normal[10]	CD[25]	UC[25]
Lamina propria	4867	6540	5778
Submucosa	1040	1920	2987

* mean total cell counts/mm^2

Table 2. Differential cell counts as expected as mean % of total cell counts

	Mucosa			Submucosa		
	Normal	CD	UC	Normal	CD	UC
Lymphocytes	15.8	34.4	38.2	0.	21.4	35.8
Plasma cells	2.7	7.3	9.8	0.	7.0	3.1
Neutrophils	0.	0.1	2.9	0.	0.	0.4
Eosinophils	0.9	3.9	3.9	0.	4.8	2.7
Spindle cells	13.6	6.9	3.0	43.6	19.8	24.1
Macrophages	67.0	47.4	42.2	56.4	47.0	33.9

Mast cell counts determined by metachromatic staining technique is shown in tables 3 and 4.

Table 3. Mast cell counts per mm^2 in the rectal mucosa

	Mean	Range	SD
Normal	33	8 - 87	26
Crohn's disease	36	1 - 126	34

Table 4. Mast cell counts per mm^2 in the muscularis mucosa and the submucosa

	Mean	Range	SD
Normal	100	43 - 259	65
Crohn's disease	134	46 - 257	61

On the basis of these mast cell counts the following conclusions were made:
1] The highest concentration of mast cells occurs in the muscularis mucosa and submucosa; 2] Cell counts of mast cells in the muscularis mucosa and submucosa are more constant and reliable than in the mucosa; 3] No significant differences were identified in the mast cell population of CD patients

compared to normal controls; 4] Mast cell counts are of no value in the determination of disease activity. Because me-tachromatic staining techniques do not identify degranulated mast cells it remains possible that the mast cell population is increased in CD in spite of these results. Dvorak (3) claims that degranulated mast cells can be recognized in electron microscope studies and that mast cells are increased in number in regional ileitis.

REFERENCES
1. Thompson H, Buchmann P. (1979) Mast cell population in rectal biopsies from patients with Crohn's disease. In: The Mast Cell. Eds. Pepys J, Edwards AM, Pitman Medical pp 697-701
2. Taylor KB, Jeffree GM. (1968) Histochem. J. 1:199
3. Dvorak AM. (1979) Mast cell hyperplasia and degranulation in Crohn's disease. In: The Mast Cell. Eds. Pepys J, Edwards AM, Pitman Medical pp 657-662

B10 Summary of Discussions relating to topics B7 to B9

Strober: I think it is important to decide whether in CD an etiologic agent, such as a virus, is causing death of epithelial cells and the immune system is reacting in a very complex fashion to that cell death, or alternatively, whether the etiologic agent is affecting primarily the immune system which is then "fooled" into killing epithelial cells. If the latter mechanism is correct, the epithelial injury is a secondary effect, and what is really important is the effect on the immune system, the lymphoid cells and the macrophages. I don't think that morphologic studies have answered this question, and I do not think that they are intrinsically able to.

Schmitz-   If it is correct that focal colitis occurs first Moormann: then you can conclude that the infiltration destroyed the epithelial cells. This could mean that epithelial cells undergo an alteration that makes them vulnerable.

Asquith: I would be cautious about over-interpreting the varied incidence of granuloma in different parts of the gut. Immunocompetent cells in the small and large intestine will react differently whatever the challenging antigen, and if the immunocompetent cells are different in those two sites, then the incidence of granulomas would indeed be different.

Chambers: I hoped the paper explained clearly why we thought length of history was the major cause of the regional variation in granuloma content in CD.

For instance, there were more granulomas in the ileum in ileocolitis than when the ileum alone was involved.

Booth: At the first International Workshop on Crohn's disease [1975] Thompson presented a paper on the occurrence of granulomas in bypassed segments of colon, and showed that there were reasonable numbers of granulomata in those bypassed segments and many years afterwards in very late CD. Does Thompson's data conflicts with the St. Mark's study.

Thompson: We did find granulomata in the by-passed colon and rectum many years after the operation. On the other hand, the disease frequently dies down in the small intestine in the bypass situation as compared to the large intestine, and it has been noted that you can reduce the severity of the disease by resting small bowel. So there does seem to be different behaviour in the two regions. The aphthous ulcers found in early CD are of great interest because they are reversible and granulomata occur in the base. The lymphatic network in the gut wall is certainly involved because you see granulomata along the lines of the lymphatics. With regard to the bypassed colon and rectum the findings suggest that the antigen is still reaching rectal mucosa, or, alternatively, we are dealing with a persistent antigen in the mucosa.

Jeejeebhoy: Could Chambers' result be explained on the basis that patients who have had a more complicated course of disease are more likely to be on steroids or immunosuppressive agents?

Chambers: There is a small reduction in the number of granulomas in patients who are on steroids, but it is not significant statistically.

Farmer: In all the series, only between 25 and 50 percent of the specimens show granulomas, depending on
whether mucosal biopsies or resected specimens are
examined. If this implies that granulomas are present early in the disease, and if granulomas are
more often associated with a good prognosis, this
seems to be a dichotomy. We found that granulomas
did not have prognostic significance.

Chambers: There were about twice as many granulomas in
patients who had a good prognosis. However, that is
a small difference compared to the difference in
granulomas in different regions.

Burnham: Chambers suggested that the presence of granulomas indicated persistence of the etiological a-
gent, and that as time went on this was eliminated,
and the granulomas disappear. Is it not surprising
therefore, that granulomas appear to have some
protective effect against subsequent recurrence
rather than the other way around? And does not this
suggest that the absence of granulomas indicates
the etiological agent is persisting?

Chambers: We are totally ignorant about the variables that
affects CD. Perhaps granuloma indicate a good prognosis because macrophages are immobile, they don't
spread so far, and hence the disease is not so
severe.

B-CELL SYSTEM AND CROHN'S DISEASE

C.J.L.M. MEIJER, P.C.M. ROSEKRANS and J. LINDEMAN

INTRODUCTION

Several reports have indicated a possible role for immunological mechanisms in the pathogenesis of Crohn's disease (1-5). For this reason it is important to analyse the cellular infiltrate in the bowel wall of patients with Crohn's disease, as this may give a clue to the type of immunological reaction involved. Literature data about the nature of the lymphoid cells in the bowel wall of Crohn's disease are inconclusive. The presence of T-cells especially in the deeper layers of the bowel wall has been stressed (6,7). This is surprising since throughout the bowel wall many lymphoid aggregates often characterized by germinal centres, can be found, structures known to contain B-cells in lymph nodes, spleen and rheumatoid synovium (8,9).

In this study we have analysed the cellular infiltrates in the bowel wall of patients with Crohn's disease for the presence of B-and Fc-receptor bearing lymphocytes with immunological and histochemical techniques. To identify the B-lymphocytes, we use three reliable independent markers: the presence of surface immunoglobulins [sIg], the presence of receptors for the activated third complement component, and the presence of membrane-bound 5-nucleotidase. We have also analyzed the population of Ig-containing cells in the bowel wall with respect to the proportion of cells belonging to each of the main Ig classes and the histological appearance of the draining regional lymph nodes. Our results indicate that in Crohn's disease the inflammatory process is composed predominantly of B-cells.

MATERIAL AND METHODS

Pieces of tissue from the affected and unaffected ilectomy and/or colectomy specimens of 10 patients with Crohn's disease and of the regional lymph nodes were either 1] snap frozen in liquid nitrogen for demonstration of surface immunoglobulins, membrane receptors and hydrolytic enzymes, 2] fixed in a sublimate formaldehyde mixture for studying the Ig containing cells or 3] fixed in buffered formaline for routine diagnostic purposes.

The diagnosis of Crohn's disease was based on criteria given by Korelitz et al.(10) for surgical specimens and on criteria described by Morson (11) and Whitehead (12) for mucosal biopsies.

As reference material for the immunological and histochemical studies unaffected ileum and colon segments of 4 bowel specimens removed for primary adeno-carcinoma were used. As reference material for the Ig-containing cells, 4 colectomy specimens from patients with ulcerative colitis were used.

The cells bearing receptors for the F_c portion of IgG [$F_c\gamma$ receptor] and for the activated third complement component [C_3 receptors] were demonstrated by the red cell overlayer-technique using sheep erythrocytes coated with rabbit IgG antibody [EA-IgG] and sheep erythrocytes coated with IgM antibody and mouse complement [EAC] respectively as described earlier (9,13,14). Sections overlayered by uncoated sheep erythrocytes or sheep erythrocytes coated by rabbit IgM antibody served as controls. Lymphocytes bearing surface IgA, IgG, IgM or IgD were demonstrated with the direct or indirect immunofluorescence technique as described earlier (13). Lymphocytes bearing surface membrane bound 5-nucleotidase were demonstrated by the method of Muller-Hermelink (15).

Alpha-naphtylacetate esterase and acid phosphatase were used as markers for mononuclear phagocytes. Demonstration of immunoglobulin-containing cells was done by the indirect immunoperoxidase technique (16). The number of Ig-containing cells in the lamina propria of three representative parts of a bowel specimen was counted per stretched mm muscularis mucosae (17). This corresponds to a mucosal unit of 1 mm width and 4 μm thick. Next the mean number of Ig containing cells per specimen was calculated.

RESULTS

The histological characteristics of the bowel of patients studied and the draining lymph nodes were typical of Crohn's disease.

The results of the membrane marker characteristics are shown in table 1. Most of the infiltrating cells were organized into follicular structures and nearly all of these cells showed diffuse ring labelling as did many of the lymphocytes scattered throughout the bowel wall. Most of the lymphocytes bore sIgM often associated with sIgD. sIgA-bearing lymphocytes were found in small numbers. sIgG-bearing lymphocytes were extremely rare. Small zones of lymphocytes, localized around the follicular structure in the submucosa, muscularis or serosa often lacked staining for sIg. The pattern of cells showing EAC adherence resembled that of sIg bearing cells. Lymphoid follicular infiltrates showed   clear

Table 1. Membrane characteristics of intestinal infiltrates in Crohn's disease

	sIg	EAC
Lamina propria		
mononuclear cells		
- diffuse	+ and -	+ and -
- follicular	++/sometimes -	++/sometimes -
Submucosa		
mononuclear cells		
- diffuse	-	-
- follicular	++	++
- perifollicular	- /sometimes +	- /sometimes +
Muscularis + serosa		
mononuclear cells		
- diffuse	-	-
- follicular	++/sometimes -	++/sometimes -
- perifollicular	+ and -	+ and -

- to ++ represent various degrees of membrane fluorescence or red cell adherence.

EAC adherence, but the margin of these infiltrates often did not show EAC adherence. Interesting was the finding that lymphoid cells surrounding epithelioid cell granulomas often showed both EAC adherence and sIg whereas the epithelioid cells showed weak EAC adherence and were negative for sIg.

5-nucleotidase staining was found in germinal centers and in most follicular infiltrates. This staining pattern corresponded roughly to the pattern of lymphocytes bearing sIg or C_3 receptors.

EA-IgG adherence in tissue sections of the bowel wall often showed background adherence on collagen and vascular lumina in submucosa and serosa. Therefore no reliable EA-IgG adherence could be obtained on diffusely infiltrated cells in the bowel wall. Clear adherence was seen on the epithelioid cells in the granulomas.

Cells in the lamina propria, at the base of ulcers or within granulomas were stained positive for acid phosphatase and alpha-naphtylacetate esterase indicating the presence of histiocytes at these locations. It appeared that the number of histocytes in the lamina propria in patients with Crohn's disease was increased as compared to control patients and patients with ulcerative colitis.

The number of Ig-containing cells in the colon is indicated in table 2. These data suggest a relation between the activity of the inflammation in the bowel wall and the number of IgA and IgG-containing cells in inflammatory bowel disease. The presence of IgG-containing cells was mainly found in the basal layers of the lamina propria. However, in contrast to the colectomy specimens from the control patients and from the patients with ulcerative colitis, colectomy specimens from patients with Crohn's disease showed a strong increase in the number of IgM-containing cells. This was found in quiescent as well as in actively inflamed parts of the bowel wall.

Table 2. Number of immunoglobulin-containing cells per mm
stretched muscularis mucosae in colectomy specimens
[mean $\pm$ SD]

	IgA	IgM	IgG
Crohn's disease[n=6] removed for toxic colon [active phase]	217 $\pm$ 31	95 $\pm$ 25	166 $\pm$ 44
Ulcerative colitis[n=4] [removed in relatively quiescent phase of the disease for strong atypia and/or carcinoma]	139 $\pm$ 25	20 $\pm$ 15	99 $\pm$ 38
Control group[n=4]	88 $\pm$ 15	9 $\pm$ 7	12 $\pm$ 8

DISCUSSION

The present study demonstrates that the lymphoid cells
in the bowel wall are mainly localized in follicular aggregates. Furthermore, B-cells, characterized by the presence
of sIg, C_3 receptors and membrane bound 5-nucleotidase and
the absence of acid phosphatase and alpha-naphtylacetate esterase were the predominant type of cells in the intestinal
infiltrates. However, the B-cells were often found in close
relation with smaller numbers of non B-cells, presumably
T-cells, which were localized in small perifollicular zones.

Although it can not be excluded that a secondary reaction
of the damaged bowel wall may be the cause of the hyperplasia
of the B-cell areas in the lymph nodes, the limited degree of
follicular hyperplasia in regional lymph nodes from patients
with extensive ulcerations complicating diverticulitis does
not support that possibility. From all these observations it
is concluded that the inflammatory process in Crohn's disease
is dominated by stimulation of the B-cell system.

It is now known that the B-cell system undergoes regulatory influences of the T-cell system (18). How this regulation takes place at tissue level is unknown. The presence of
small numbers of non B-cells localized scattered throughout
the bowel wall and perifollicularly, possibly existing mainly
of T-cells, may indicate that these cells have a modulating
influence on the B-cell system.

Although the finding of large numbers of T-cells especially in the deeper layers of the bowel wall by Strickland et al. (7) and Meuwissen et al. (6) from methodological point of view do rise some questions, even the presence of small numbers of T-cells indicates the involvement of the T-cell system. However, we believe that based upon the findings of these authors the role of the T-cell system in the pathogenesis of Crohn's disease has been overemphasized in the past.

Also the increase of the total number of plasma cells, the end stage of the differentiation of the B-cells, in the intestinal infiltrate supports the view that the inflammatory process in Crohn's disease is dominated by a B-cell response, probably modulated by non-B, mainly T-cells. In addition it is remarkable that also in the colectomy specimens the findings of Rosekrans et al. (17), that the number of IgM-containing cells in the lamina propria is increased, could be confirmed. Probably in the future this finding may be of diagnostic help in the differential diagnosis between Crohn's disease and ulcerative colitis.

REFERENCES
1. Jones J, Housley J, Ashurst PM, Hawkins CF. (1969) Development of delayed hypersensitivity to dinitrochlorobenzene in patients with Crohn's disease. Gut 10:52-56
2. Meuwissen SGM, Schellekens PThA, Huismans L, Tijtgat GNJ. (1977) Impaired amnestic cellular immune response in patients with Crohn's disease. Gut 16:854-861
3. Skinner SF, Whitehead R. (1974) The plasmacells in inflammatory bowel disease of the colon; a quantitative study. J.Clin.Pathol. 27:643-646
4. Stobo JD, Tomasi TB, Huizenga KA, Spencer RJ, Shorter RG. (1976) In vitro studies of inflammatory bowel disease. Surface receptors of the mononuclear cell required to lyse allogeneic colonic epithelial cells. Gastroenterology 70:171-176
5. Auer IO. (1979) Immunology in Crohn's disease. Z.Gastroenterol. 17: suppl. 83-93
6. Meuwissen SGM, Feltkamp-Vroom ThM, Brutel de la Riviere A, Borne van den AEG, Tijtgat GNJ. (1976) Analysis of the lympho-plasmacytic infiltrate in Crohn's disease, with special reference to identification of lymphocyte subpopulations. Gut 17:770-780
7. Strickland RG, Husby G, Black WC, Williams RC Jr. (1975) Peripheral blood and intestinal lymphocyte subpopulations in Crohn's disease. Gut 16:847-853

8. Nieuwenhuis P. (1974) On the origin and fate of immuno-
    logically competent cells. PH.D. Thesis, Groningen, The
    Netherlands
9. Meijer CJLM, Putte van de LBA, Eulderink F, Kleinjan R,
    Lafeber G, Bots GThAM. (1977) Characteristics of mononu-
    clear cell populations in chronically inflamed synovial
    membrane. J.Pathol. 121:1-14
10. Korelitz BI, Present DM, Alpert LI, Marshak RH, Janowitz
    HD. (1972) Recurrent regional ileitis after ileostomy and
    colectomy for granulomatous colitis. New Engl.J.Med.
    287:110-114
11. Morson BC, Dawson IMP. (1972) In: Gastrointestinal Patho-
    logy, Oxford Blackwell Scientific Publ. pp 269-274
12. Whitehead R. (1973) Mucosal biopsy of the gastrointesti-
    nal tract. WB Saunders Company Ltd. London pp 139-165
13. Meijer CJLM, Bosman FT, Lindeman J. (1979) Evidence for
    predominant involvement of the B-cell system in Crohn's
    disease. Scand.J.Gastroenterol. 14:21-32
14. Jansen J, Schuit HRE, Zwet van ThL, Meijer CJLM, Hymans
    W. (1979) Hairy cell leukaemia: a B lymphocytic disorder.
    Brit.J.Heamatol. 42:21-33
15. Muller-Hermelink HK. (1974) Characterization of the
    B-cell and T-cell regions of human lymphatic tissue
    through enzyme histochemical demonstration of ATPase and
    5-nucleotidase activities. Virchows Arch. B Cell. Path.
    16:371-378
16. Bosman FT, Kreuning J, Wal van der AM, Kuiper I, Lindeman
    J. (1977) The influence of fixation on immunoperoxidase
    staining of plasma cells in paraffin sections of intesti-
    nal biopsy specimens. Histochemistry 53:57-62
17. Rosekrans PCM, Meijer CJLM, Lindeman J. (1980) Immunoglo-
    bulin-containing cells in Crohn's disease of the colon
    and rectum. These proceedings
18. Reinherz EL, Schlossman SF. (1980) Current concepts in
    Immunology: Regulation of the immune response-inducer and
    suppressor T-lymphocyte subsets in human beings. New
    Engl.J.Med. 303:370-372

IMMUNOGLOBULIN-CONTAINING CELLS IN COLONIC AND RECTAL MUCOSA
IN CROHN'S DISEASE

P.C.M. ROSEKRANS, C.J.L.M. MEIJER and J. LINDEMAN

INTRODUCTION

The large number of plasma cells and lymphocytes in the
lamina propria of the large bowel mucosa in patients with
Crohn's disease suggests that an immunological mechanism
plays a role in the pathogenesis of this disease. Earlier
studies on immunoglobulin-containing cells in Crohn's disease
were performed with immunofluorescence techniques (1,2,3).
Skinner and Whitehead (2) and Baklien and Brandtzaeg (3)
showed that in Crohn's disease of the colon the increase was
greatest for IgG and IgM. O'Donoghue and Kumar (4) found in
ulcerative colitis and Crohn's disease a marked increase in
IgE-containing cells in rectal mucosa.

The purpose of the present work was to determine the
number of immunoglobulin-containing cells in colonic mucosa
of patients with Crohn's disease [CD] and to compare these
numbers with those found in patients with ulcerative colitis
[UC] and in patients without any sign of colitis.

MATERIALS AND METHODS

Three groups of patients were studied:
-Ten patients with ulcerative colitis [average age, 37]. The
diagnosis was based on the presence of typical clinical,
radiological, endoscopical and histological findings (5). All
patients had a severe inflamed mucosa in sigmoid and rectum.
-Ten patients with Crohn's disease of the colon [average age
34]. The diagnosis was based on the presence of clinical,
radiological, endoscopical and histological findings (6).
Because of the segmental involvement of the colon in Crohn's
disease, in a number of cases there were only minor signs of
inflammation in the distal part of the colon. In seven pa-

tients we compared the biopsy findings from the rectum and sigmoid with areas of more active inflammation in the transverse or descending colon.

-Ten patients without any sign of colitis in which a colonoscopy was done because of a single polyp or the irritable colon syndrome [control group, average age, 35].

In every patient at least two biopsy specimens were obtained during endoscopical examination, one biopsy from the sigmoid and another from the rectum. The biopsy specimens were fixed in a sublimate formaldehyde mixture, and embedded in paraplast. Tissue sections were cut 4μ m thick, perpendicular to the luminal surface. Using the indirect immunoperoxidase staining technique, the sections were specifically stained for IgA, IgG, IgM and IgE. The specificity of the antisera and control staining procedures have already been reported (7). From the IgA, IgG, IgM and IgE stained sections the lamina propria area was measured per millimetre mucosal length. We counted the immunoglobulin-containing cells in three consecutive sections per millimeter mucosal length, that is in a "mucosal tissue unit" defined as a block of tissue, 4μ m thick and 1 mm width, from the surface epithelium to the muscularis mucosae (8).

RESULTS

In controls: IgA-containing cells were predominant while those containing IgG and IgM were in a small minority.

In patients with Crohn's disease the most important immunoglobulin-containing cell class was IgA. The number of the IgM-containing cells per millimeter mucosal length was significantly increased compared with the control group and the patients with ulcerative colitis [Fig.1, 2a and 2b]

The number of IgG-containing cells varied with the degree of colonic inflammation. In seven of the ten patients with Crohn's disease we found in actively inflamed mucosa of the

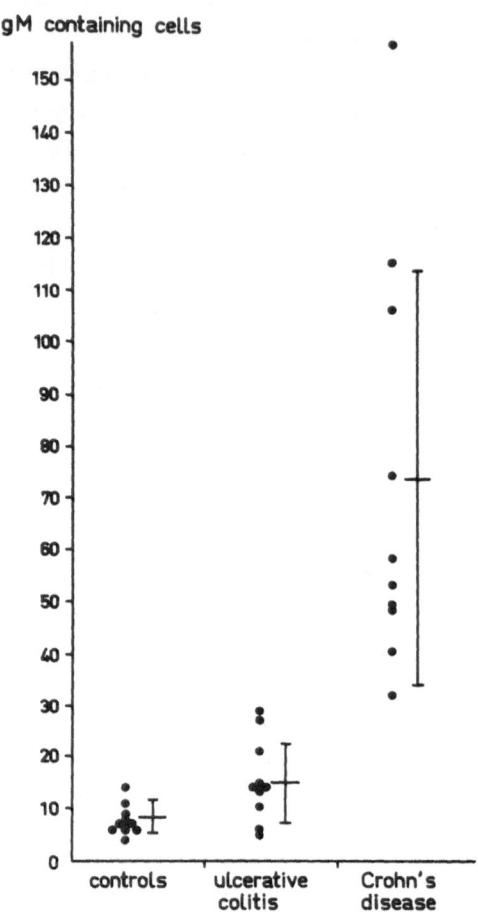

Figure 1. Number of IgM-containing cells per millimetre mucosal length in rectal mucosa in 10 controls, 10
patients with UC and 10 patients with CD

transverse or descending part of the colon the same high
number of IgG-containing cells as in active ulcerative colitis. The number of IgM-containing cells per millimeter mucosal length was increased, independing on the degree of activity of the inflammation [Table 1].

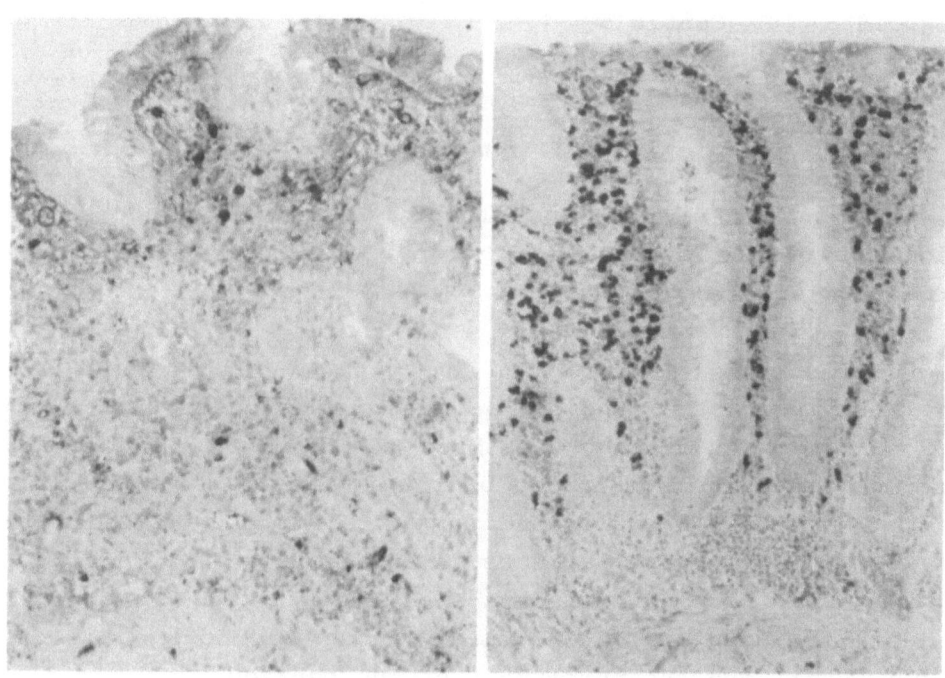

Figure 2a. IgM staining of rectal biopsy in patient with UC [x120]

Figure 2b. IgM staining of rectal biopsy in patient with CD [x120]

In patients with ulcerative colitis the IgG-containing cells formed an important proportion of the lamina propria cellular infiltrate, but the IgA-containing cells remained the major cell class. The degree of activity of inflammation seemed to correlate with the number of IgG-containing cells per millimetre mucosal length. The number of IgM-containing cells was almost the same as in the control group [Table 1].

Table 1. Number of IgA, IgG and IgM-containing cells per millimeter mucosal length in biopsy specimens [mean]

		IgA	IgG	IgM
Rectum	Controls	88	14	8
	UC	173	118	15
	CD	154	46	73
Sigmoid	Controls	81	12	7
	UC	164	97	15
	CD	161	36	68
Transverse or descending colon	CD [active inflammation]	181	105	59

The number of IgE-containing cells in the rectal and sigmoid colonic mucosa were very low in the three patient groups we studied.

DISCUSSION

Most previous studies about immunoglobulin-containing cells in Crohn's disease have been performed with immunofluorescence techniques. Because of the impermanence of the frozen sections and the limited possibilities for screening of these sections, quantitative studies are relatively difficult to perform with immunofluorescence staining. The immunoperoxidase staining technique has the advantage of the histological detail and the permanence of the section.

In Crohn's disease and ulcerative colitis we found, compared with controls, a marked absolute increase in immunoglobulin-containing cells, associated with a relative decrease of IgA-containing cells. The number of IgG-containing cells is increased and seemed to correlate with the degree of active inflammation of the bowel wall. In our opinion, the local increase of IgG-containing cells is a secondary reaction to mucosal destruction and the penetration of antigens or mitogens from the gut lumen. The number of IgM-containing cells was significantly increased in both quiescent and active parts of the colonic mucosa in Crohn's disease, as compared with numbers of IgM-containing cells in controls and ulcerative colitis specimens. Also, in colectomy specimens of patients with Crohn's disease (6) the number of IgM-containing cells is increased as compared to those of patients with ulcerative colitis. Therefore we believe that the increase of IgM-containing cells in patients with Crohn's disease may be of diagnostic help to differentiate the histology of inflammatory bowel disease.

REFERENCES
1. Crabbe PA, Heremans JF. (1966) The distribution of immunoglobulin-containing cells along the human gastrointestinal tract. Gastroenterology 51:305-316
2. Skinner JM, Whitehead R. (1974) The plasma cells in inflammatory bowel disease of the colon. A quantitative study. J.Clin.Pathol. 27:643-646
3. Baklien K, Brandtzaeg P. (1975) Comparative mapping of the local distribution of immunoglobulin-containing cells in ulcerative colitis and Crohn's disease of the colon. Clin.Exp.Immunol. 22:197-209
4. O'Donoghue DP, Kumar P. (1979) Rectal IgE-cells in inflammatory bowel disease. Gut 20:149-153
5. Morson BC. (1974) In:Pathology Annual.Ed. Sommers SC. Appleton-Century Crofts New York pp. 209-230
6. Meijer CJLM, Rosekrans PCM, Lindeman J. (1980) B-cell system and Crohn's disease. These proceedings
7. Rosekrans PCM, Meijer CJLM, Wal van der AM, Cornelisse CJ, Lindeman J. (1980) Immunoglobulin-containing cells in inflammatory bowel disease of the colon (A morphometric and immunohistochemical study) Gut, in press
8. Brandtzaeg P, Baklien K, Fausa O, Hoel PS. (1974) Immunohistochemical characterization of local immunoglobulin formation in ulcerative colitis. Gastroenterology 66: 1123-1136

B13 Summary of Discussions relating to topics B11 to B12

Strober: I wonder if Meijer characterized cells in early lesions, namely the small collections of lymphoid cells around crypts.

Meijer: These infiltrates are always B-cells, especially in the upper lamina propria, which bear mostly surface IgM and Fc receptors.

Strober: There have been some reports of reduced immuno-globulin-containing cells in areas adjacent to lesions. Could that be confirmed?

Das: I could not confirm that.

Rosekrans: There was an increase in the IgG-containing cells adjacent to lesions.

Meijer: You must distinguish between surface membrane immunologlobulins on lymphocytes, and IgG-containing cells. IgG-containing cells are probably secondary, because they are found only in active disease.

Fielding: Do these studies make it possible to differentiate between CD and UC where other methods have failed?

Meijer: So far I only have studied one example of UC. However, there were increased B-cells, so I do not think that the B-cell response is specific for CD.

Meuwissen: Meijer has emphasized that the B-cell line is increased in CD and in UC. We showed a few years ago in CD that T-cells were not present in follicular infiltrates, but in the transmural infiltrate. We found a very heavy, scattered increase of T lymphocytes. I think that we are looking at a reaction of both T and B lymphocytes.

Meijer: In the follicular infiltrates we found B-cells in the center while the perifollicular areas were negative, and we think that these were T-cells forming a reaction border to the follicular B-cells.

Van Tongeren: Did you find any differences during treatment or during follow-up in the number or distribution of lymphocytes with IgM, IgA, or IgG on the cell surface?

Rosekrans: We have followed some patients after treatment, and the total number of immunoglobulin-containing cells decreased after treatment. In some patients from both UC and CD groups the infiltrates became almost normal after local treatment.

Jewell: We have done studies with highly specific T-cell antisera, and the result are very similar to Meuwissen. There was an overall increase of both T- and B-cells and there also seemed to be an increased number of null cells.

Shorter: Did the two speakers examined surgical specimens that showed analogous chronic inflammation, for example in long-standing chronic diverticulitis, rather than just so-called normals?

Rosekrans: We have seen two specimens from patients with diverticulitis and we found increased IgG-containing cells in the inflamed mucosa. Other areas were normal.

Elson: Did you verify your techniques with purified B cells or T-cells from peripheral blood?

Meijer: The C_3 receptor technique detects at the most about 3 percent of T cells and a small proportion of what we think is a non-T, non-B population. Furthermore, we used four different markers including 5-nucleotidase with which many of the follicular infiltrates were positive, adenosine triphosphatase, C_3 receptors, and surface membrane immunoglobulins. It is hard to believe that all of these markers were wrong.

TISSUE MAST CELLS IN CROHN'S DISEASE AND ULCERATIVE COLITIS

K. MATSUEDA, J.J. RIMPILA, H.E. FORD, B. LEVIN and S.C. KRAFT

INTRODUCTION

The possible role of mast cells in mediating the tissue lesions of Crohn's disease [CD] and ulcerative colitis [UC] has been considered by numerous investigators over the last two decades (1-12). That view is fostered by more recent knowledge of the cell biology of the mast cell, e.g., observations that a] its surface contains receptors having a high affinity for the Fc portion of IgE, b] the interaction of the Fab portion of the bound IgE with certain multivalent antigens triggers mast-cell degranulation, and c] the resulting release of chemical mediators directly influences immediate hypersensitivity, tissue repair, and adjacent cellular elements.

The purposes of this study were to quantify mast cells in the different layers of the intestinal wall in inflammatory bowel disease and control surgical specimens, and to compare the distribution of mast cells and immunoglobulin-containing lymphoid cells, with special reference to IgE cells.

PROCEDURE

We studied 20 specimens from patients with Crohn's disease [11 ileum; 9 colon], 7 colons involved with chronic ulcerative colitis, and 19 normal [uninvolved segment resected for neoplasm] or inflamed [e.g., ischemia, diverticulitis] control tissues [8 ileum; 11 colon]. The tissues were freshly frozen in liquid nitrogen, stored at -196°C, and cut transmurally at a thickness of 4-6µ in a cryostat at -30°C. Coded serial sections were either stained for immunoglobulin heavy chains using the direct fluorescent antibody technique, or for mast cells using the polychrome methylene blue stain [Unna's method]. For each stained slide, at least 10 differ-

ent high-power fields of the lamina propria were photograped;
for mast cells, the submucosa and muscularis propria were
similarly photographed. Cell density indices were calculated
as the number of cells per mm^2 of tissue, using a planimetric
modifcation of the method described by Gelzayd et al. (13).
Differences between groups were analyzed by the Student's
t-test.

RESULTS

Mast cells were identified most prominently in the submucosa where they often were located near the muscularis mucosa
and about blood vessels, frequently in close proximity to
plasma cells and lymphocytes. In the colonic lamina propria
[Table 1], only the mean mast-cell index in Crohn's disease
was significantly decreased in comparison to the normal controls [p<0.02]. No striking differences were noted between
six of these patients who were receiving corticosteroids at
the time of surgery and three who were not. The lamina proprial mast-cell counts in ulcerative colitis also tended to
be reduced, but varied more. In the submucosa and muscularis
propria, on the other hand, there was a trend towards higher
mean mast-cell indices in both disorders.

Table 1. Quantitation of mast cells in the colon

Tissue	No.	Lamina propria	Submucosa	Muscularis propria
Normal control	7	60.0 + 33.0[*]	68.2 + 21.9	20.2 + 30.0
Inflamed control	4	48.0 + 16.4	74.5 + 8.9	16.4 + 17.8
Crohn's disease	9	30.6 + 6.7	77.8 + 28.9	41.3 + 35.2
Ulcerative colitis	7	32.0 + 16.7	92.7 + 62.9	30.3 + 15.8

* Mean cell density index per mm^2 + 1 standard deviation.

In the ileum [Table 2], mast-cell numbers did not differ
significantly among the three groups of subjects, although
there was a trend towards more mast cells in the muscularis
propria in the presence of inflammation of any etiology.

Immunoglobulin-containing lymphoid cells of each isotype
were prominent in the lamina propria of the inflamed colon in

both Crohn's disease and ulcerative colitis, and in ileal Crohn's disease. In addition, these cells occasionally were

Table 2. Quantitation of mast cells in the ileum

Tissue	No.	Lamina propria	Submucosa	Muscularis propria
Normal control	6	67.7 + 26.0*	113.9 + 67.3	43.8 + 30.7
Inflamed control	2	42.6 + 11.9	51.8 + 3.2	65.4 + 6.4
Crohn's disease	11	47.4 + 21.5	117.7 + 8.3	62.1 + 47.3

* Mean cell density index per mm^2 + 1 standard deviation.

identified in the deeper bowel layers, especially in the pre-sence of inflammation. Statistical analyses failed to demon-strate significant differences in this phase of the study. Interestingly, in the colonic lamina propria of individual patients with Crohn's disease, somewhat increased numbers of IgE cells often appeared to correlate with the reduced num-bers of mast cells observed at this site.

DISCUSSION

When other workers (1,3-7) have counted or otherwise graded mast cells in inflamed tissues obtained from patients with either CD or UC, mast cells generally have been more prevalent than in normal control tissues. Although the report by Lloyd et al. (8) described an almost total absence of stainable mast cells in affected areas of the bowel in CD, they suggested that this was due to degranulation of these cells, leading to the loss of their recognition on light microscopy. They pointed out that the electron microscopic study of Ranlov et al. (6) had shown many degranulated mast cells in the inflammatory lesions of CD, a phenomenon sub-sequently emphasized by Dvorak et al. (11).

Numerous investigators have studied immunoglobulin-con-taining cells in tissues from patients with IBD with varied results (14). As regards IgE-containing cells, O'Donoghue and Kumar (15) reported a marked increase in the number of IgE cells in inflamed rectal biopsy specimens from patients with either CD or UC. Their data were consistent with an earlier biopsy study by Heatley et al. (16) using patients with either active or quiescent ulcerative proctitis.

CONCLUSIONS

Although we observed mast cells and IgE cells in the inflamed tissues resected from patients with CD and UC, the counts generally did not differ appreciably from those in subjects with specific types of inflammation. Nevertheless, these limited observations, coupled with those cited from the literature, are consistent with the possibility that antigen-induced interaction between IgE and mast cells may play a role in the pathogenesis of the tissue reaction in inflammatory bowel disease.

Hypothetically, an undefined antigen may stimulate immunocytes committed to IgE synthesis. Specific IgE then localizes on the mast-cell membrane. When the same or a cross-reacting antigen comes in contact with the sensitized mast cell, degranulation occurs and potent chemical mediators of inflammation are released into the tissue. For example, if proteolytic enzymes were liberated deep within the bowel wall, this could conceivably contribute to the formation of fistulas in CD. In the above situation, the mast cell would be serving an immune-effector function. This type of reasoning has led some workers to initiate clinical trials of the efficacy of various mast-cell stabilizers in patients with idiopathic inflammatory bowel disease (12,17-20). Of course, mast cells also may play an important role in protective responses to local tissue injury of many sorts.

ACKNOWLEDGEMENTS

This work was supported in part by research grants from the National Institutes of Health, U.S.P.H.S. (#CA-14,599), and the National Foundation for Ileitis and Colitis, Inc., New York, N.Y.

REFERENCES
1. McGovern VJ, Archer GT. (1957) The pathogenesis of ulcerative colitis. Australas Ann.Med 6:68-74
2. Kraft SC, Kirsner JB. (1960) Mast cells and the gastrointestinal tract: a review. Gastroenterology 39:764-770
3. McAuley RL, Sommers SC. (1961) Mast cells in nonspecific ulcerative colitis. Am.J.Dig.Dis. 6:233-236
4. Hiatt RB, Katz L. (1962) Mast cells in inflammatory conditions of the gastrointestinal tract. Am.J.Gastroenterol. 37:541-545
5. Bercovitz ZT, Sommers SC. (1966) Altered inflammatory reaction in nonspecific ulcerative colitis. Arch.Intern.Med. 117:504-510
6. Ranlov P, Nielsen MH, Wanstrup J. (1972) Ultrastructure of the ileum in Crohn's disease: immune lesions and mastocytosis. Scand.J.Gastroenterol. 7:471-476
7. Rao SN. (1973) Mast cells as a component of the granuloma in Crohn's disease. J.Pathol. 109:79-82
8. Lloyd G, Green FHY, Fox H, Mani V, Turnberg LA. (1975) Mast cells and immunoglobulin E in inflammatory bowel disease. Gut 16:861-866
9. Korelitz BI, and Sommers SC. (1976) Responses to drug therapy in ulcerative colitis: evaluation by rectal biopsy and mucosal cell counts. Am.J.Dig.Dis 21:441-447
10. Kubo K. (1976) A clinico-pathological study of ulcerative colitis. J.Wakayama.Med.Soc 27:227-244
11. Dvorak AM, Monahan RA, Osage JE, Dickersin GR. (1978) Mast cell degranulation in Crohn's disease. Lancet 1:498
12. Piovatnetti Y, Kocoshis SA, Sheahan DG, Gryboski JD. (1978) Effects of cromolyn on inflammatory bowel disease. Pediatr.Res. 12:440
13. Gelzayd EA, Kraft SC, Kirsner JB. (1968) The distribution of immunoglobulins in human rectal mucosa. I. Normal control subjects. Gastroenterology 54:334-340
14. Kraft SC. (1979) Inflammatory bowel disease [ulcerative colitis and Crohn's disease]. In: Immunology of the gastrointestinal tract, Ed. Asquith P. Edinburgh, Churchill Livingstone. pp 95-128
15. O'Donoghue DP, Kumar P. (1979) Rectal IgE cells in inflammatory bowel disease. Gut 20:149-153
16. Heatley RV, Rhodes J, Calcraft BJ, Whitehead RH, Fifield R, Newcombe RG. (1975) Immunoglobulin E in rectal mucosa of patients with proctitis. Lancet 2:1010-1012
17. Heatley RV, Calcraft BJ, Rhodes J, Owen E, Evans BK. (1975) Disodium cromoglycate in the treatment of chronic proctitis. Gut 16:559-563
18. Mani V, Lloyd G, Green FHY, Fox H, Turnberg LA. (1976) Treatment of ulcerative colitis with oral disodium cromoglycate: a double-blind controlled trial.Lancet 1:439-441
19. Dronfield MW, Langman MJS. (1977) Controlled comparison of sodium cromoglycate and sulphasalazine in the maintenance of remission in ulcerative colitis. Gut 18:A973
20. Davies PS, Rhodes J, Counsell B, Heatley RV, Newcombe RG. (1979) A nitroindanedione mast cell stabiliser in the treatment of ulcerative colitis: a controlled trial. Clin. Allergy 9:373-376

B15 Summary of Discussions relating to topic B14

Lindeman: How did you differentiate between IgE plasma
               cells, IgE on mast cells, and mononuclear eosino-
               phils. The last have a strong non-specific binding
               to FITC.

Kraft: We could not demonstrate IgE on the mast cells.
               Eosinophils have a rather characteristic appearance
               and the mast cells tend to be bigger cells.

Rosekrans: We have found a large number of IgE-containing
               cells in allergic proctitis, and in our opinion
               this is a clinical and histopathological entity
               which is different from UC. In the UC group we did
               not find increased IgE-containing cells.

Kraft: We too did not find significantly increased
               numbers of IgE cells.

Binder: As part of a controlled study on disodiumchro-
               moglycate, we did mast cell counts in patients with
               active as well as inactive UC. We found that with
               active disease mast cell counts showed a median
               value of 35 per square millimetre while in quies-
               cent patients (60 in all) the median was 70. These
               values are in agreement with Kraft's results.

Kraft: Virtually any substance which leads to in-
               creased accumulation of cyclic AMP in mast cells
               will prevent degranulation.

Thompson: Does the trauma of surgical resection induces
               mast-cell degranulation and leads to a reduced

population of these cells?

Kraft: There is no question that trauma can cause mast-cell degranulation, and perhaps it does make it more difficult to show differences between groups.

Meijer: You expressed your mast cells per square millimetre of lamina propria. Brandtzaeg described in 1974 a "mucosal tissue unit" which is histologically comparable even with an increase in the lamina propria area. Is it possible that the total number of mast cells is normal because the increase in the area of the lamina propria was not taken into account?

Kraft: We do know that our method is quite comparable in terms of cells per square millimetre with those described by Lloyd in 1975, and we're not saying that mast cells are statistically increased.

ELECTRONMICROSCOPY IN CROHN'S DISEASE

G.N. TIJTGAT, A. VAN MINNEN and T. VERHOEVEN

INTRODUCTION

Surprisingly few EM studies have been performed on tissue obtained from patients with Crohn's disease (1-9). The purpose of this EM study was to find out whether EM could provide any clues to the etiology or pathogenesis of CD.

MATERIALS AND METHODS

Tissue specimens from 100 patients, mean age 31.6, with active Crohn's disease were studied. Involvement of colon, terminal ileum, rectum and stomach was present in respectively 62,22,15 and 1 patient. Multiple biopsies were obtained in 40 patients before they ever had any medical treatment. 32 patients only received sulfasalazine, 14 sulfasalazine and prednisone whereas the remaining patients received various combinations of sulfasalazine at the time of biopsy.

Following regions of interest were selected for study: giant cells 51, epithelioid collections 25, lymphoid follicles 33, focal edema and tissue necrosis 24, focal crypt cell degeneration 26, aphthoid ulcers 15, areas of chronic inflammation 86, granulation tissue 17, lymphatic vessel walls 12 and normal and abnormal looking epithelial cells.

After screening 3252 1μ sections, obtained from 2159 biopsies, 330 regions of interest were selected for ultrathin sectioning and detailed EM analysis.

RESULTS

Search for viral particles

All regions of interest were carefully studied for EM evidence of viral structures. Nothing was seen which could be construed confidently as viral particles. Confusing structures were occasionally seen within nuclei and in the perinu-

clear area, the latter presumably corresponding to nuclear
pores. Furthermore confusing aggregates of tubuloreticular
structures inside the cytoplasm and microvesicular structures
inside and outside the cell contours were occasionally observed, presumably representing breakdown products of cell
organelles. All these confusing images were not identified as
viral particles although they may have been called 'virus-
like' particles by others in the past.

Search for microorganisms

Microorganisms were observed in 13 patients. They occurred in variable size, shape and structure. Usually different
types of bacteria were detected within the same biopsy specimen, which suggested that microbial invasion was probably the
result of actual or previous epithelial disruption. Large
collections of microorganisms were usually found, along the
edges of intramural fissures. Areas of focal edema and necrosis in specimens, covered with an apparently intact epithelial layer were characterized by a monotonous amorphous precipitate, subdivided by empty looking spaces. Careful search
in serial sections of such areas occasionally revealed a rare
microorganism. Rarely, single microorganisms were detected in
areas of fibrosis.

EM study of the epithelial and subepithelial layer

Normal and abnormal looking epithelial cell layers were
extensively investigated for evidence of intra-or interepi-
thelial presence or passage of identifiable structures. However, recognizable structures were never detected, even when
epithelial cells in close proximity to aphthoid erosions were
studied. Epithelial cells which appeared damaged, permeated
by degenerated inflammatory cells, or containing conspicuous
phagolysosomes also did not contain recognizable structures.
Microvesicular structures in the area of the microvillus layers were considered a nonspecific vesicular breakdown of the
luminal cell membrane. There was no evidence of alteration of
the tight junctions nor of the desmosomal structures [Fig.1].

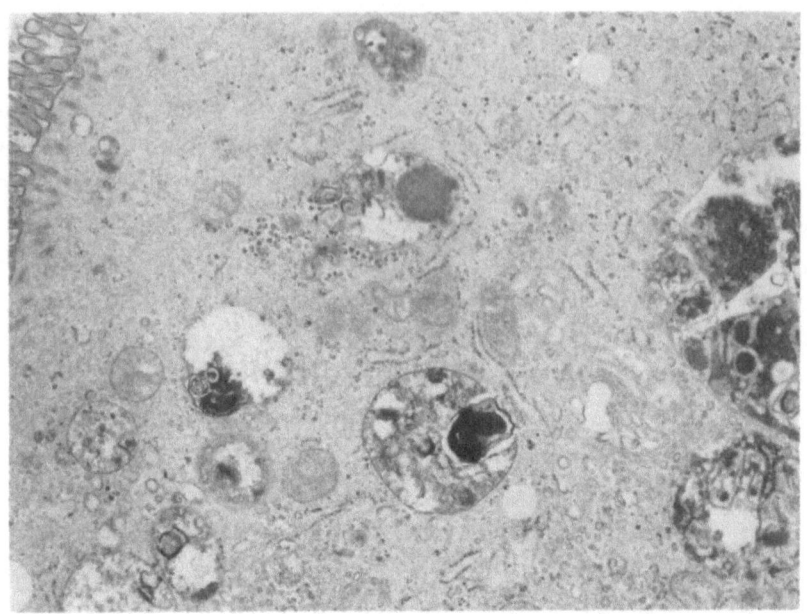

Figure 1. Epithelial cell with vesiculation of the microvillus layer and phagolysosomes in the cytoplasm,
showing only degenerated organelles.

EM study of epithelial cells and giant cells

Epithelioid cell granulomas with giant cells were found
in 16 patients. All except 1 of the 53 epithelioid cell granulomas were seen in rectal or colonic biopsies. In 4 of the
16 patients, microorganisms of variable morphology were detected elsewhere in the biopsy material.

Mature epithelioid cells were rather large [20-40μ] with
an eccentric nucleus and usually a prominent nucleolus. Most
conspicuous were the many characteristic membrane-lined vesicles, either electron-lucent, clear and debris free or containing a fine granular content. The peripheral cell contours
were usually irregular, exhibiting numerous interdigated long
and slender filiform processes. Usually small amounts of
amorphous or granular material were detectable within the va-
cuolated honeycomb-like network, but truly identifiable
structures were never observed.

Giant cells were either of the foreign body type or of

the Langhan's type. The overall appearance of the giant cells was somewhat heterogenous, suggesting various phases of maturation. The appearance of the cytoplasm was similar to that of the epithelioid cells. Most conspicuous was the prescence of a high number of vesicles, which were either empty-looking or filled with a fine granular material. In none of the many serially sectioned giant cells was there any recognizable viral, microbial or parasitic structures, neither in the giant cells which contained asteroid or Schaumann bodies [Fig.2].

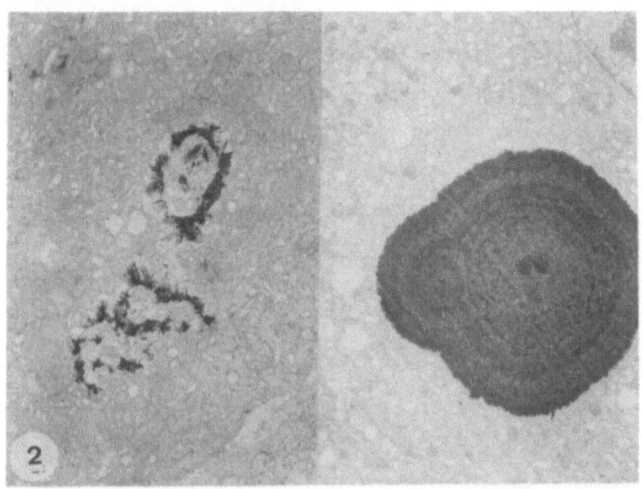

Figure 2. Lamellated concretions [left] and Schaumann body
[right] with concentric lamellations in giant cell.

Quite often fibrin strands, as suggested by 21 nm periodicity, could be identified in close proximity to the giant cell plasma membrane. Occasionally such fibrinous material appeared to be engulfed within pinocytotic vesicles [Fig. 3].

EM study of aphthoid ulcers

Aphthoid ulcers were extensively studied in 5 untreated patients with active CD. No evidence of viral microbial structures could ever be detected.

EM analysis of other regions of interest

Extensive EM analysis of the other regions of interest did not reveal relevant abnormalities nor evidence or identifiable particulate material.

114

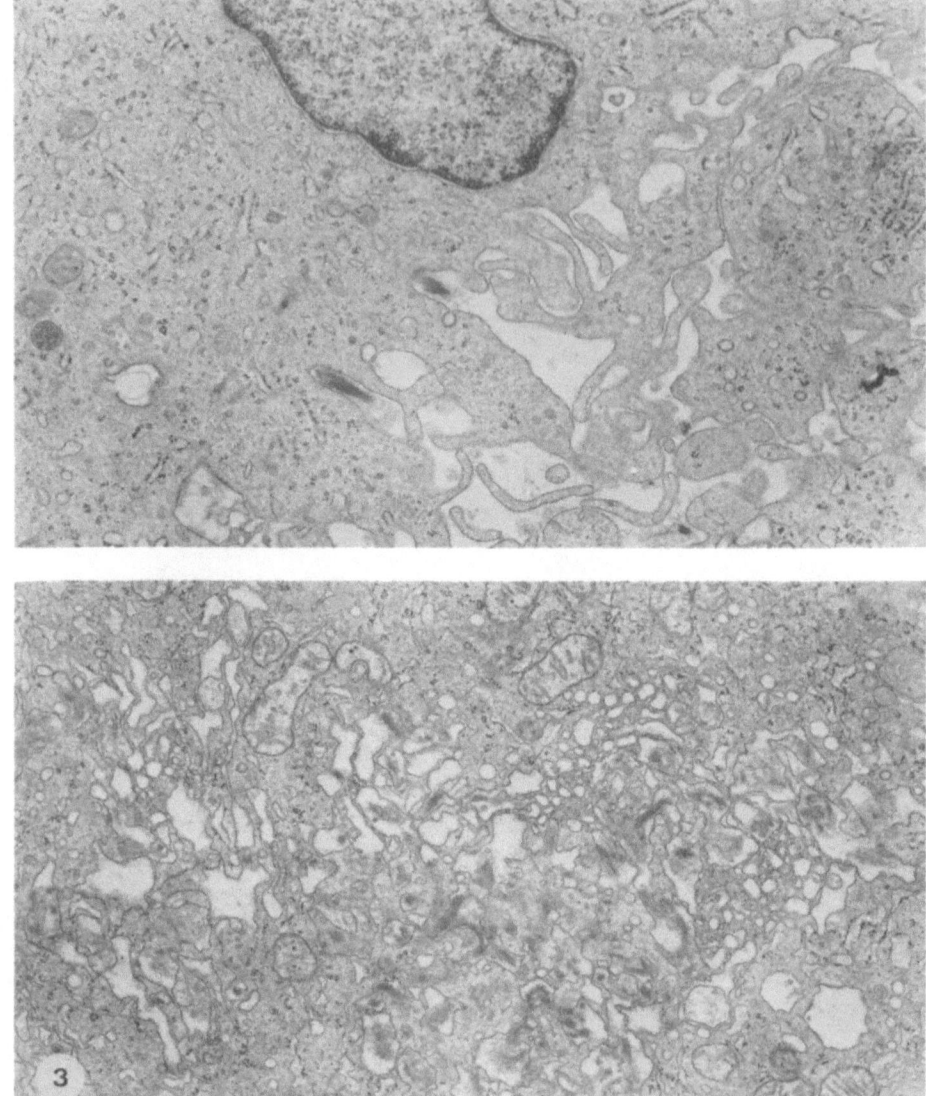

Figure 3. Fibrinous material in close proximity of giant cell
plasma membrane [upper] and perhaps engulfed within
giant cell [lower].

DISCUSSION

Many investigators have tried to find a causal relationship between a particular infective agent and CD. From our detailed electronmicroscopic study, of a large group of CD patients, often before they received any medical treatment, no support could be derived for a possible viral, microbial or parasitic etiology. Many microorganisms have been identified but this probably reflects secondary or opportunistic infection of a damaged mucosa. Crohn's disease therefore appears to differ from many other granulomatous diseases where there is evidence of some non-degradable particular material inside the macrophage-epithelioid cell system. In general, granulomas are thought to arise when macrophages cannot adequately degrade ingested foreign material (10,11). Macrophages apparently turn into epithelioid cells when phagocytosis or pinocytosis leads to incomplete elimination of the particle. The persistence of particulate or antigenic material may then result in damage of the surrounding tissues by the release of toxic lysosomal enzymes from macrophages and epithelioid cells (12-18).

Much experimental work still has to be done to find out whether particulate or antigenic material enters the lamina propria through a 'leaky'? epithelial layer and to find out whether such material finally leads to the focal granulomatous response in Crohn's disease.

REFERENCES
1. Albot G, Parturier-Albot M, Camilleri JP, Diebold J. (1970) La maladie de Crohn colique. IV. Etude cytologique et ultrastructurale des infiltrants inflammatoires plasmocytaires et epithelio-giganto-cellulaires. Sem. Hôp. Paris 46:1545-1566
2. Aluwihare APR.(1971) Electron microscopy in Crohn's disease. Gut 12:509-518
3. Aluwihare APR.(1971) The ultrastructure of the colon in Crohn's disease. Proc. Roy. Soc. Med. 64:162-164
4. Aluwihare APR. (1976) Clin. Gastroenterol. 5:279
5. Cook MG, Turnbull GJ.(1975) A hypothesis for the pathogenesis of Crohn's disease based on an ultrastructural study. Virchows Arch. A [Pathol.Anat.] 365:327-336
6. Dourmashkin RR, Davies H, Wells C. Shah D, Price A, O'Morain C, Levi J, Hall Th.A. (1980) These proceedings

7. Gebbers JO, Otto HF. (1980) Immuno- and ultracytochemical observations in Crohn's disease. These proceedings
8. Ranlov P, Nielsen MH, Wanstrup J.(1972) Ultrastructure of ileum in Crohn's disease. Scand.J.Gastroenterol.7:471-476
9. Riemann JF.(1977) Further electronmicroscopic evidence of Virus-like particles in Crohn's disease. Acta Hepato-Gastroenterol. 24:116-118
10. Epstein WL.(1967) Granulomatous hypersensitivity. Progr. Allerg. 11:36-88
11. Spector WG.(1976) Immunologic components of granuloma formation. Epithelioid cells, giant cells, and sarcoidosis. Ann. N.Y. Acad. Sci. 278:3-6
12. Cardella CJ, Davies P, Alloson AC.(1974) Immune complexes induce selective release of lysosomal hydrolases from macrophages. Nature 247:46-48
13. Dingle JT, Poole AR, Lazarus GS, Barrett AJ.(1973) Immunoinhibition of intracellular protein digestion in macrophages. J. Exp. Med. 137:1124-1141
14. Tytgat GN, van Minnen A, Verhoeven A. (1979) Electronen microscopisch onderzoek van granuloma bij de ziekte van Crohn. Tijdschr. Gastroenterol. 21:465-480
15. Cohn ZA, Benson B.(1965) The diffentiation of mononuclear phagocytes. J.Exp.Med. 121:153-169
16. Klockars M, Reitamo S, Reitamo JJ, Möller C.(1977) Immunohistochemical identification of lysozyme in intestinal lesions in ulcerative colitis and Crohn's disease. Gut 18:377-381
17. Sutton JS, Weiss L.(1966) Transformation of monocytes in tissue culture into macrophages, epithelioid cells, and multinucleated giant cells. An electronmicroscopic study. J.Cell Biol. 28:303-332
18. Williams D, Williams JW, Williams JE.(1969) Enzyme histochemistry of epithelioid cells in sarcoid-like granulomas. J.Path. 97:705-709

EARLY EPITHELIAL LESIONS IN CROHN'S DISEASE, REVEALED BY ELECTRON MICROSCOPY

R.R. DOURMASHKIN, H. DAVIES, C. WELLS, D. SHAH, A. PRICE, C. O'MORAIN, J. LEVI and TH.A. HALL

INTRODUCTION

Although the pathology of Crohn's disease [CD] is characterized by well-defined regions of gross inflammation, it has long been recognised that it is a widely disseminated disease of the gut. Brooke first described "aphthoid ulcers" in the mucosa of otherwise uninflamed intestine of CD in 1953 (1). Morson (2) found that these lesions consisted of lymphoid follicles that were involved in the granulomatous inflammation of CD with break-down and pin-point mucosal ulceration. Recently Dvorak (3) and Rickert et al. (4) have correlated these ulcers with their surface appearance by scanning electron microscopy, in addition pointing out the considerable enhancement of mucous secretion and the villous fusion in "unaffected" areas that can be observed using this technique.

A number of investigators have commented on the absence of virus-like particles in electron microscope studies of CD (3,5). Without surveying the literature extensively we will describe epithelial lesions in "unaffected" areas of CD that may represent a stage earlier than that of the aphthous ulcer, and also attempts to identify particles of microbial origin in material from CD patients.

PROCUDURE

Fixation of tissues

Surgical specimens of bowel both from areas affected with inflammation and from areas close to the resection margin, were fixed by immersion without rinsing the mucosa, in either 3% glutaraldehyde in 0.1 M cacodylate buffer, pH 7.4 + 5% sucrose, or alternatively, 3% glutaraldehyde + 1% tannic acid in the same buffer for two hours at room temperature. The cut pieces of tissue were rinsed in the same cacodylate buffer, fixed in 1% OsO_4 + 0.1 M cacodylate, pH 7.4 at 4^oC for 1 hour then rinsed in distilled water, dehydrated with acetone and propylene oxide, and embedded in Spurr resin. 1μm sections were mounted on glass slides and stained with Toluidine blue for histological examination. Ultrathin sections of the whole block face were cut and stained with uranyl acetate and lead citrate. Adjacent specimens were embedded for histology in the usual way.

Rectal biopsies were collected and immersed in 3% glutaraldehyde fixative in a manner so as not to damage the surface epithelium. Nearby biopsies were taken for histology and for the specimens used in the blind trial, both the pathologist and electron microscopist received the samples by number only and had no contact with the patient at the time of biopsy. Otherwise the preparation of 1 μm and ultrathin sections was identical to that above.

Bowel washings

Patients were prepared for surgery or colonoscopy by perfusing 10 litres hypotonic saline perfusate [Fenning Ltd.] via a jejunal tube. The first clear fluid was collected. 100 ml was centrifuged at 3000g for 20 min., the supernatant centrifuged at 10,000g for 30 min. and that supernatant centrifuged at 100,000g for 1 hr. The resulting pellet was carefully collected in distilled water and layered onto a caesium chloride solution [1.39g/ml] in 6.5 ml swing out buckets and centrifuged as an isopycnic equilibrium gradient at 100,000g for 16 hrs. 13-drop fractions were collected and their density measured in an Abbe refractometer. The fractions were concentrated and also depleted of salt by layering a drop onto a 3 mm^3 cube of 2% agar in water, then applying a parlodion-carbon coated grid and allowing the fluid to diffuse into the agar. The grids were negatively charged in 2% sodium phosphotungstate pH 6.5 and examined in the electron microscope [EM]. Similar fractions were collected, diluted with distilled water, pelleted at 100,000g for 1 hr, and fixed for embedding and sectioning in the manner described above.

X-ray microanalysis

Rectal biopsies from patients with active rectal CD were fixed and embedded for X-ray microanalysis according to the method of Yarom (6).

RESULTS

Surgical specimens

There were two findings arising from the examination of surgical specimens of bowel excised for CD. Firstly, there was a characteristic lesion of the epithelium found in both large and small bowel in tissue distant from regions of inflammation as well as in the inflamed region itself. The lesion consisted of necrosis of small patches of epithelial cells, often of one cell alone, which we have termed "patchy necrosis" [PN]. The damage to the cells was very localised; completely normal cells being adjacent to those that showed damage. The density of stain of the damaged cells varied greatly, some being very pale, whereas others were more dense than usual. This difference in density was most noticeable in the 1 μm sections stained for light microscopy. Generally only the superficial epithelium was involved, the crypts (in the large intestine) being free.

Secondly, in the ileum of resected bowel for CD, we found an interesting abnormality of the microvilli. In regions of patchy necrosis the microvilli often showed densely staining buds at their tips, and sometimes along their sides. In some areas, the buds would separate from the stems of the microvilli and be swept into the bowel lumen as particles. In other areas, the budding appeared to be directly from the epithelial cell membrane. Alkaline phosphatase staining showed diminished enzyme in the areas of microvillous damage. However, similar changes in microvilli were found in other conditions, although to a lesser extent; in addition, the changes were observed only in the mucosa of the ileum and not in the large intestine. For these reasons we concluded that these were not related to virus particles. However, further evidence in this regard will be discussed in the section on the examination of bowel washings.

Rectal biopsies

The finding of patchy necrosis in the rectal biopsies was identical to that observed in the surgical specimens. The addition of tannic acid in the fixative was omitted for this series, as occasionally the tissue did not infiltrate well with resin. The results are presented in table 1.

Table 1. Results of the double blind study on rectal biopsies

EM diagnosis	PN[a]	Inflam-mation	Histological diagnosis	Clinical diagnosis
1. uninvolved CD	2+	–	normal	ileal CD + skip area in colon
2. UC[b]	–	4+	UC	UC
3. healing UC	2+	3+	UC	UC
4. UC	2+	4+	UC	UC
5. normal	+/–	–	normal	CD in SB[c], normal rectum
6. Intestinal spirochaetosis	–	–	?Spirochae-tosis	normal
7. active CD	3+	2+	?proctitis, ?UC, ?CD	rectal CD
8. uninvolved CD	1-2+	?	UC	rectal CD
9. active CD	3+	2+	CD,?resolving infection	CD in SB and colon
10. ?normal or ?healing CD	1+	–	crushed, probably normal	normal
11. normal or healing UC	1+	–	normal	normal
12. UC	–	4+	UC	UC
13. healed UC	1+	–	normal	CD in SB and colon
14. normal	+/–	–	normal	normal
15. normal; lipid inclusions in epithelium	–	–	no specimen	CD in SB and colon

a] PN: "Patchy necrosis" up to 1+ was assessed as normal
b] UC: ulcerative colitis
c] SB: small bowel

It was clear that the most consistent correlation of the EM data in CD was the finding of greater than 1+ patchy necrosis with a mild or moderate degree of inflammation in the lamina propria [Table 2].

Table 2. Summary of the results of the double blind-study on rectal biopsy specimen

Inflammation even or greater than PN	: 4/4 UC
PN greater than inflammation	: 4/4 CD
Neither PN nor inflammation	: 4/7 normal
	: 3/7 CD

The finding of 1+ patchy necrosis [about one damaged cell per slide] probably represents the normal process of epithelial replacement. In this way UC was clearly distinguished from CD. Three cases of CD were not diagnosed, one of which showed widespread lipid inclusions in the epithelium. This case is under further study. It is to be emphasized that most of the observations were made from the 1μm sections for light microscopy, although the illustrations of patchy necrosis are best shown in electron micrographs. There was no correlation of patchy necrosis with the medical therapy.

Bowel washings

Particles were observed in density gradient separation of bowel washings, that ranged from 70 - 200nm in diameter, had a "fuzz" around their periphery, and a dense core on section. These particles sedimented at densities of 1.40 - 1.44g/ml, too dense for cytoplasmic debris. However, a few similar particles could be observed in bowel washings from other conditions, and so the interpretation of these particles remained in doubt [Fig. 1].

DISCUSSION AND CONCLUSIONS

The correlation of patchy necrosis with CD in a blind trial of rectal biopsies demonstrates the significance of this finding. Moreover, the presence of epithelial damage with little or no inflammation in the adjacent lamina propria, suggest that the earliest lesion in CD is in the epithelial cells. The aphthous ulcers previously described (1,2) show considerable localized inflammation, and so probably

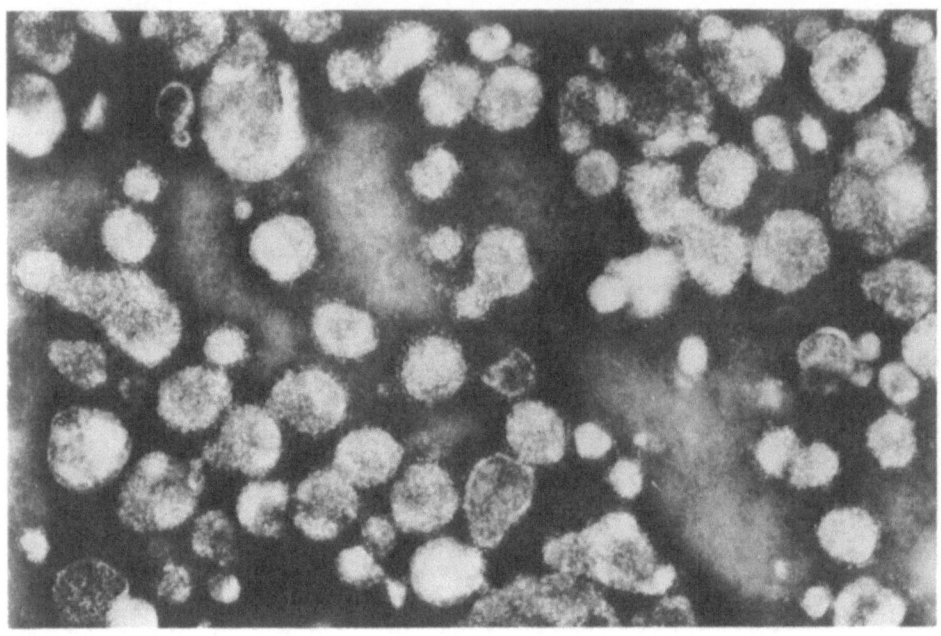

Figure 1. Particles from density gradient of bowel washings of Crohn's disease density = 1.4 g/ml Magnification x 150,000. Micrograph by H. Davis

represent a later stage in the disease.

In addition, the finding of patchy necrosis might be useful in diagnosing CD. However, we have not as yet examined other conditions, such as acute colitis.

The observation of particles in the ileal mucosa and bowel washings must be interpreted with caution, in view of their presence in control material.

REFERENCES
1. Brooke BN. (1953) What is ulcerative colitis? Lancet 1:
    1220-1225
2. Morson BC. (1972) The early histological lesion of
    Crohn's disease. Proc.Roy.Soc.Med. 65:71-72
3. Dvorak HM, Dickersin GR, Osage JC, Monahan RA.(1978)
    Absence of virus structures in Crohn's disease tissues
    studied by electron microscopy. Lancet 1:328-
4. Rickert RR, Carter HW. (1977) The gross light microscopic
    and scanning electron microscopy appearance of the early
    lesions of Crohn's disease. Scanning Electron Microscopy
    II:179-186
5. Tytgat GN, Minnen van A, Verhoeven A. (1979) Electronen
    microscopisch onderzoek van granulomen bij de ziekte van
    Crohn. Tijdschr.Gastroenterol. 21:465-480
6. Yarom R, Maunder C, Scripps M, Hall TA, Dubowitz VA.
    (1975) A simplified preparation for X-ray microanalysis
    of muscle and blood cells. Histochemistry 45:49-59

LIGHT- AND ELECTRONMICROSCOPICAL STUDIES ON THE DISTRIBUTION
OF VARIOUS CELL TYPES IN THE SIGMOID COLON OF NORMAL SUBJECTS
AND IN PATIENTS WITH CROHN'S DISEASE

L.A. GINSEL, HELEN P. LIEPMAN AND IRENE T. WETERMAN

INTRODUCTION

Studies on the characterization and distribution of cell
populations in normal human intestine and in the intestine of
patients with Crohn's disease [CD] are mainly based on light-
microscopical investigations. Since light-microscopical studies alone are insufficient for complete characterization and
quantification of cell populations, we studied by means of
comparative light-microscopical [LM] and electron-microscopi-
cal [EM] photomontages the distribution of cell populations
in the sigmoid colon for normal controls and for patients
with CD.

PROCEDURE

"Normal" biopsy specimens were obtained from the sigmoid
colon of five patients undergoing routine observations for
complaints such as irritable colon and unexplainable diarrhoea. The classification as CD [three patients] was made on
basis of LM diagnosis at the Pathological Laboratory [Univer-
sity Hospital Leiden]. Two biopsies from the sigmoid area of
the colon were obtained from each patient. The biopsy specimens were divided into small blocks and fixed at 4°C for 60
minutes in 1% osmium tetroxide buffered with phosphate to pH
7.2. The fixative had a final osmolality of 320 mOsm. Dehy-
dration and embedding were performed according to standard
techniques.

About 0.75 µm thick LM-sections were cut passing from
surface epithelium of the sigmoid colon, through the lamina
propria, muscularis mucosa and submucosa. The sections were
stained with toluidine blue. Ultrathin sections were cut from

the same area and stained with uranyl acetate and with lead
hydroxide. LM- and EM-photomontages were made of two specific
areas of the lamina propria: the "upper" third below the
epithelial layer and the "lower" third above the muscularis
mucosa. The LM- and EM photo montages were examined, cells
identified and quantified in the two areas. The density of
cells [number/mm^2 tissue] was calculated by inserting a
counting grid into the ocular of the lightmicroscope. Statistical comparison of absolute cell numbers was made by the
Student's t-test.

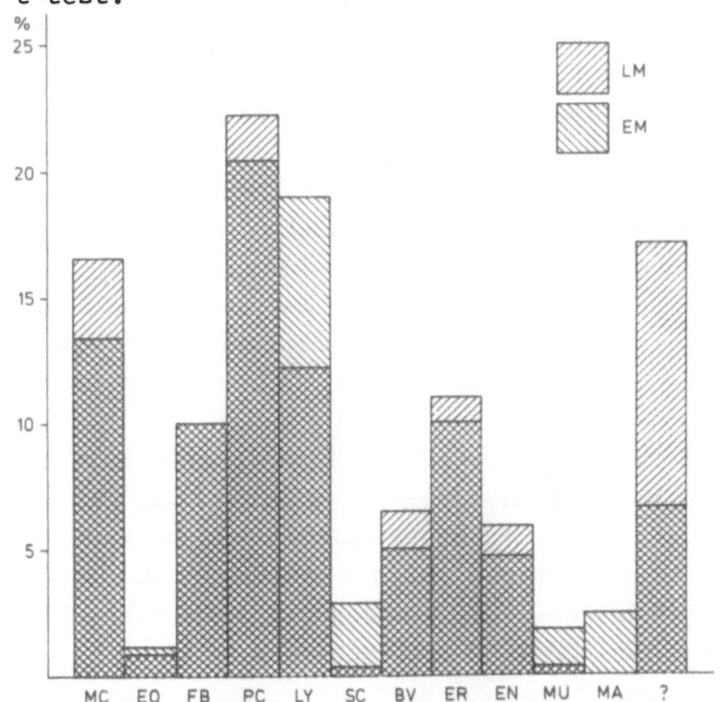

Figure 1. Frequency distribution of cells as observed on LM-
and EM-photomontages [MC-macrophage, EO-eosino-
phil, FB-fibroblast, PC-plasma cell, LY-lymphocyte, SC-Schwann cell, BV-blood vessel, ER-ery-
throcyte, EN-endothelial cell, MK-muscle cell,
MA-mast cell, ?-unidentifiable cell].

RESULTS

The comparative LM- and EM-photomontage study shows that the latter give a more accurate impression of the cellular build up of the sigmoid colon [Fig. 1], and about 10% more cells are identifiable, i.e., lymphocytes [7%], Schwann cells [1.5%], mast cells [1%] and muscle cells [0.5%]. Nevertheless, even on EM-photomontages 6.5% of the cells remain unrecognizable.

The study of cells in two regions of the lamina propria of the sigmoid colon, one below the epithelium and one above the muscularis mucosa reveals that their distribution is not random [Tables 1, 2 and 3]. The "upper" region of the lamina propria of normal sigmoid colon had more macrophages and eosinophils than the lower part. In the "lower" region of the lamina propria of patients with CD and of controls the total number of cells is unchanged [Table 1]. However, a decrease in the number of fibroblasts and an increase of neutrophils was found [Tables 2 and 3]. The other cell types, i.e., macrophages, plasma cells, lymphocytes, eosinophils, mast cells, muscle cells and Schwann cells are not significantly changed in number.

The "lower" region of the lamina propria of the patients with CD contained significantly more cells [Table 1]. Significantly more macrophages, plasma cells, eosinophils, and neutrophils were found in this region [Fig. 2, Table 2]. The number of Schwann cells was reduced [Table 3]. The other cell types were not significantly changed.

Table 1. Total number of cells/mm^2 + s.d. in the lamina propria of the sigmoid colon from normal controls and patients with Crohn's disease

Lamina propria	controls	Crohn's patients	t-test
Upper	8.040 + 1080	7.620 + 1260	n.s
Lower	6.360 + 1140	10.080 + 840	p<0.025

Tables 2 and 3. Means and standard deviations of the number of cells/mm^2 tissue from the lamina propria of the sigmoid colon from normal controls and patients with CD. Cell numbers were compared with the t-test [n.s. = not significant]

Table 2.

Lamina propria	MC*	PC	LY	EO	NE
Upper-controls	1800+ 570	1370+ 160	1280+280	180+ 80	0
-CD	1790+1030	1210+ 550	970+310	170+160	80+70
-t-test	n.s.	n.s.	n.s.	n.s.	p<0.025
Lower-controls	410+230	1130+ 420	1260+240	40+ 50	0
-CD	890+230	4370+1430	1160+170	420+440	140+160
-t-test	p<0.025	p<0.005	n.s.	p<0.05	p<0.025

Table 3.

Lamina propria	FB	MA	MK	EN	SC
Upper-controls	1010+420	50+ 60	30+ 30	360+190	130+160
-CD	290+110	40+ 60	100+ 70	360+140	20+ 20
-t-test	p<0.025	n.s.	n.s.	n.s.	n.s.
Lower-controls	1200+600	140+ 80	120+ 80	280+130	260+100
-CD	950+520	120+ 140	100+ 90	220+150	30+ 20
-t-test	n.s.	n.s.	n.s.	n.s.	p<0.005

* Abbreviations, see subscript fig.1. NE-Neutrophil

DISCUSSION

The study of the distribution of various cell types in the lamina propria of the sigmoid colon of normal controls and in patients with CD by means of LM- and EM- photomontages indicates that the latter method improves cell recognition and about 10% more cells are identifiable.

In our study the division of the lamina propria into "upper" and "lower" area has confirmed the findings in previous studies (1,2) that certain cells are most likely to be positioned in a particular area within the lamina propria. Since other reports do not make the distinction between the two areas it is only possible to compare our quantitative results with "observations" made in the literature (3,4,5).

All authors who view the lamina propria from the sigmoid colon classified as "normal" report on a close collection of macrophages just below the epithelium surrounding superficial blood vessels and fibroblast projections. It is just under

this region that the other cell types are found, i.e. lymphocytes, plasma cells, eosinophils, nerve cells, muscle cells
and mast cells. Fibroblasts are characterized by their peri-
cryptical formation, and as expected muscle cells are located
in lower regions in the proximity of the muscularis mucosa,
along with mast cells which are reported as being most abundant in the submucosa.

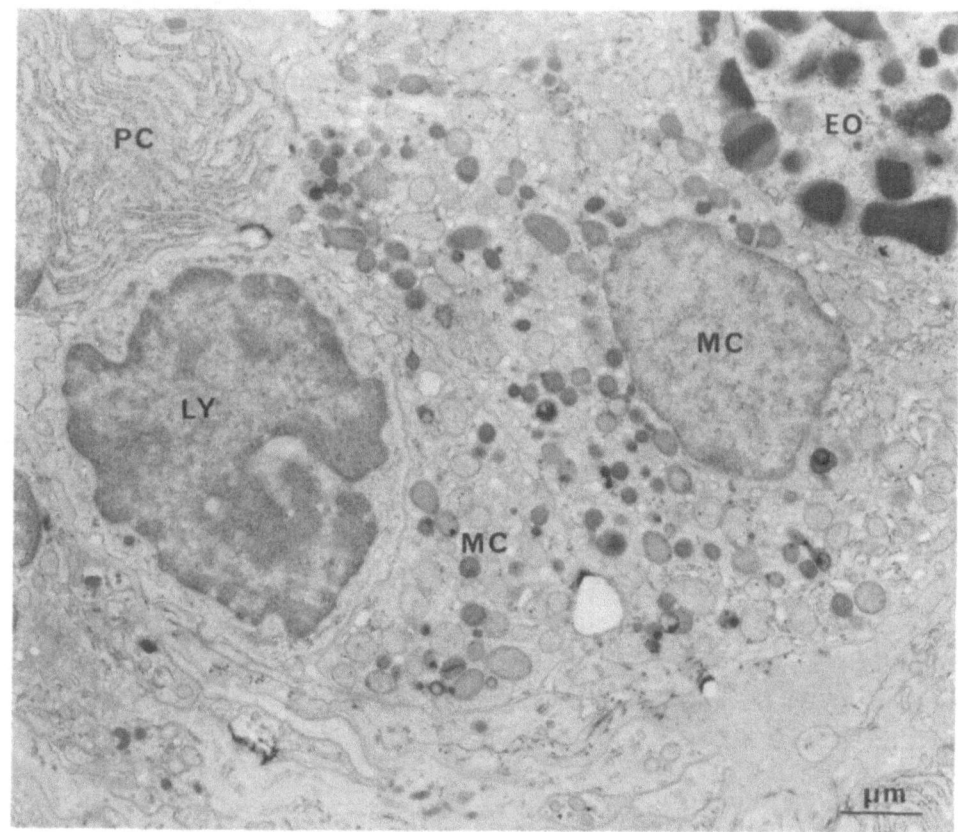

Figure 2. Part of the "lower" lamina propria of a patient
with Crohn's disease. Numerous macrophages[MC],
plasma cells[PC] and eosinophils[EO] are present.
LY-lymphocyte

The results reported here are not in conflict with these,
but merely strengthen them. Macrophages and eosinophils were
found to be significantly more in the "upper" area and mast
and muscle cells in the "lower" region.

Although we could only present some preliminary data on the distribution of the various cell types in the sigmoid colon of patients with CD, some characteristic differences were noticed in comparison of the controls. Specifically in the "lower" region of the lamina propria increased number of macrophages, plasma cells, eosinophils and neutrophils were found [Fig. 2]. However, an inflammatory infiltrate of plasma cells, eosinophils and neutrophils seems not only to be characteristic of CD, since similar findings have been made in patients with UC (5).

Increased numbers of macrophages in Crohn's disease were also proven quantitatively by Korelitz and Sommers (5). Since granulomas are predominantly found in the deeper region of the lamina propria (6), the observed increase in the number of macrophages specifically in this area may be related to a function in granuloma formation, which needs further investigation (7).

CONCLUSIONS

1. Investigation of the lamina propria of the sigmoid colon from controls and patients with CD by means of EM photomontages improves cell recognition.

2. The distribution of cells in the normal lamina propria of the sigmoid colon is not random. Significantly more macrophages and eosinophils are found in the "upper" region of the lamina propria, whereas more mast and muscle cells are found in the "lower" region.

3. The "lower" region of the lamina propria of patients with CD contained significantly more cells. It seems that there is a specific infiltration of macrophages, plasma cells, eosiniphils and neutrophils into this lower area.

ACKNOWLEDGEMENTS

The authors acknowledge the technical assistence of J.J.M. Onderwater, L.D.C. Verschragen, P.H. Cambier and J.J. Magdelijns; and are greatly indebted to Prof. W.Th. Daems for valuable criticism.

REFERENCES

1. Donnellan WL. (1965) The structure of the colonic mucosa.
    Gastroenterology 49:496-513
2. Eidelman S, Lagunoff D. (1972) The morphology of the
    normal human rectal biopsy. Hum.Pathol. 3:389-401
3. Nagle GJ, Kurtz SM. (1967) The electron microscopy of the
    human rectal mucosa. Am.J.Dig.Dis. 12:541-567
4. Binder V. (1970) Cell density in lamina propria of the
    colon: A quantitative method applied to normal subjects
    and ulcerative colitis patients. Scand.J.Gastroenterol.
    5:485-490
5. Korelitz BI, Sommers SC. (1974) Differential diagnosis of
    ulcerative colitis and granulomatous colitis by sigmoido-
    scopy, rectal biopsy and cell counts of rectal mucosa.
    Am.J.Gastroenterol. 61:460-469
6. Rotterdam H, Korelitz BI, Sommers SC. (1977) Microgranu-
    lomas in grossly normal rectal mucosa in Crohn's disease.
    Am.J.Clin.Pathol. 67:550-554
7. Ward M. (1979) Phagocytic function in Crohn's disease.
    Z.Gastroenterol. 17:116-124

B19 Summary of Discussions relating to topics B16 to B18

Hermon-   The membrane-coated vesicles described by Dour-
Taylor: mashkin might either be messenger RNA endogenous to
the enterocyte, which is dying and being released
into the lumen, or they might be some foreign
agent. One way out would be to put them into an in
vitro translation system and see what they produce.
Have such studies been done or proposed?

Dourmashkin: Our plan is first to see whether they contain
nucleic acids, and then to see if they have any
particular function.

Daems: The plasma membrane of animal cells is thicker
than the membranes of the endoplasmic reticulum and
nuclear envelope and so on. Did Dourmashkin measure
the thickness of the membrane of the particles he
found after isolation?

Dourmashkin: I think they correspond simply to the thickness of the external cell membrane, but on the
other hand many virus particles such as the myxo-
virus group have external membranes identical to
the lipid layer of cell membranes. I did find a
few particles in the controls. We have not established them to be viral agents.

de Dombal: Ginsel's data were clearly non-parametric.
There were figures of 80 ± 90 and 90 ± 120, and yet
I think that Student's t-test was used for the analysis. You might get better separation between
groups using non-parametric tests.

Ginsel: I think you are correct. These data were the results of preliminary studies.

Yardley: Dourmashkin, were the epithelial cells changes limited to the surface epithelium or were they also found in crypts? Furthermore, did the patients receive an enema preparation before biopsy? Enemas, can cause mucosal damage.

Dourmashkin: The patchy lesions were almost invariably in the surface epithelium, and there was no enema preparation. Also, there was no relationship with medication such as Salazopyrine and steroids.

Hermon-   Does Dourmashkin think that those manifestly
Taylor: dying enterocytes are normal cells being shed from the apex of a villus, or could the findings be related to parasitization with some microorganism?

Dourmashkin: The quantitative studies make it clear that this is not a normal shedding of epithelial cells. As we showed by the blind trial, we could pick up the cases of CD from the patchy necrosis of the epithelial cells.

Asquith: Scanning EM may be a better way of picking up the surface changes. Mura Kami and colleagues in Japan did scanning EM on rectal biopsies in IBD and specific infections. They suggest that there are differences between CD and UC [microvillus changes], but they would not say that they were unique for IBD. They also occurred in specific gut infections.

Tijtgat: I would urge caution about looking at the vesicular break-up of microvilli since it is seen in all sorts of diseases and in normal people, and it may depend on the fixative used. In fact, I think that it is largely artifact.

Elson: Did Tijtgat and Dourmashkin look at mesenteric lymph nodes which are the tissue being used for studies in experimental animals, and did Tijtgat look at the epithelial cells. Also, what does he think of the possible viral particles described by Dourmashkin?

Tijtgat: I only looked at a small number of mesenteric lymph nodes, and I didn't see anything in particular. I would agree that there is more epithelial shedding and damage overall in CD as compared to controls, although I never counted this specifically. I do not accept that what has been shown has anything to do with viral particles. I think there are many pictures in the literature of so-called virxus-like particles which are just breakdown products of cellular components, nothing more. I very carefully examined normal looking epithelial cells, damaged epithelial cells, epithelial cells close to aphthoid ulcers etc., and in none of these areas I could find convincing pictures of viral structures or replication.

Dourmashkin: I was of the same opinion as Tijtgat after I had looked at the sections. I thought that they represented degenerating microvilli, especially since we found them in the controls. The thing that surprised me was that density gradient studies of the bowel washings showed that those particles had a density of 1.4-1.44 g/ml. This is very dense and could only be due to a dense material such as nucleic acid. I don't think that you would find such material after breakdown of cellular products.

Daems: I agree with those who question the significance of these observations, and I think we should
not leave the impression that a viral origin has
been established. Nor do I believe Dourmashkin
wants to leave that impression. I have one question: Did you try to demonstrate nucleic acids in
these vesicles?

Dourmashkin: No, we did Feulgen stains, but they weren't
sensitive enough. This has to be done in the future, to see whether in fact they do contain nucleic acid.

Daems: Don't you think that the differences in shape
and size are contrary to the assumption that these
are virus particles?

Dourmashkin: No. The particles I showed demonstrate fuzz
around their edges and they could be similar, for
example, to picorna virus in size and shape. The
variation in size was also not against a virus.
But again, I don't want to say I am making a claim
for anything. I think we can only establish this by
infectivity studies.

Booth: If we look at any faecal sample we find viruses. What is different here is a claim by Dourmashkin that there is a difference between controls
and Crohn's. How many did you do?

Dourmashkin: We have four control patients and 2 with CD.
There were a few vesicles in the controls which
were not like the particles found CD.

Strober: Dourmashkin said that the areas associated with
the decaying epithelial cells were not associated
with inflammation. Did he attempt to actually quan-

titate or look at those subjacent areas? After all, if this is an early lesion then it would contain only very small increases in lymphoid cells.

Dourmashkin: That is quite right. The fact that we did not see an increase in polymorphs or lymphocytes does not necessarily mean that there is not an immunological process going on.

Das: Another technique which might be very helpful is immuno-electronmicroscopy. It might even help in establishing specificity, particularly using the serum from patients with CD. We have used immunofluorescent technique to study Crohn's disease in a separate model system.

Daems: A lot has been said about macrophages being involved in CD, and Tijtgat stated that in his material giant cells were derived from epithelioid cells. What data does he have for this assumption? Giant cells may derive from monocytes or from macrophages without the intermediate step of the epithelioid cell.

Tijtgat: We saw often intermediate stages in macrophage morphology like those seen in sarcoidosis, so I presume that the same process goes on in CD in the formation of giant cells. The majority are formed by fusion of epithelioid cells - although there might be an alternative.

IMMUNOHISTO- AND ULTRACYTOCHEMICAL OBSERVATIONS IN CROHN'S DISEASE

J.-O. GEBBERS   and H.F. OTTO

INTRODUCTION

There is increasing acceptance that immunological mechanisms are implicated in the pathogenesis of Crohn's disease [CD]. This is particularly concluded from clinical observations and from findings indicating changes of the systemic immune apparatus and of the gut-associated lymphoid system. Therefore, the local immune response is of interest.

In the present study we have studied the local inflammatory process and we have looked for indications 1] of a local involvement of the complement system, 2] of the degree and pattern of the local plasma cell response and 3] of the functional activities of macrophages, granulocytes, and granuloma associated cells to attempt a characterization of the local immune response and to evaluate its possible pathogenetic significance. Additionally, we have looked for epithelial changes and for viral or bacterial particles.

MATERIAL AND METHODS

Surgical and biopsy specimens were obtained from 28 patients suffering from CD of the ileum [23] and colon [5].

We applied the unlabeled antibody enzyme technique [indirect immunoperoxidase [PAP] method] and the indirect and direct immunofluorescence method on paraffin wax embedded sections of Bouin or formaldehyde-sublimate fixed tissue. IgA, IgE, IgG, IgM, C1q, C3, lysozyme, secretory component and coliantigen [by polyvalent anti-OK-coli sera, BEHRING Institute] were demonstrated. In parallel, electron microscopy and ultracytochemistry were done for demonstration of acid phosphatase and peroxidase. The class pattern of immunoglobulin-containing cells were quantitatively determined.

RESULTS AND DISCUSSION

The secretory component was demonstrated in the epithelial cells of non-ulcerated mucosa and the microvilli were
ultra-structurally intact unlike to findings in ulcerative
colitis.

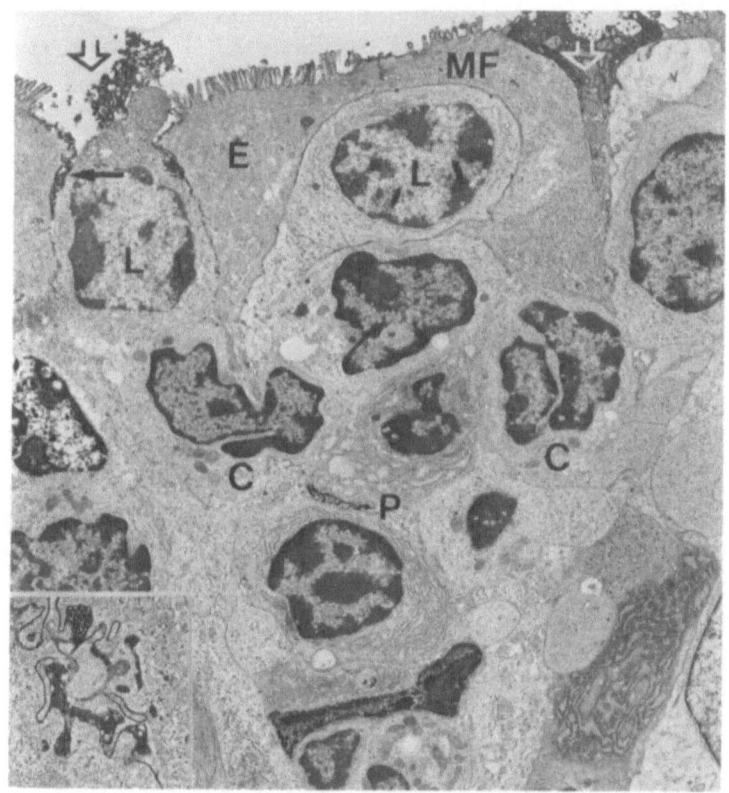

Figure 1. Electron micrograph of the dome of Peyer's patch in
CD: Micro-ulcerations [white arrows] as early lesions. Interstitial deposits of ruthenium red indicating the possible pathway of the antigenic influx
[black arrows and inset].
MF = microfold epithelial cell, E = enterocyte, C =
cerebriform nuclei of [T?] lymphocytes, P = plasma-
cytic cells. Ruthenium red - OsO4.

The earliest histological changes in CD of the small intestine consisted in a marked hyperplasia of Peyer's patches
and in aphthous ulcers. Electron microscopically epithelial
defects and microulcerations were often seen at the dome of

Peyer's patches [Fig. 1]. In addition to small lymphocytes, lymphoid cells with cerebriform nuclei and plasmacytoid cells were frequently seen in the vicinity of microfold epithelial cells [Fig. 1].

The early B-cell response [in non-ulcerated mucosa] was characterized by a balanced augmentation of the number of plasma cells with IgA, IgG or IgM [Table 1]. This corresponds to a typical humoral immune response. In the course of the disease and in relationship to the degree of inflammatory changes, there was a progressive increase of IgG-positive cells [Table 1]. The ratio of the two plasma cell classes IgA/IgG decreases from the normal value of 14.3 to 0.7 in the severely inflamed mucosa.

Table 1. Quantitative-qualitative analysis of the plasma cell populations in the ileal mucosa of 15 patients with CD and of 11 normal controls.

IMMUNOGLOBULIN-CONTAINING CELLS IN ILEAL MUCOSA*

| | Controls | CROHN's disease | | |
		slightly inflamed	severe non-ulcerated	severe ulcerated
Plasma cell number*	53	161	595	1031
IgA	81%	79%	57%	36%
IgM	13%	14%	11%	11%
IgG	6%	7%	32%	53%
IgA/IgG ratio	14.3	11.5	1.8	0.7

* in a defined "mucosal unit"

Similar changes were seen in diseased segments of the large intestine, akin to those seen in ulcerative colitis. The crypt epithelium of non-ulcerated mucosa contained IgM and in that of ulcerated mucosa IgG is demonstrable. Signs of transmural inflammation were typically seen in advanced stages of CD. In the deeper layers, i.e., the tunica muscularis and the subserosa, we found increased proportions of IgG-positive plasma cells. The latter consituted about 90% of all

Ig-positive cells in these areas. A marked infiltration of
IgE-containing cells was observed within severely inflamed
mucosa particularly around ulcerations. This observation
points to the possibilility of local hypersensitivity reactions, which would correspond to the electron microscopic
finding of degranulated mast cells in the severely inflamed
mucosa. The development of the heteromorphous "Crohn granulomas" was related to the degree of inflammatory changes. The
core of the granulomas contained free interstitial IgG [Fig.
2].

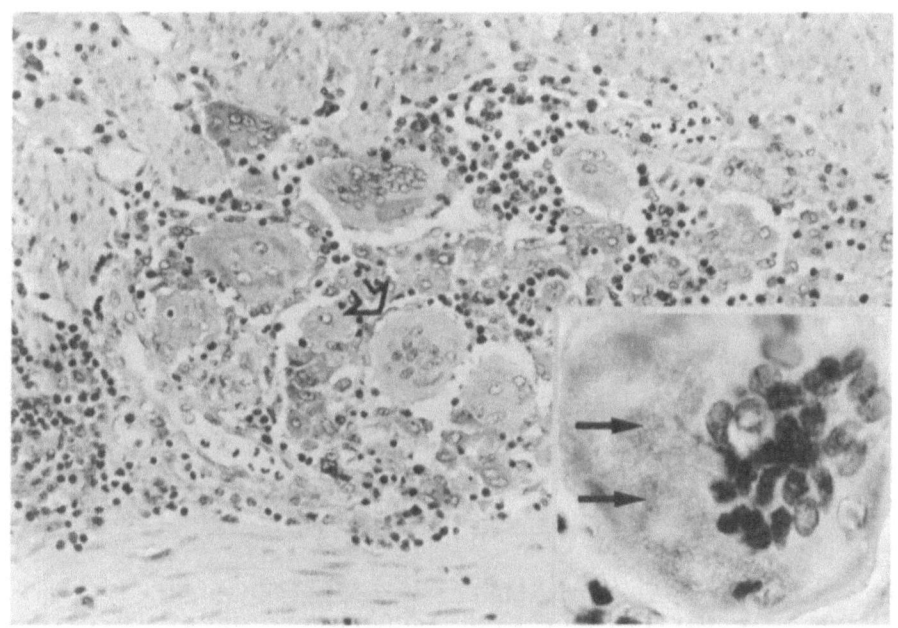

Figure 2. Photomicrograph of a granuloma in CD with multinucleated giant cells and interstitial IgG [arrow]
Inset: Intracellular IgG in a giant cell [arrows].
Immunoperoxidase [PAP] Diaminobenzidine, Haematoxylin.

Membrane-associated and intracellular IgG was also found
in some macrophages and granulocytes, and in multinucleated
giant cells. Smaller giant cells with few nuclei contained
more IgG than larger [older ?] cells with many nuclei. Lysozyme was demonstrable in many monocytes and macrophages in
the inflammatory infiltrate but not in the multinucleated

giant cells. Ultracytochemically, there was a conspicuous positivity for extracellular peroxidase within the granulomas [Fig. 3a,b]. Since peroxidase is a marker enzyme for lysosomal enzymes its positivity was associated to the presence of acid phosphatase [Fig. 3c]. Controversely, peroxidase was virtually absent in macrophages, multinucleated giant cells, epithelioid cells and granulocytes associated with the granulomas.

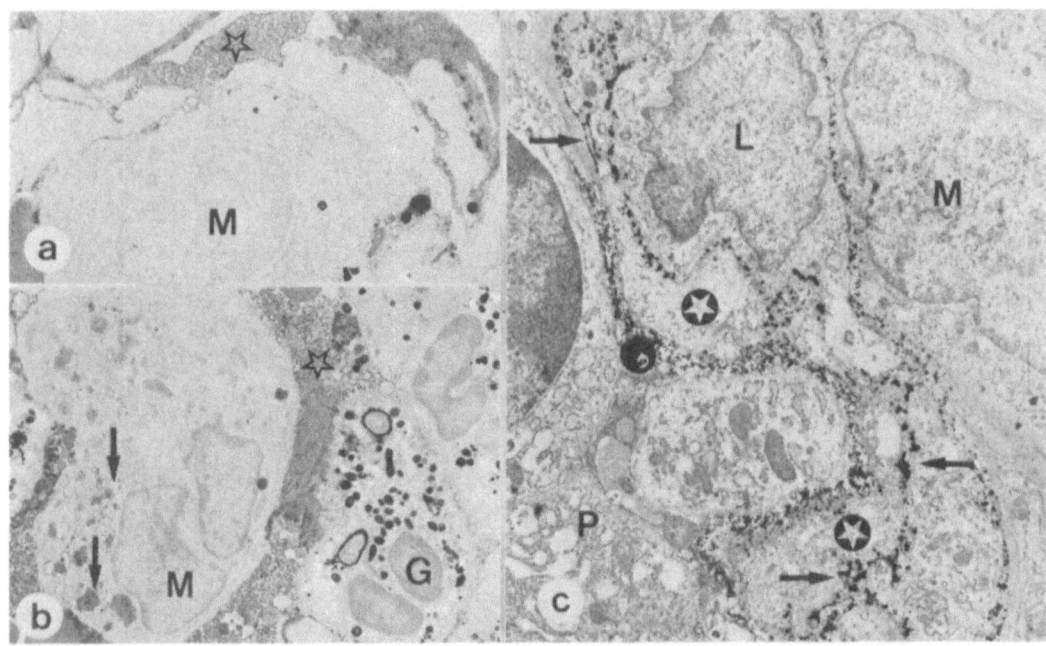

Figure 3. Electron micrographs of granulomas in CD.
a,b: Ultracytochemical demonstration of peroxidase in the interstice [*] and in cytoplasmic vesicles [arrows] of macrophages [M] and of a granulocyte [G].
c: Ultracytochemical demonstration of acid phosphatase in the interstice [arrows] around necrotic material [*].

Intracellular OK-coli antigen could be detected in many granulocytes and in some macrophages in ulcerated mucosa and in the deeper bowel layers.

We were not able to demonstrate C3 or C1q bound to epithelial or vascular basement membranes, and no electron dense deposits were found. Viral particles or bacteria in any of the specimens were not demonstrated by electron microscopy.

CONCLUSIONS

There is no evidence for a primary mucosa block defect. The findings indicate an initial intense local B-cell response with a proportional increase of IgA-, IgG-and IgM-cells in the non-ulcerated mucosa. It seems likely, therefore, that a primary defect of the secretory immunoglobulin system cannot explain the development of the disease; but a definite conclusion needs further characterization of the quality of the local IgA response.

The micro-ulcerations of the dome epithelium of Peyer's patches could be interpreted as an early lesion where luminal antigens gain uncontrolled access to this primary immunologic contact organ. This could lead to an overstimulation of the local immune system, causing a disturbed local immune homeostasis with an imbalanced local Ig-production. The latter is indicated by the disproportional increase of IgG-[IgE-] cells. The imbalance of the immunoglobulin class pattern with IgG-overproduction could cause the formation of granulomas, since there is evidence that the tissue response which produces granulomas is sometimes dependent on the presence of antigen-antibody complexes in antibody excess.

The simultaneous occurrence of coli-antigen and IgG in granulocytes provides evidence for the phagocytosis of immune complexes. This process could also explain the membrane associated and intra-cellular IgG in some macrophages and in multinucleated giant cells. During their phagocytic activities these cells may have lost lysosomal enzymes, which could explain the findings of extracellular peroxidase and acid phosphatase [as lysosomal marker enzymes]. The occurrence of extracellular lysosomal enzymes could be of pathogenetic significance, since they could be responsible for the cell and tissue damage.

ACKNOWLEDGEMENTS

We thank Professor J.A. Laissue for his criticisms and suggestions. We also thank Miss Mary Economou and Miss Cornelia Schürmann for excellent technical assistance. This work was in part supported by a grant of the Deutsche Forschungsgemeinschaft [Ot 53/4-6].

B21 Summary of Discussions relating to topic B20

Peña: Did you study the dome epithelium of the Pey-
               er's patches? Owen has described epithelial "M"
               cells in that location which might be important in
               antigen uptake and its transport in the immune
               system.

Gebbers: In one electron-micrograph I showed the dome
               epithelium of the Peyer's patch and indicated an
               M-cell. That M-cell was intact. We saw micro-
               ulcerations in the dome epithelium which might be
               the door through which the antigens might be ab-
               sorbed into the Peyer's patches.

Jewell: The work of Owen and others seems to show that
               when antigens are absorbed through the Peyer's
               patch you get sensitization of both T- and B-cells,
               the B-cells then recirculate and home back into the
               intestine and develop into plasma cells, and al-
               though they predominantly go to the small intes-
               tine, they do, in fact, distribute throughout the
               whole gastrointestinal tract. If there is ulcera-
               tion of the Peyer's patch this may allow increased
               absorption of antigen into that Peyer's patch. The
               result could be an increase in lymphocytes and
               plasma cells up and down the gastrointestinal
               tract, providing an explanation for the generalized
               abnormality of the gastrointestinal tract.

Gebbers: That is our hypothesis as well. In addition, we
               have seen plasma cells in the dome epithelium of
               Peyer's patches, which is seen neither in control
               patient material nor in animal tissues. So it might

be that antigenic response is occurring within the dome epithelium with differentiation of some lymphocytes into plasma cells.

Asquith: I wonder if you can give further details of the coli antigen. I think it was implied that this antigen might be producing the immunological disturbances which you describe.

Gebbers: We only used a polyvalent antibody against OK-coli antigen [Behring Institute]. We didn't characterize our results because we don't have the necessary special antigens and antisera. I am not sure whether this is a primary defect or only an epiphenomenon. In three cases of UC we found granulocytes stained for coli antigen, but only in the vicinity of ulcers.

Yardley: I believe that increased IgG cells in the mucosa in active CD is a very non-specific reaction. The same thing is seen in other inflammatory conditions such as infections. My own assumption would be that many antigens enter when you break-down the mucosal barrier. If so, increased IgG cells may be unrelated to the specific etiology and pathogenesis in CD, or UC, except to the degree that it may indicate direct access of bowel antigens into the lamina propria.

Gebbers: We don't think increased IgG cells are specific either, because we find the same increase in UC.

Douwes: Has OK-0127 coli antigen also been found in patients with diseases other than CD? All kinds of antigens will pass a damaged mucosa. Did you study patients with, for example, bacterial colitis for OK antigen?

Gebbers: No, not for bacterial colitis. Our controls were especially from malignant diseases, but we saw in CD granulocytes staining for coli antigen were also occurring in non-ulcerated areas and in the deeper layers of the bowel wall.

Lloyd-Still: Have you noted abnormalities in platelet aggregation? Donnellen in one of the earlier studies of UC by EM emphasized platelet aggregation.

Dourmashkin: We found platelet aggregates in the capillaries, but a few platelets are found in normal biopsies as well, so I don't know what it means.

Daems: I would like to close with a comment about the cytochemical evidence for release of lysosomal enzymes. I want to plead for caution. The cytochemical demonstration of acid phosphatase activity with the lead method is tricky. More often than not you find lead precipitate which is due to causes other than enzyme activity. The same holds true for peroxidase, which is often seen in circumstances other than CD and is especially positive in the neighbourhood of eosinophils.

B 22   General Discussion and Conclusions

Reported by J.H. Yardley and W.Th. Daems

MORPHOLOGICAL ASPECTS

Studies presented at the workshop strongly emphasized that histological changes in Crohn's disease [CD] are found throughout the gastrointestinal tract, including the oral cavity. Morphometric methods also indicate that subtle, albeit non-specific increases are found in total number of inflammatory cells and there is a characteristic increase in macrophages. However, diagnosis of CD and its differentiation from other forms of inflammatory bowel disease remains inexact. Except for granulomas, and to a much lesser degree, focal non-specific inflammation, the inflammatory lesions in Crohn's disease have no important distinguishing features.

The earliest mucosal lesion in CD is often focal and development of "aphthoid ulcers" could well be a related phenomenon. At the Workshop, Schmitz-Moormann and Beckers described an initial focal cryptitis and made the interesting suggestion that the granuloma appears as a latter manifestion in the inflammatory sequence. The observation by Chambers and Morson that there are distributional differences in granulomas, with the largest numbers being found in the anal region and the least in the ileum, provoked much discussion and general agreement that further studies of this type are needed. Those authors also presented good evidence that granulomas are more common in early than in late stages of CD.

From a practical standpoint, histopathology can play a useful role in managing patients with various types of IBD by helping in assessment of disease activity. However, because of the much more focal character of the inflammatory changes in CD, this is not as straightforward as successful for CD as it is for ulcerative colitis [UC]. The need for a better contribution by histopathology to an overall activity index in CD was emphasized at the Workshop. Some improvement in this direction may be found in systematic counting of various cell types, combined with computerized statistical analysis as described by Schmitz-Moormann et al. However, considerable refinement and simplification in the methods and verification of reliability would be needed for regular use. Automated cell counting techniques may also be essential to any practical application.

The observation by Gebbers and Otto that cells in the epithelial dome over Peyer's patches show evidence of injury were among the more intriguing investigations presented. A basic fact still to be established, however, is whether the injury is associated with entry of the etiologic agent or whether it only represents a secondary occurrence [epiphenomenon]. Questions were also raised as to whether the evidence of injury to dome epithelium is related to Dourmashkin's observation of injured surface epithelial cells. It is also noteworthy that Tijtgat et al. did not confirm those findings in their meticulous and thorough study. Epithelial injury should be further explored by using rectal biopsy tissue, with emphasis on epithelium over lympoid nodules which are readily found in the rectum.

Several mechanisms of tissue injury in Crohn's disease were proposed during the Workshop, including: 1] Initiation by presence of immune complexes, 2] Degranulation of mast cells mediated through the IgE route, 3] Release of lysosomal enzyme after inflammation becomes established. While further exploration of these possible mechanisms is indicated, there was general skepticism that any significant role has yet been shown for them.

This workshop made it clear that meaningful integration of light-and electron-microscopic studies is so far largely lacking. In addition, data from the electron microscopy studies reported - although highly interesting - were not conclusive, and results obtained by different investigators were in part contradictory. They merit, however, further studies, especially with respect to the etiology and pathogenesis of CD.

It should be emphasized that in CD electron microscopy cannot be expected to become a routine method for pathologists. Its use for diagnostic purposes, if there is any, is extremely limited. However, electron microscopy should be applied in fundamental studies on the etiology and pathogenesis of CD, and it can expect to be of great help in the characterization and identification of the various types of cells involved in CD. Electron microscopy can potentially overcome difficulties in cell characterization even better when combined with cytochemical methods, including enzyme cytochemistry and immunocytochemistry. Differentiation of populations and subpopulations of cells at the site of the inflammatory process, including the monocyte/macrophage series and lymphoid cells, can be followed. Moreover, electron microscopy could eventually provide important information on the topographical relation between cells, and especially on cell contacts and transport of information between cells. Use of isolated cells in fundamental studies on cell identification should be considered.

Scepticism was expressed during the Workshop at the ultimate role of morphology in establishing the pathogenesis and etiology of CD. The limited, tentative, and controversial character of the data presented certainly makes this scepticism understandable. Nonetheless, there is conviction that continued efforts to apply morphologic techniques, combining them with immunochemical, histochemical and other parameters, could ultimately still play a key role in our understanding of the etiology and pathogenesis of CD. An analogous situation occurred with infectious hepatitis, a disease where for many years an infectious agent had been known from epidemiological and other evidence to cause the condition. Yet from a morphological standpoint nothing more than the inflammatory and injurious aspects of the disease were noted using all of the most modern morphologic techniques. Following discovery of the Australian antigen, however, with subsequent observa-

tions on particulate material from serum and improved understanding of the relationships between injury in the liver and
presence of infectious agents, it became possible to visua-
lize the etiologic agent in hepatitis. Thus the experience
with hepatitis confirms the belief that current failure to
see clear-cut primary elements in the etiology and pathogenesis of CD does not mean they are absent, nor does it mean
that some day they won't be demonstrated morphologically.
Current failure is in all likelihood only evidence that we do
not yet know what we are looking for or where and how to look
for it. Clearly, such efforts should continue.

SECTION C

EPIDEMIOLOGY

Section Editor: M.J.S. Langman

THE EPIDEMIOLOGY OF CROHN'S DISEASE, TRENDS AND CLUES

T. GILAT and P. ROZEN

INTRODUCTION

Epidemiologic studies performed by numerous investigators, many of them present here, have produced data which may be of help in elucidating the etiology of Crohn's disease. In recent decades medical research was focussed on possible endogenous causes; now the pendulum has swung again and the search is on for possible exogenous causes. I would like to submit that available epidemiological information supports the predominance of exogenous or environmental factors in the causation of Crohn's disease. This evidence may be grouped under 3 headings: a] Rapidly increasing incidence of the disease in defined populations, b] study of a migrant populations Ashkenazi Jews and c] the very low [and rising] incidence in several developing populations.

RESULTS AND DISCUSSION

a] Rapidly increasing incidence of the disease in defined populations. Table 1 shows the results of population studies in 10 different geographic locations.

Table 1. Rising incidence of Crohn's disease

Area	Period		Incidence/10^5	
	from	to	from	to
Cardiff(1)	1936–40	1971–75	0.18	4.83
Aberdeen(2)	1955–61	1962–68	1.7	2.6
Nottingham(3)	1958–60	1970–77	0.73	3.63
Uppsala(4)	1956–61	1968–73	1.7	5.0
Goteborg(5)	1951–60	1961–70	1.4	6.3
Malmo(6)	1958–65	1966–73	3.5	6.0
Copenhagen(7)	1961–65	1966–69	0.7	1.9
Basel(8)	1960–66	1967–69	1.1	2.6
Tel-Aviv(9)	1970–72	1975–76	0.7	1.9
Cape Town(10)	1956–66	1970–74	Fourfold increase	

The impressive finding is that in all of them the incidence of the disease has risen sharply within the last decades. In many of them the increase was very marked, from fourfold, to more than tenfold. The prevailing opinion is that this represents a true increase and not merely better detection. The genetic material, i.e., the population in each of these studies was relatively constant. The sharply rising incidence thus indicates the effect of environmental factors. It is noteworthy that all these studies come from developed industrialized countries.

b] Study of a migrant population Ashkenazi Jews.

Ashkenazi Jews comprise, a group of individuals who following exile to ancient Rome, were dispersed in various European countries. Together with these European populations some of them eventually migrated to America, Australia and Southern Africa. They were thus exposed for generations to local environmental influences.

Following early reports from the U.S.A. (11-15) of an increased incidence of ulcerative colitis and Crohn's disease in Jews, this particular group was intensively studied for the incidence of inflammatory bowel disease [IBD] in many parts of the world. Table 2 shows the incidence of Crohn's disease in Ashkenazi Jews in several geographic locations. For comparison table 3 shows the distribution of a genetic trait, primary adult lactase deficiency, in Ashkenazi Jews in Israel, the U.S.A. and Canada.

Table 2. Incidence [per 10^5] of Crohn's disease in Ashkenazi Jews and general population

Area	Period	Ashkenazi Jews	General Population
Tel-Aviv(9)	1970-76	1.6	1.2
Basel(8)	1960-69	2.2	1.6
Cape Town(10)	1970-74	2.8	0.8
Baltimore(11)	1960-63	7.2	2.5
Malmo(6)	1958-73	24.0	4.8

Table 3. Adult lactase deficiency in Jews

Area	% With deficiency
Tel-Aviv(16)	66
Connecticut, U.S.A.(17)	71
Vancouver, Canada(18)	69

The contrast is striking. While the prevalence of lactase deficiency is almost identical in all three locations, there is a more than tenfold variation in the incidence of Crohn's disease. There may be inaccuracies in these figures due to the small numbers of Jews in some of these locations: nevertheless, the overall picture is quite suggestive of strong environmental influences. It also seems that the incidence varies according to the general incidence of Crohn's disease in the local population.

It may be recalled that studies of another migrant population, Japanese, were a major piece of evidence incriminating environmental factors [as yet unidentified] in the etiology of colon cancer.

c] The very low [and rising] incidence in several developing populations.

Studies from Cape Town (10), Johannesburg (19), and Kampala (20) indicate that the disease is almost nonexistent in Black Africans, particularly Bantus. It is not a question of underdiagnosis, since in all three centers there are experienced investigators well familiar with the disease which is present in the white population in these areas. Crohn's disease was and is relatively rare in Asians (21). Lately, cases have been reported from India and more particularly in Indians residing in Britain (22). Very recently initial single cases of IBD have been reported in urbanized middle class Bantus in Johannesburg (19). This is reminiscent of the natural course of diverticulosis of the colon in that same population.

It may also be pertinent to note the results of the Organisation Mondiale de Gastroenterologie survey of IBD (23). This survey conducted in many different centers around the globe found good agreement in diagnostic criteria for Crohn's disease and ulcerative colitis among the different centers. Yet the ratio of Crohn's disease to ulcerative colitis in different parts of the world varied markedly from 3/1 to 1/8.

Environmental and genetic factors are, however, not mutually exclusive. Both have been quite convincingly implicated in colon cancer. In several studies in the U.S.A. Crohn's disease and IBD in general were shown to be more frequent in Jews than in other whites (11,12,15). The same was found in Cape Town (10) and Malmo (6).

The difference in the incidence of Crohn's disease between Jews and other whites in these areas may be due to genetic factors, while the differences between Jews in the U.S.A. and in Israel may reflect environmental influences (24,25).

CONCLUSION

Epidemiologic data from various parts of the world show a markedly rising incidence of Crohn's disease. Variations in incidence have been noted in migrant populations. The data are compatible with the predominance of exogenous environmental factors in the causation of the disease. These putative factors may be particularly active in an urban industrialized milieu. Genetic factors may coexist in particular groups.

REFERENCES
1. Mayberry J, Rhodes J, Hughes LE. (1979) Epidemiology. Incidence of Crohn's disease in Cardiff between 1934 and 1977. Gut 20:602-608
2. Kyle J. (1971) An epidemiological study of Crohn's disease in northeast Scotland. Gastroenterology 61:826-833
3. Miller DS, Keighley AC, Langman MJS. (1974) Changing patterns in epidemiology of Crohn's disease. Lancet 2:691-693
4. Bergman L, Krause U. (1975) The incidence of Crohn's disease in central Sweden. Scand.J.Gastroenterol. 10:725-729
5. Kewenter J, Hulten L, Kock NG. (1974) The relationship and epidemiology of acute terminal ileitis and Crohn's disease. Gut 15:801-804
6. Brahme F, Lindstrom C, Wenckert A. (1975) Crohn's disease in a defined population. An epidemiological study of incidence, prevalence, mortality, and secular trends in the city of Malmo, Sweden. Gastroenterology 69:342-351

7. Hoj L, Jensen PB, Bonnevie O, Riis P. (1973) An epidemiological study of regional enteritis and acute ileitis in Copenhagen County. Scand.J.Gastroenterol. 8:381-384

8. Fahrlander H, Baerlocher C. (1971) Clinical features and epidemiological data on Crohn's disease in the Basle area. Scand.J.Gastroenterol. 6:657-662

9. Rozen P, Zonis J, Yekutiel P, Gilat T. (1979) Crohn's disease in the Jewish population of Tel-Aviv-Yafo. Gastroenterology 76:25-30

10. Novis BH, Marks IN, Bank S, Louw JH. (1975) Incidence of Crohn's Disease at Groote Schuur Hospital during 1970-1974. S.Afr.Med.J. 49:693-697

11. Monk M, Mendeloff AI, Siegel CI, Lilienfeld A. (1967) An epidemiological study of ulcerative colitis and regional enteritis among adults in Baltimore. I. Hospital incidence and prevalence, 1960 to 1963. Gastroenterology 53:198-210

12. Acheson ED. (1960) The distribution of ulcerative colitis and regional enteritis in United States veterans with particular reference to the Jewish religion. Gut 1:291-293

13. Weiner HA, Lewis CM. (1960) Some notes on the epidemiology of nonspecific ulcerative colitis. An apparent increase in incidence in Jews. Am.J.Dig.Dis. 5:406-418

14. Nefzger MD, Acheson ED. (1963) Ulcerative colitis in the United States Army in 1944. Follow-up with particular reference to mortality in cases and controls. Gut 4:183-192

15. Rogers BHG, Clark LM, Kirsner JB. (1971) The epidemiologic and demographic characteristics of inflammatory bowel disease: an analysis of a computerized file of 1,400 patients. J.Chron.Dis. 24:743-773

16. Gilat T. (1979) Lactase Deficiency: The world pattern today. Isr. J.Med.Sci. 15:369

17. Tandon R, Mandell H, Spiro HM, Thayer WR.Jr. (1971) Lactose intolerance in Jewish patients with ulcerative colitis. Am.J.Dig.Dis. 16:845-848

18. Leichter J. (1971) Lactose tolerance in a Jewish population. Am.J.Dig.Dis. 16:1123-1126

19. Walker ARP, Segal I. (1979) Epidemiology of non-infective intestinal diseases in various ethnic groups in South Africa. Isr.J.Med.Sci. 15:309-313

20. Hutt MSR. (1979) Epidemiology of chronic intestinal disease in middle Africa. Isr.J.Med.Sci. 15:314-317

21. Lee SK. (1974) Crohn's disease in Singapore. Med.J.Aust. 1:266-269

22. Das SK, Montgomery RD. (1978) Chronic inflammatory bowel disease in Asian immigrants. Practitioner 221:747-749

23. Myren J, Bouchier IAD, Watkinson G, deDombal FT. (1979) Inflammatory bowel disease an OMGE survey. Scand.J.Gastroenterol. 14 (Suppl.)56:1-29

24. Gilat T, Rozen P. (1979) Epidemiology of Crohn's disease and ulcerative colitis: etiologic implications. Isr.J. Med.Sci. 15:305-308

25. Gilat T. (1979) Etiology of inflammatory bowel disease. J.Clin.Gastroenterol. 1:299

SOME EPIDEMIOLOGICAL ASPECTS OF CROHN'S DISEASE IN STOCKHOLM
COUNTY 1955-1979

G. HELLERS

INTRODUCTION

About a year ago, in Cape Town, South Africa, I reported
on a 20-year study of the epidemiology of Crohn's disease
[CD] in Stockholm County (1). The study covered the period
1955-74 and included 826 cases. Today I am going to give an
update of this study including data collected through 1979.

PATIENTS, RESULTS AND DISCUSSION

During the 25-year period 1955-79, the county of Stockholm's population has increased from about 1.2 million in
1955 to 1.5 million in 1972, and has since then remained
stable. We have obtained data on 1133 patients, 523 males
and 610 females; this gives a male-female ratio 1:1.17 which
is not significantly different from the expected 1:1.08.

The absolute number of cases divided chronologically in
five-year periods is shown in table 1.

Table 1. Absolute number of Crohn's disease cases divided in
five years periods.

| | Five-year period | | | | | |
	1955-59	1960-64	1965-69	1970-74	1975-79	All
Males	36	66	120	157	144	523
Females	57	79	133	178	163	610
Both	93	145	253	335	307	1133

The incidence [calculated as the annual number of new
cases per 100,000 mean population] has increased up to 1970,
but is again decreasing during the late seventies [Table 2].

Table 2. Incidence of Crohn's disease in the county of Stock-
         holm [new cases per 100,000]

| Five-year period | | | | | |
1955-59	1960-64	1965-69	1970-74	1975-79	All
Males 1.3	2.1	3.5	4.4	4.0	3.1
Females 1.8	2.3	3.7	4.7	4.2	3.3
Both 1.5	2.2	3.6	4.5	4.1	3.2

The increase was rather slow up to 1966, becoming rapid
between 1966 and 1969, forming a plateau during the early
seventies and finally slowly decreasing during the late seventies [Fig 1]

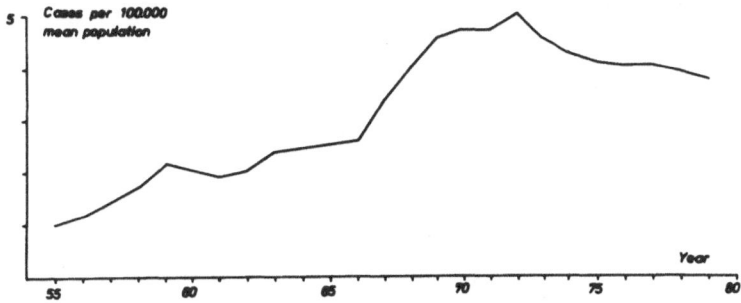

Figure 1. Graphical illustration of increase in incidence of
          Crohn's disease in the county of Stockholm.

Such an increase in incidence may be, at least partly, be
caused by a shortening of this time between onset and definite diagnosis. The time-interval was 3.0 years in the beginning of the study, but decreased significantly during the
years 1965-69, and has since then remained stable.

It is of some interest to determine the incidence of in
relation to the age of the patient at time of diagnosis [Fig.
2]. During the first five-year period 1955-59, there is no
obvious pattern. In the next period, 1960-64, the incidence
is increasing in younger age-groups only, and these age-
groups account for the overall increase in incidence. In the
next five-year period, this pattern is more pronounced with a

sharp peak in the age-group 15-19 years. During the next
period, 1970-74, the peak is a little lower and wider, and
the top of the peak is in the age-group 20-24 years. Finally,
in the last period 1975-79, the peak is even wider and lower,
and the top of the peak is in the age-group 25-29 years.

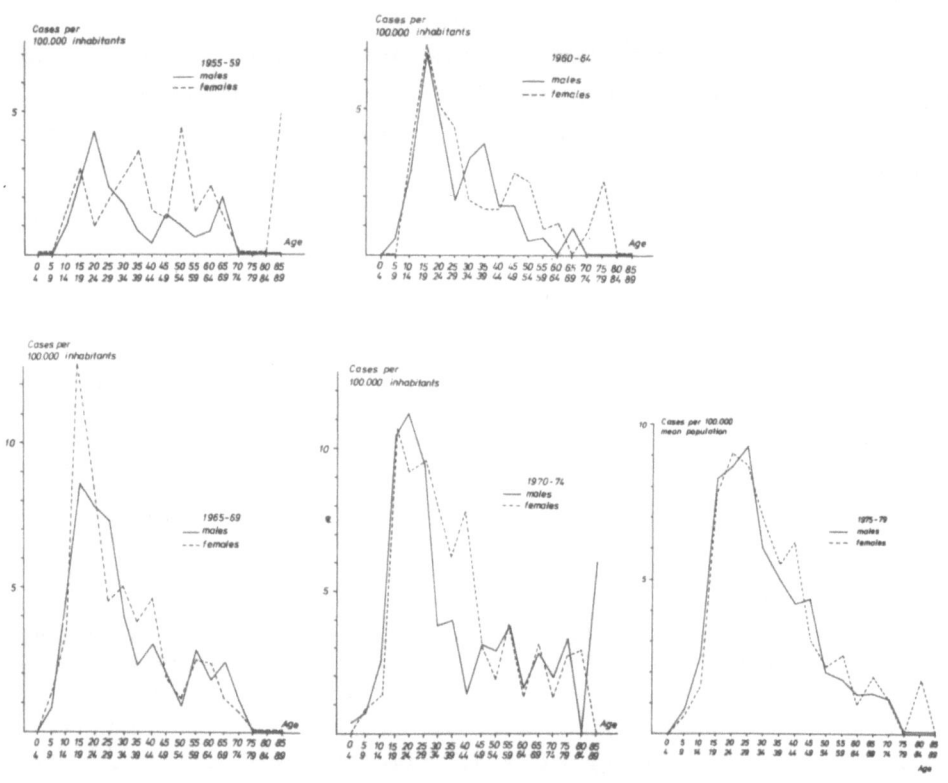

Figure 2. Incidence of Crohn's disease in relation to the age
of the patient at the time of diagnosis in five-
year periods from 1955 to 1979

These results could be explained if we assume that a
single cohort of individuals of a given age range has a greater susceptibility to CD and gradually moving up in age
through the population. The patients group at risk were born
primarily during the period 1945-55: patients born earlier or

later do not seem to get CD at the same rate. An example: the incidence among 15-19-year-olds in 1979 is only 40 percent of the incidence in the same age-group in 1969; in addition, the mean age for the whole patient group has increased by approximately 3.5 years in each of the last five-year periods. If we project five years ahead, we will get a lower incidence, and the dominant age-group will be 30-34 years. If we extrapolate 20 years ahead, perhaps CD will have disappeared by the year 2000! More likely however the incidence of CD will return to a lower baseline.

We are now faced with an obvious question: What happened during the period 1945-55? Did some environmental factors change, or was some change taking place later that affected only individuals born between 1945 and 1955?

DIETARY FACTORS

One possible environmental factor in the causation of CD is that these patients differed with respect to breast-feeding. We have therefore determined the length of breast-feeding during infancy in patients later in life developing CD compared with controls matched in pairs. The matched controls were selected at random from the Stockholm county population registry and were chosen so that they were of the same sex, and were born on the same day and in the same area of Sweden as the patients to which they were matched. Both patients and controls were asked for how long a period they had been breast-fed, in months, during their infancy. The information given had to be checked with the parents or some other reliable source; if the information could not be checked the individual was excluded from further analysis.

The study started with 826 cases of CD, but a number of patients were not, for various reasons, available for study. In the end there were 308 complete pairs, that is, pairs in which both patient and control were able to produce adequate answers [incomplete pairs, where one or both in the pair could not give an adequate answer, were excluded from further study]. The difference in the length of the breastfeeding period between patients and matched controls for the whole material, and in relation to time of diagnosis and age-group is shown in table 3.

Table 3. Differences in the length of breast-feeding period in months between patients and controls in relation to time of diagnosis and age-groups.

Time-period		Age-interval							
		0-9	10-19	20-29	30-39	40-49	50-59	60-	All
55-59	Mean	0.00	-0.29	-0.25	-6.25	-6.00	0.00	0.00	-2.14
	SE	0.00	1.81	1.52	2.84	3.46	0.00	0.00	1.14
	N	0	7	8	4	3	0	0	22
60-64	Mean	0.00	-2.15[a]	-1.59	2.25	-9.00	0.00	0.00	-1.73[a]
	SE	0.00	0.79	1.31	4.27	0.00	0.00	0.00	0.73
	N	0	27	17	4	1	0	0	49
65-69	Mean	-2.20	-1.94[b]	-1.28[a]	0.50	1.75	0.00	0.00	-1.27[b]
	SE	1.36	0.69	0.63	1.42	2.02	0.00	0.00	0.42
	N	5	36	46	10	4	0	0	101
70-74	Mean	0.67	-0.53	-1.33[b]	-0.71	1.44	-0.33	8.00	-0.73[a]
	SE	0.33	0.63	0.47	1.13	1.47	1.45	0.00	0.36
	N	3	30	66	24	9	3	1	136
All	Mean	-1.13	-1.46[b]	-1.28[b]	-0.67	-0.41	-0.33	8.00	-1.17[b]
	SE	0.97	0.40	0.36	0.89	1.35	1.45	0.00	0.25
	N	8	100	137	42	17	3	1	308

a: Significance p<0.025
b: Significance p<0.005

For the whole material, the difference is 1.17 months with the individuals later developing CD having been breast-fed for a shorter period of time. Additionally, the greater differences seem to appear among patients born between 1945 and 1955, i.e., the cohort of individuals with a greater than average prevalence of CD.

There are strong indications that breast milk is of major importance for protection against infection and for the normal development of the infant. These studies suggest that it may even play a role in the development of Crohn's disease.

REFERENCE

1. Hellers G. (1980) Epidemiology of Crohn's disease in Stockholm county. In: Crohn's disease. A global assessment. Ed. Lee E. HM-M Publishers, Aylesbury, England, in press

STUDIES ON THE INCIDENCE, PREVALENCE, MORTALITY AND DIETARY
HISTORY OF PATIENTS WITH CROHN'S DISEASE

J.F. MAYBERRY and J. RHODES

INTRODUCTION

During the last decade several epidemiological studies of
Crohn's disease have suggested that the condition has increased in frequency. We have examined the incidence in
Cardiff over the last 40 years and considered a possible
explanation for the rise in incidence. Although some centres
have reported urban clustering of cases, others have been
unable to show this. Clustering suggests that infection or
an environmental agent may be important in the aetiology of
the disease. We have also examined the distribution of 1098
patients with Crohn's disease throughout Wales and the prevalence of inflammatory bowel disease in 1st degree relatives
of patients with the disease. During the last 5 years the
role of diet in the aetiology of Crohn's disease has attracted considerable attention; for this reason dietary differences between patients with Crohn's disease, ulcerative colitis and normal controls were also assessed.

RESULTS AND DISCUSSION
Changes in the incidence of Crohn's disease in Cardiff between 1934 and 1977 (1).

Hospital admissions have been recorded in Cardiff since
the Dispensary was opened in 1822. Actual case records have
been retained from 1926 until the present. Consequently, a
long term retrospective study of Crohn's disease in Cardiff
was possible. 264 patients were identified and the notes of
256 retrieved. The diagnosis of Crohn's disease was confirmed in 232 patients by histology or radiology. The date and
method of diagnosis were recorded, together with the patient's age; from this data the annual incidence was derived.

The incidence rose from $0.18/10^5$/year during 1931-1935 to $4.83/10^5$/year during 1971-1975, with a maximum value of $5.95/10^5$/year in 1973. This increase in incidence could not be attributed to:

1] Greater recognition of Crohn's colitis: between 1960 and 1970 there was an increase in the frequency of the disease affecting small bowel as well as the ileocaecal area and colon.

2] More accurate diagnosis and detection of milder cases by radiology: surgical detection and diagnosis increased throughout the period 1934 to 1977 and the standardised mortality ratio [SMR] has remained constant.

3] Early confusion of Crohn's disease with typhoid fever, tuberculosis of the bowel or ulcerative colitis.

4] Better retrieval and identification of recent cases: a similar increase in incidence was not seen for patients with achalasia retrieved from identical sources (2).

It would appear that the rise in incidence of Crohn's disease is real rather than apparent.

Mortality in Crohn's disease. A study based on Cardiff residents (3).

The state of health on December 31st, 1976 was established in 218 of the 219 patients diagnosed between 1934 and 1976; 40 had died. The study was conducted at the end of 1978 to allow a 2 year period for mortality data to emerge. Sources of information included: patients' notes, families or neighbours, family doctors and the National Health Service Central Register, Southport, England.

The expected mortality for each patient was calculated each year during the study according to sex and age and compared with the observed mortality. In addition, expected mortality was derived for disease at different anatomical sites and dates of diagnosis. The standardised mortality ratio [SMR] for the 219 patients was 2.16 relative to the population of Cardiff [χ^2 =24.98;p<0.001]. The SMR for the 90 male patients was 2.02 and for the 129 female patients

2.29. The SMR varied with the site of the disease; it was greatest for extensive disease involving several sites [SMR = 2.88] and least for colonic involvement [SMR = 0.86].

Young patients aged 10-19 were at particular risk of death [SMR = 11.04]. The highest mortality was seen in the first 3 years after diagnosis and again after about 13 years of illness. This may reflect early death of several ill patients and later the effects of multiple surgical procedures and prolonged treatment with steroids. During the last 40 years drugs and surgery have controlled symptoms without improving the prognosis.

Prevalence of inflammatory bowel disease in first degree relatives and spouses of patients with Crohn's disease (4).

In 1977, 156 patients with Crohn's disease were living in Cardiff [prevalence = $55.7/10^5$]. Of the 147 alive in 1979, 139 completed a questionnaire about family size and the occurrence of ulcerative colitis or Crohn's disease in 1st degree relatives and spouses. Thirteen had at least one affected relative in whom the diagnosis was confirmed by radiology or histology. The commonest association was of sibling pairs, 7 of 437 siblings had Crohn's disease and 4 had ulcerative colitis. The risk of siblings developing the disease is about 30 times that in the total population. Such an increased risk is not high enough to indicate a disease of simple Mendelian inheritance with high penetrance, but suggests that an external factor such as infection or diet may be responsible for the condition in susceptible individuals.

The period prevalence of Crohn's disease throughout Wales, 1967-1976 (5).

1098 patients from Wales were admitted to hospital between 1967 and 1976 with a diagnosis of Crohn's disease, which gives a period prevalence of $40.2/10^5$. The condition was most common in South Wales with a period prevalence in South Glamorgan of $54.1/10^5$, in West Glamorgan $46.1/10^5$ and in Gwent $40.1/10^5$. Independent of this observation it was found that patients came predominantly from urban [period prevalence = $47.6/10^5$] rather than rural areas [period prevalence = $31.4/10^5$].

Patients in this study were identified from a computer index held by the Welsh Office and its accuracy was assessed from independent data held from Cardiff. In 90% of cases the diagnosis was confirmed by histology or radiology; about 10% of patients in Cardiff were treated entirely as outpatients during this period and were not on the computer record. Consequently although the data is limited the differences in period prevalence between the north and south and between urban and rural areas are probable real and add further support to a possible role for environmental agents in the aetiology of this condition.

Dietary studies

Diet has recently been examined in Crohn's disease and the observed differences may be of importance in the aetiology or simply reflect secondary changes. We have undertaken several dietary studies and reviewed the possible role of breakfast cereals (6), sugar (7) and milk (8) in the aetiology of Crohn's disease. In the first study (9) which included 100 patients with Crohn's disease and 100 age-and-sex matched controls, a questionnaire was completed and showed no difference in the consumption of breakfast cereals but patients used more sugar than controls. Since the difference may simply reflect chronic ill health we then asked 120 different patients with Crohn's disease, 100 with ulcerative colitis and age-and-sex matched controls to complete a questionnaire about current and past dietary habits. More patients with Crohn's disease added sugar to their beverages [76%] and cereals [63%] than controls [56% and 35% respectively], and the quantity of sugar used daily by patients with Crohn's disease [66g] was significantly greater than in ulcerative colitis [39g] or controls [38g]. The difference in sugar consumption does not appear to be simple a consequence of ill health and diarrhoea. In a third study an attempt was made to exclude the effect of medical advice by questioning 32 newly diagnosed patients. Their current consumption of sugar [49g] was significantly greater than by matched controls [24g]. Similarly, patients ate each day significantly more foods which contained sugar compared with controls. The rise in incidence of Crohn's disease has not been associated with a marked change in sugar consumption which makes it more likely that the association is a secondary rather than a causal one.

CONCLUSION

The incidence of Crohn's disease has increased significantly in recent years. It is more common in 1st degree relatives than non-relatives and in towns rather than country areas. These findings would suggest that an environmental factor such as infection or diet may be important in the aetiology of Crohn's disease. Dietary studies have demonstrated an increased intake of sugar by patients with Crohn's disease, but these findings are probably secondary associations and the aetiology of Crohn's disease remains unknown.

REFERENCES
1. Mayberry JF, Rhodes J, Hughes LE. (1979) Incidence of Crohn's disease in Cardiff between 1934 and 1977. Gut 20:602-608
2. Mayberry JF, Rhodes J. (1980) Achalasia in the City of Cardiff from 1926 to 1977. Digestion 20:248-252
3. Mayberry JF, Newcombe RG, Rhodes J. (1980) Mortality in Crohn's disease. Quart.J.Med. 49:63-68
4. Mayberry JF, Rhodes J, Newcombe RG. (1980) Familial prevalence of inflammatory bowel disease in relatives of patients with Crohn's disease. Brit.Med.J. 1:84
5. Mayberry JF, Rhodes J, Newcombe RG. (1980) Crohn's disease in Wales, 1967-76; an epidemiological Survey based on hospital admissions. Postgrad.Med.J. 56:336-341
6. James AH. (1977) Breakfast and Crohn's disease. Brit.Med. J. 1:943-945
7. Martini GA, Brandes JW. (1976) Increased Consumption of Refined Carbohydrates. Klin.Wschr. 54:367-371
8. Warthin T. (1969) Some epidemiological observations on the etiology of regional enteritis. Trans.Am.Clin.Climatol.Assoc. 80:116-124
9. Mayberry JF, Rhodes JF, Newcombe RG. (1978) Breakfast and dietary aspects of Crohn's disease. Brit.Med.J. 2:1401

CROHN'S DISEASE IN THE CENTRAL AREA OF SPAIN

J. GARCIA PAREDES and J.M. PAJARES GARCIA

INTRODUCTION

The aim of this retrospective study was to obtain epidemiological information about Crohn's disease in the Central Area of Spain. The incidence and certain clinical characteristics of patients with well established Crohn's disease have been studied.

MATERIALS AND METHODS

Eleven general hospitals* participated in the present study. These hospitals provide the medical care of 80% of the population of the province of Madrid and surroundings. 394 patients with CD have been collected. The diagnosis was established following histo-pathological criteria [including typical radiological findings]. In order to get homogenous data, the same questionnaire was used in all collaborating centres. This questionnaire included age, sex, place of birth, date of diagnosis, antecedents, profession, localization of the lesions, mode of presentation of the disease and complications. The data were obtained by collaboration of the Services of Internal Medicine, Gastroenterology, General and Digestive Surgery in every hospital. Data from children hospitals are not included. To study the frequency of new cases we have considered only those patients who had lived in the province of Madrid for two years before the diagnosis was made. 256 patients fulfilled these criteria.

---

* Puerta de Hierro [110], Clinico Universitario [84], La Concepcion [54], 1º Octubre [42], Gran Hospital [36], La Paz [25], Ciudad Sanitaria Provincial [18], Gastroenterology School [6], Ramon Y Cajal [10], Cruz Roja [10], Military Hospitals [13] - In brackets the number of patients seen.

RESULTS

The incidence of new cases per one million inhabitants in
the province of Madrid from 1965 to 1979 is shown in fig. 1.

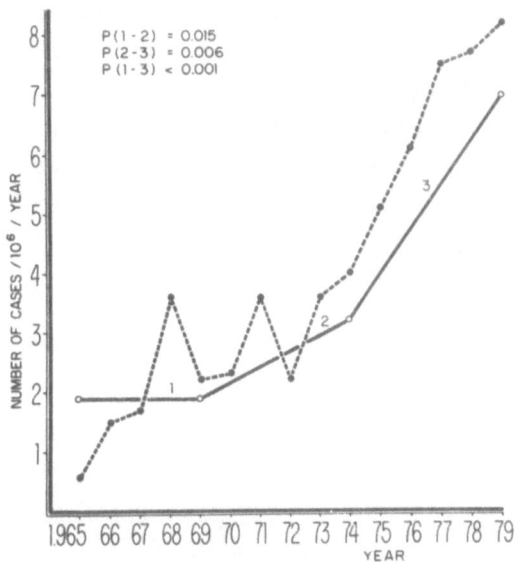

Figure 1.   New cases of Crohn's disease in the area of Madrid
during 1965-79 [n=256] Mean incidence over each
five year period [————].

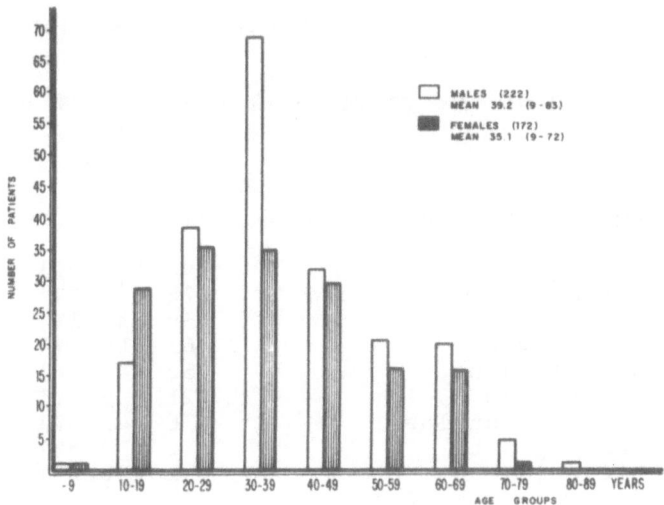

Figure 2. Age at onset of symptoms in 394 patients with
Crohn's disease.

From the 394 Crohn's patients, 222 were men [56.4%] and 172 were women [43.6%] [Ratio = 1.3/1]. 22% of the patients were white collar workers; [72.9% of this group were students]. 29.1% were unskilled; 48.9% were semi-skilled and 30% of this group were housewives. 94.2% from the patients came from urban zones and only 5.8% of them from rural areas.

The main areas affected with CD are shown in Fig.3;23.5% of the patients had more than one affected area.

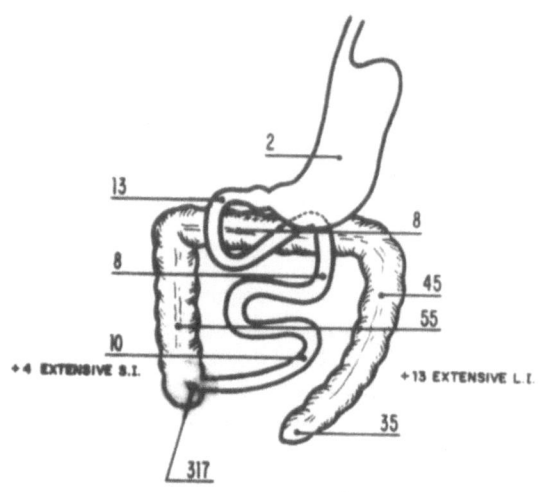

Figure 3. Localization of disease in 394 patients with Crohn's disease.

The symptoms of the patients at the time of diagnosis are shown in table 1.

Table 1. Crohn's disease in Madrid area, mode of presentation

Diarrhoea	296	[75.5%]
Recurrent abdominal pain	278	[70.9%]
Fever	150	[38.3%]
Acute abdomen	63	[16.1%]
Rectal bleeding	52	[13.3%]
Malabsorption	21	[5.4%]
Abdominal fistulae	6	[1.5%]
Retarded growth	2	[0.5%]
Septicaemia	1	[0.3%]

The local and systemic complications presented by 185 [47.2%] and 71 [18.1%] patients respectively can be seen in table 2.

Table 2. Crohn's disease in Madrid area - Local and systemic
complications

Fistula	133	[33.8%]
Perianal Lesions	40	[10.2%]
Abscesses	36	[9.2%]
Intestinal obstruction	35	[8.9%]
Perforation	16	[4.1%]
Stenosis	8	[2.0%]
Carcinoma	1	[0.3%]
Arthritis	39	[9.9%]
Ankylosing spondylitis	9	[2.3%]
Erythema nodosum	22	[5.6%]
Aphthous ulcers in the mouth	6	[1.5%]

DISCUSSION

This study shows that the incidence of new cases of CD
diagnosed in the province of Madrid has increased in the last
15 years, especially during the last 10 years. In certain
areas in other countries the incidence of CD seems to have
been stabilized, for example in Sweden, (1) or disminished,
as in Scotland (2). As the incidence of new cases in countries like Holland, England, Sweden, Denmark, Ireland, Norway
and U.S.A. (3,4,5,6,7,8,9,10) is very much higher than in
Spain, we can expect a further rise of incidence. The higher
incidence of Crohn's disease in the area of Madrid might be
due to the urbanization of the area of Madrid in the last 20
years. Another factor might be, the growing medical interest
in this disease, and improved diagnosis.

The mean age of onset of symptoms in our patients [37.3
years] seems to be higher than in other series (1,3,11), but
this could be due to the fact that children were not included
in the present study. We have not found a second "peak" in
the presentation of the disease after 40 years of age like
other authors (12). The age of presentation was the same for
both sexes. We have observed more males then females as opposed to other series (1, 11).

It is interesting that 94.2% of the patients came from
industrial areas. However, we have to consider that the inhabitants of Madrid have only developed an industrial way of
life during the last 15 years. The mode of presentation is

very similar to other series (3,11) with the only difference that in our study diarrhoea is the most frequent symptom [75.5%] and fever the third one [38.3%]. The local complications presented by our patients are similar to those reported in other series (3,11).

ACKNOWLEDGEMENTS

The following colleagues from the hospitals mentioned earlier provided the data. We gratefully acknowledge their participation. J. Abad, L. Abreu, R. Alcala-Santaella, L. Barbosa, R. Campos, C. Chantar, H. Duran Sacristan, J.M. Esteban, F. Pacheco, C. Hernandez-Guio, J. Garcia-Aguilar, A. Garcia Plaza, J.G. Lobo, M. Gutierrez, I. Jimenez, L. Tonkin, L. Molina, A.P. Mota, J. Muro, Rodriquez-Zapata, J.S. Herruzo, J.M. de la Torre, A.R. de Aguiar, C.V. Thorbeck and J.M. Vilches.

REFERENCES

1. Hellers G. (1979) Crohn's disease in Stockholm County 1955-1974. Acta Chir.Scand. [Suppl]. 490
2. Kyle J, Stark G (1980) Fall in the incidence of Crohn's disease. Gut 21:340-343
3 Weterman IT. (1976) Course and long-term prognosis of Crohn's disease. M.D. Thesis. Leiden
4. Mayberry J. Rhodes J, Hughes LE. (1979) Incidence of Crohn's disease in Cardiff between 1934 and 1977. Gut 20:602-608
5. Brahme F, Lindström C, Wenckert A. (1975) Crohn's disease in a defined population. An epidemiological study of incidence, prevalence, mortality and secular trends in the city of Malmo Sweden. Gastroenterology 69:342-351
6. Norlén BJ, Krause U, Bergman L. (1970) An epidemiological study of Crohn's disease. Scand.J.Gastroenterol. 5:385-390
7. Höj L, Brix Jensen P, Bonnevie O, Riis P. (1973) An epidemiological study of regional enteritis and acute ileitis in Copenhagen County. Scand.J.Gastroenterol. 8:381-384
8. Humphreys WG, Parks TG. (1975) Crohn's disease in Northern Ireland - a retrospective study of 159 cases. Irish J.Med.Sci. 144: 437-446
9. Myren J. (1976) Epidemiology of Crohn's disease. In: The management of Crohn's disease. Eds. Weterman IT, Peña AS, Booth CC. Excerpta Medica, Amsterdam, pp 32-34

10. Monk M, Mendeloff AI, Siegel CI, Lilienfeld A. (1967) An epidemiological study of ulcerative colitis and regional enteritis among adults in Baltimore - 1. Hospital incidence and prevalence, 1960-1963. Gastroenterology 53:198-210
11. Truelove SC, Peña AS. (1976) Course and prognosis of Crohn's disease. Gut 17:192-201
12. Mekhjian HS, Switz DM, Melnyk CS, Rankin GB, Brooks RK. (1979) Clinical features and natural history of Crohn's disease. Gastroenterology 77:898-906

C5 Summary of Discussions relating to topics C1 to C4

Booth: What is the incidence of CD in the Sephardic population in Israel? They came from North Africa after 1948 and would therefore come into a comparable period to the Stockholm group.

Gilat: The disease is more frequent in Jews born in Europe and America than in Asia and Africa. Now we do not know what happens after living in Israel. If environmental factors are important, the differences between communities coming from different areas will disappear.

Riis: Could low incidence or prevalence rates in Africa reflect socio-economic levels and poor access to medical services?
              Secondly, in conducting family studies one must remember that members of families are much more aware of any disease when having a relative with it.

Gilat: In Israel, medical help and diagnostic opportunities are equivalent in all Jewish communities so that I think our differences are real. In Cape Town, at Groote Schuur hospital doctors are certainly familiar with CD which is seen in white and in Cape coloured populations of the area but not in the Bantu. The same is true for the Baragwanath hospital in Johannesburg.

Jeejeebhoy: Have there been any study of the incidence of CD in Japanese immigrants to the USA? Secondly, the desire to eat sugar might be related to mixed-feeding of the child, and therefore a reduced frequency of breast-feeding, so Mayberry's findings [on increased sugar consumption in CD] and Hellers on breast-feeding may be related.

Langman: Crohn's disease is well decribed in Japan.

Mayberry: The Chinese have apparently described about 50 cases of CD in Shanghai over the last 20 years. There are suggestions that patients with Crohn's disease may be zinc deficient and may be unable to taste sweet things.

de Dombal: In Leeds we found in a study of 465 patients that the incidence of CD in siblings was ten times what you would expect in the general population.

Langman: Did anyone want to comment on the curious cohort phenomenon from Sweden?

Truelove: Twenty years ago Acheson and I found that patients with UC were significantly more often likely to have been weaned from the breast within the first month of life. Recently, Whorwell in Southampton has found the same thing but Singleton who was working in Oxford has failed to confirm it. When you have a cohort phenomenon, such as appears to be the case with Hellers' patients in Stockholm, one wonders whether common habits might not be the explanation of it.

Valkenburg: In the 40's - 50's breastfeeding was uncommon in Sweden like it was in most countries. It has increased considerably since then untill the seventies.

Hellers: Immediately after the war the habit of breast-feeding children decreased greatly. This has since then changed back. However, as in many other European countries there have also been great changes in our way of preparing food and storing food.

Fielding: Garcia Paredes' figures are typical of any area that becomes interested for the first time in CD. Is this a true phenomenon?

Lloyd-Still: There have been other changes, for example in poliomyelitis immunization and other variables, I think that we ought to know those figures as well. Intestinal protection may be important.

Jarnerot: Up to 1945 during the war there was rationing of sugar which afterwards was readily available.

Asquith: Am I correct that Mayberry did consider sugar added to beverages. What about other carbohydrates? In the prospective study was UC used as a control?

Mayberry: We initially studied sugar added to beverages and cereals. In the later study of 16 patients and 16 controls, we persuaded people to record details of what they ate. We did not include any patients with ulcerative colitis. There was no difference in intake between carbohydrates and total disaccharides and monosaccharides, in complete contrast to Heaton's in Bristol where his group of patients with CD had a higher intake of refined sugars. We think we simply see a secondary non causal phenomenon but worthwhile following up.

Asquith: But this would tend to negate the link-up between the breast-feeding story and your added sugar data.

Mayberry: Yes.

Thayer: Could a switch from a private health-care sys-
            tem to a socialized health-care system explain
            Hellers' result? Secondly, there has apparently
            been a tremendous increase in dental caries in some
            of the native populations of the U.S. like the
            Eskimos and Indians which they blamed on an in-
            crease of the refined carbohydrates in their diet.
            To my knowledge there has been no increase, or even
            any patient, with IBD, described in those popula-
            tions.

Hellers: In 1970 when the incidence started to decrease
            we had a socialized system. There are about 45.000
            Laps in Sweden and they all live in the North.

van Tongeren: Hellers suggested that probably between 1945
            and 1955 there was less breast-feeding. Another
            possibility is, that between 1945 and 1955 anti-
            biotics were introduced.

Douwes: In the period of the increase in CD did Hellers
            notice a decrease in UC?

Hellers: The incidence of UC is about 5 new cases per
            100,000 per year and it has been pretty stable.

MALIGNANCY IN CROHN'S DISEASE

H. THOMPSON, S. GYDE and R.N. ALLAN

INTRODUCTION

Since the first analysis of Crohn's material in Birmingham by Fielding and Cooke (1) and the pathological assessment of intestinal cancer in Crohn's disease (2) we have been able to enlarge the clinical series and determine more accurately the cancer risk in Crohn's disease (3).

MATERIAL

The extended Birmingham series includes 513 patients [243 males and 270 females] who have been under long-term review between 1944 and 1976. The mean interval from diagnosis was 14.5 years. The mean age of onset was 29.3 years and the mean age at diagnosis was 31.8 years. The average period between onset and diagnosis was 2.5 years. The male female ratio was 0.9.

Almost half the patients [45%] had involvement of the ileum with or without extension into the right colon while a third had extensive involvement of the colon with or without distal ileal involvement [34%].

METHODS

Special care has been exercised in this series to discriminate between Crohn's disease [CD] and ulcerative colitis [UC]. All patients with inflammatory bowel disease under the care of the gastro-intestinal unit have recently been reviewed. Follow-up is complete apart from 9 patients.

The majority of patients had been resident in the West Midlands region for the duration of their illness and the cancer incidence rates for the region have therefore been used to assess the level of the risk of cancer.

The survival experienced by the series was expressed as

patient years at risk grouped by sex, age at diagnosis and interval from diagnosis. By applying the appropriate age and sex specific incidence rates to the patient years at risk, the number of tumours that might be expected to occur in this series was computed. The corresponding observed number of tumours were ascertained from the clinical records of the patients with CD corroborated by scanning the Registry files. The Poisson distribution was used to test the significance of the differences between observed and expected numbers. The probability of the observed number or more occurring by chance was then calculated.

RESULTS

A total of 31 patients developed malignancies in the series. These comprised 18 cases in the digestive system: 9 in colon, 4 in stomach, 1 in small intestine, 1 in oesophagus, 1 in pancreas, 1 in pharynx and 1 in parotid gland. There was a two fold excess mortality rate among patients with CD matched with the general population [Table 1]. In addition, the deaths were predominantly due to complications in the digestive system [Table 2].

Table 1. Deaths from CD

	Expected [E]	Observed [O]	O/E
Males	31.6	63	2.0
Females	20.2	39	1.9
Total	51.8	102	2.0

Table 2. Digestive system-related deaths from CD

	Expected [E]	Observed [O]	O/E
Males	0.9	29	32.2
Females	0.6	17	28.3
Total	1.5	46	30.7

Cancer morbidity in the upper and lower tracts is in excess of what would be expected [Table 3].

Table 3. Digestive cancer morbidity in 513 patients with CD

Site	Total Number of Cancers		p value
	Expected	Observed	
Digestive system	5.396	17	<0.001
Upper tract	2.525	8	<0.01
Lower tract	2.273	8	<0.01
Liver, gall bladder and pancreas	0.798	1	n.s.

The increased incidence in the upper tract occurred in the stomach and oesophagus remote from the site of macroscopic disease. The significant excess in the lower tract involved the large intestine in which cancer usually occurred at the site of macroscopic disease and in patients with extensive colitis of longstanding. There is a four fold increased incidence of carcinoma of the colon and rectum.

Panprotocolectomy had been carried out in 17.3% of patients and colectomy with ileorectal anastomosis in 9.4%. Correction of the statistics for surgical resection increased the cancer risk but not greatly [Table 4].

Table 4. Cancer morbidity - 513 patients in series

Patient years at risk	Cancers			p value
	Expected [E]	Observed [O]	O/E	
All	2.26	9	4.0	<0.001
Adjusted for colectomy	2.07	9	4.3	<0.001

Correction of the statistics for extensive colitis greatly increases the incidence and emphasises the importance of extensive colitis as a cancer risk in CD [Table 5].

Table 5. Cancer morbidity in patients with extensive colonic
involvement [n = 174]

Patient years at risk	Cancers			
	Expected [E]	Observed [O]	O/E	p value
All	0.39	5	12.8	<0.001
Adjusted for colectomy	0.21	5	23.8	<0.001

DISCUSSION

This extended study shows a statistically significant
association between CD and cancer of the upper and lower
digestive tract. The increased incidence was predominant in
the large intestine, stomach and oesophagus. We have not
been able to confirm the earlier suggestion that there may be
an increased cancer risk in the pancreas and small intestine.
There was only one case of cancer of the small intestine but
it must be emphasised that the figures for this site are not
sufficiently large to be statistically conclusive and that
the surgical policy of right hemicolectomy for stenosing
regional ileitis undoubtedly reduced the number of possible
malignancies .

Only 2 of the 9 patients developing cancer of the large
intestine are still alive [2 and 8 years later]. Four of
them died from metastatic disease at intervals of 1 and 4
years after resection and two others died of incidental causes 9 and 18 years later. All but two of the patients presented with symptoms related to the cancer.

There was no excess deaths from cancer outside the digestive tract and there was no statistical evidence of an increased incidence of lymphoma although one patient in the
series was diagnosed concurrently as having CD and lymphoma
of the caecum.

Some of the tumours were occult, diffusely infiltrating
lesions and were only discovered after extensive examination
of the specimen but all showed the characteristic appearances
of infiltrating adenocarcinoma. An endometriosis like pat-

tern described by some workers (4) was a feature of 2 cases in the series. Precancerous changes in rectal biopsies of patients with CD was occasionally encountered in this series (2).

The absolute numbers of patients developing cancer remains small. It should be noted, however, that since this study closed we have observed 2 further cancers in the upper digestive tract and three in the large intestine among the study patients.

Weedon et al.(5) and Greenstein et al.(6) have also found an increased incidence of carcinoma in large series of patients with CD. In addition, various case reports of CD and cancer are found in the medical literature (7-11).

CONCLUSION

Statistical analysis of the Birmingham Crohn's series shows an increased incidence of carcinoma in the digestive system. Patients with extensive colitis of longstanding are at greatest risk.

REFERENCES
1. Fielding JF, Prior P, Waterhouse JA, Cooke WT. (1972) Malignancy in CD. Scand.J.Gastroenterol. 7:3-5
2. Thompson H. (1976) Malignancy in Crohn's disease. In: The management of Crohn's disease Eds. Weterman IT, Peña AS, Booth CC. Excerpta Medica, Amsterdam pp 146-149
3. Gyde SN, Prior P, Macartney JC, Thompson H, Waterhouse JAH, Allan RN. (1980) Gut, in press
4. Fleming KA, Pollock AC. (1975) A case of "Crohn's Carcinoma". Gut 16:533-537
5. Weedon DW, Shorter RG, Ilstrup DM, Huizenga KA, Taylor WF. (1973) CD and cancer. New Engl.J.Med. 289:1099-1103
6. Greenstein AJ, Sachar D, Pucillo A et al. (1978) Cancer in CD after diversionary surgery. Am.J.Surg. 135:86-96
7. Darke SG, Parks AG, Grogono JL, Pollock DJ. (1973) Adenocarcinoma and Crohn's disease. A report of 2 cases and analysis of the literature. Brit.J.Surg. 60:169-175
8. Perrett AD, Truelove SC, Massarella GR. (1968) Crohn's disease and carcinoma of the colon. Brit.Med.J. 2:466-468
9. Chevrel B. (1974) Maladie de Crohn et transformation maligne. Med.Chir.Dig. 3:431-436
10. Lightdale CJ, Sternberg SS, Posner G, Sherlock P. (1975) Carcinoma complicating CD. Am.J.Med.59:262-268
11. Sheil FO'M, Clark CG, Goligher JC. (1968) Adenocarcinoma associated with Crohn's disease. Brit.J.Surg. 55:53-58

C7 Summary of Discussions relating to topic C6

Valkenburg: Why are the cancers located at the two ends of the GI tract mainly.

Thompson: I do not know.

Strober: Do you have data on the relatives of patients?

Thompson: No

Korelitz: Did cancers in the lower GI tract occur in by-passed loops and so forth.

Thompson: Two were in by-pass loops of large intestine. Two were multiple cancers. We have also seen cancer developing at the site of fistulae.

Peña: Does resecting the disease area diminish the risk of cancer?

Thompson: Yes, hemicolectomy seems to reduce the cancer risk in regional ileitis.

Hodgson: What about dysplastic changes elsewhere in the bowel in resected specimens?

Thompson: Dysplastic changes are rare in CD. I have seen this in about five patients, three of whom were described in the previous workshop. Finding precancerous change in one patient led to the discovery of three minicancers in the colon.

Thayer: What is the risk of cancer in CD viz à viz the risk in UC?

Thompson: The risk for UC is between 3% and 4%, is mainly in patients with total colitis or extensive colitis as it is in CD. The incidence in CD appears to be lower than that in UC.

C8 General Discussion and Conclusions

Reported by T. Gilat

Available epidemiologic evidence and data presented here strongly implicate environmental factors in the causation of CD. The evidence may be summarized as follows:

1. There is a rising incidence of the disease in recent decades in developed as well as developing countries. This rise seems to be too rapid to explain by genetic changes.
2. Changes in the incidence of the disease have occurred in migrant populations such as Ashkenazi Jews.
3. The incidence of the disease in populations of developing countries has risen with urbanization and industrialization or with migration to such areas.

Environmental and genetic factors are not mutually exclusive and have been reported to coexist in several other diseases. The higher incidence of the disease in Ashkenazi Jews in several parts of the world may point to the coexistence of genetic factors, at least in some population groups.

Which environmental factors are important? Crohn's disease starts in most people at an early age in the second or third decade. Since the disease is unlikely to be an infection with a short incubation period events occurring in childhood have been investigated. Hellers has found a negative correlation with breast-feeding. The relationship of nutrition, infection, vaccinations, immunity and allergy to the disease are clearly areas for future research. A questionnaire for patients with early onset of Crohn's disease and controls is to be established by Langman and Gilat. This will be forwarded to all interested investigators.

SECTION D

GENETICS

Section Editor: R.B. McConnell

HISTOCOMPATIBILITY ANTIGENS IN PATIENTS WITH CROHN'S
DISEASE

Z. COHEN, P. McCULLOCH, M.K. LEUNG and H. MERVART

INTRODUCTION

Recent work on the pathogenesis of Crohn's disease has
focused attention largely on immunological mechanisms (1,2)
and on the possible role of a transmissible agent (3). It
has been suggested that a virus is the most likely source of
antigen[s] initiating the immunological reaction (4). If one
assumes that these transmissible agents are ubiquitous, why
then should Crohn's disease develop in only a minority of the
population? Genetic characteristics might influence individual susceptibility to Crohn's disease. The involvement of
genetic factors is suggested by a familial tendency (5) as
well as by immunological abnormalities found in both Crohn's
disease patients and their families (6).

The distribution of HLA alloantigens in Crohn's disease
has been investigated by several people (7-9). Weak and
unconfirmed antigenic associations have been found. In recent studies, some disorders, notably multiple sclerosis and
coeliac disease, have shown a closer association with B-cell
alloantigens [DR] (10-11).

This study was undertaken to determine the frequency of
HLA-A,-B, and -DR alloantigens in two Crohn's disease populations.

PROCEDURE

Material and methods

Patient populations. Forty-eight European Crohn's disease patients were compared with 561 European controls at the
HLA-A and -B loci. Forty-seven Toronto Crohn's disease
patients were compared with 100 Toronto random controls
[blood donors] at the DR locus. One patient in the European

Crohn's disease group had ankylosing spondylitis. There were no statistically significant differences between the ethnic origins of the Crohn's disease patients and the controls in either group.

Tissue typing. Peripheral blood lymphocytes were separated on a Ficoll-Hypaque density gradient. HLA-A and -B phenotypes were determined using the standard NIH microlymphocytotoxicity test. For HLA-DR typing, two techniques were compared:

[i] The technique performed for the 8th International Histocompatibility Workshop [B lymphocytes separated by the nylon wool method and microlymphocytotoxicity].

[ii]Two-colour immunofluorescent cytotoxicity (12). HLA-A, -B, and -DR antisera selected to type for all the specificities recognized in the 7th International Histocompatibility Workshop were either reference sera used in the 8th International Histocompatibility Workshop or American Workshops, or sera highly correlated with them.

Statistical analyses. χ^2 values were calculated from two by two tables using Yates' correction.

Table 1. HLA antigens in patient with Crohn's disease and in controls

	Controls (561)		Crohn's (48) patients	
	no.	%	no.	%
A1	183	32.62	17	35.42
A2	288	51.34	26	54.17
A28	56	9.98	3	6.25
A3	163	29.06	13	27.08
A11	69	12.30	3	6.25
Aw23	7	1.25	-	-
Aw24	83	14.80	7	14.58
A25	12	2.14	1	2.08
A26	26	4.63	3	6.25
Aw34	-	-	-	-
Aw33	6	1.07	1	2.08
A29	58	10.34	3	6.25
Aw30	28	4.99	5	10.42
Aw31	16	2.85	1	2.08
Aw32	38	6.77	2	4.17
X	88	15.69	11	22.92

Table 1 continued

	Controls (561) no.	%	Crohn's (48) patients no.	%
B5	44	7.84	3	6.25
Bw51	–	NC	3	(6.25)
Bw52	–	NC	–	–
B7	135	24.06	8	16.67
Bw47	6	1.07	1	2.08
B8	140	24.96	14	29.17
B12	170	30.30	14	29.17
Bw45	–	NC	1	2.08
B13	18	3.21	3	6.25
B14	58	10.34	5	10.42
B15	83	14.80	5	10.42
Bw16	39	6.95	1	2.08
(Bw38)	–	NC	–	NC
(Bw39)	–	NC	–	NC
B17	58	10.34	3	6.25
B18	30	5.35	6	12.50
Bw21	22	3.92	2	4.17
Bw22	26	4.63	–	NC
B27	50	8.91	4	8.33
B40	62	11.05	6	12.50
Bw35	90	16.04	6	12.50
B37	20	3.57	4	8.33
TT	–	NC	1	2.08

p Value 0.995

Table 2. DR typing results

	Controls n=100	Crohn's patients n=47	χ^2 (3.84=p<0.05)
DR1	20	4	2.31
DR2	26	12	0.02
DR3	26	11	0.02
DR4	27	18	1.43
DR5	25	12	0.02
DRw6	16	4	0.96
DR7	26	13	0.00015
DRw8	–	–	–
DRw9	–	–	–
DRw10	–	–	–

RESULTS

HLA A and B. As can be seen from table 1, the frequency of Aw30, B13, B18, and B37 was increased, and that of A11 and Bw16 decreased. However, there was no significant difference when this frequency was compared to that in the control group following correction for the number of comparisons. The one ankylosing spondylitis patient was B27 positive.

HLA-DR. No statistically significant associations were found. Testing for DRw 8, 9, and 10, as defined in the 8th International Histocompatibility Workshop was not done.

DISCUSSION

Our findings agree with most reports in that no significant differences have been found in studying HLA-A and -B locus antigenic frequencies in Crohn's disease (9,13,14). Gleeson et al. (15) found a significant association with A3 but only 18 Crohn's disease patients were studied. Asquith (7) reported A9 to be increased in his 56 Crohn's patients. Our data does not confirm either of these associations. Van den Berg-Loonen et al.(8) reported a raised incidence of B18 [χ^2 =12.21] in 51 patients. In our data, the percentage of B18 was more than double that of controls but did not reach statistical significance when corrected for the number of comparisons. If any association exists between HLA-A and -B locus antigens and Crohn's disease, it is extremely weak. It is therefore unlikely to have any clinical prognostic value.

Genes in the HLA-DR region in man and in the homologous I region in the mouse H-2 system have been shown to code for important parts of the immune response and for sensitivity to certain antigens (16). It therefore did not seem unreasonable to assume that the HLA-DR locus might be of some importance in the pathogenesis of Crohn's disease, either by coding for an abnormal immune reactivity or for susceptibility to a transmissible agent. However, in the 47 Toronto Crohn's disease patients studied, no statistically significant associations were found with DR antigens. It is possible that further definition of DR alloantigens will allow a more conclusive evaluation.

CONCLUSIONS

Two populations of Crohn's disease patients have been studied. No significant associations have been found between Crohn's disease and any of the HLA-A,-B, or -DR alloantigens tested.

ACKNOWLEDGEMENTS

This work was supported by the Canadian Foundation for Ileitis and Colitis and the Canadian Red Cross. Our thanks to H. Festenstein and E. Woolf.

REFERENCES
1. Strickland RG, Miller WC, Volpicelli NA, Gaeke RF, Wilson ID, Kirsner JB, Williams RC.Jr. (1977) Lymphocytotoxic antibodies in patients with inflammatory bowel disease and their spouses - evidence for a transmissible agent. Clin.Exp.Immunol. 30:188-192
2. Kagnoff MF. (1978) On the etiology of Crohn's disease. Gastroenterology 75:526-527
3. Cave DR, Mitchell DN, Brooke BN. (1975) Observations on the transmissibility of Crohn's disease and ulcerative colitis. Gastroenterology 68:871
4. Gitnick GL, Rosen VJ, Arthur MH, Hertweck SA. (1979) Evidence for the isolation of a new virus from ulcerative colitis patients. Comparison with virus derived from Crohn's disease. Dig.Dis.Sci. 24:609-619
5. Lewkonia RM, McConnell RB. (1976) Familial IBD - heredity or environment? Gut 17:235-243
6. Watson DW, Shorter RG. (1975) The immunology of ulcerative colitis and Crohn's disease: Cell mediated immune responses. In: Inflammatory Bowel Disease. Eds. Kirsner JB, Shorter RG. Lea and Febiger, Philadelphia, pp 81-98
7. Asquith P, Mackintosh P, Stokes PL, Holmes GKT, Cooke WT. (1974) Histocompatibility antigens in patients with inflammatory bowel disease. Lancet 1:113-115
8. Berg van den-Loonen EM, Dekker-Saeys BJ, Meuwissen SGM, Nijenhuis LE, Engelfriet CP. (1976) Histocompatibility antigens and other genetic markers in ankylosing spondylitis and IBD. J.Immunogenet. 4:167-175
9. Delpre G, Kadish U, Gazit E, Joshua H, Zamit R. (1980) HLA antigens in ulcerative colitis and Crohn's disease in Israel. Gastroenterology 78:1452-1457
10. Compston DA, Batchelor JR, McDonald WI. (1976) B-Lymphocyte alloantigens associated with multiple sclerosis. Lancet 2:1261-1265

11. Mann DL, Katz SI, Nelson DL, Abelson LB, Strober W. (1976) Specific B-cell antigens associated with gluten sensitive enteropathy and dermatitis herpetiformis. Lancet 1:110-111
12. Rood van JJ, Leeuwen van A, Ploem JS. (1976) Simultaneous detection of two cell populations by two-colour fluorescence and application to the recognition of B-cell determinants. Nature 262:795-797
13. Thorsby E, Lie SO. (1971) Relationship between the HL-A system and susceptibility to diseases. Trans.Proc. 3:1305-1307
14. Jacoby RK, Jayson MI. (1974) HL-A 27 in Crohn's disease. Ann.Rheum.Dis. 33:422-424
15. Gleeson MH, Walker JS, Wentzel J, Chapman JA, Harris R. (1972) Human leucocyte antigens in Crohn's disease and ulcerative colitis. Gut 13:438-440
16. In: The role of products of the histocompatibility gene complex in the immune response. Eds. Katz DA, Benacerraf B. Acad.Press, New York(1980)

HLA-D RELATED ANTIGENS IN INFLAMMATORY BOWEL DISEASE

W.R. BURNHAM, K. GELSTHORPE and M.J.S. LANGMAN

INTRODUCTION

There is good evidence that genetic as well as environmental factors are important in the aetiology of inflammatory bowel disease (1). However, studies of HLA-A and -B specificities have not shown consistent differences between patients and controls. Nevertheless an investigation of the HLA-D related [DR] antigens in such patients would be of interest for two reasons. Firstly an association has been found in some diseases such as rheumatoid arthritis (2) with HLA-DR alloantigens when little or no association was seen with HLA-A and -B antigens. Secondly studies in mice and humans suggest that HLA-DR genes may be associated with genes which control the immune response (3). A genetically mediated abnormality of the immune response might result in susceptibility to an environmental agent leading in turn to the development of inflammatory bowel disease.

MATERIALS AND METHODS

a] Tissue Typing

'B' Lymphocytes were isolated from peripheral blood lymphocyte suspensions by removal of T-lymphocyte-SRBC rosettes on Ficoll-Triosil, using techniques already described. The resulting 'B' lymphocyte rich suspension was then tested in a modified two step microcytotoxicity test against 60 different antisera capable of defining eight different HLA-DR specificities (4) [-DR 1-7, -DRw 4 x 5]. 120 antisera were used to define HLA-A and -B specificities. All samples were assessed without knowledge of their origin.

b] Subjects tested

142 patients with inflammatory bowel disease were studied. Seventy-five had ulcerative colitis and 67 had Crohn's

disease. All were out-patients or in-patients at Nottingham
City Hospital. The diagnosis in each case was based on clinical, radiological and where possible, histological evidence. Three siblings pairs [two Crohn's disease, one ulcerative colitis] were examined. Three other patients with
Crohn's disease and one with ulcerative colitis gave a family
history of inflammatory bowel disease.

500 controls were taken from healthy blood transfusion
donors for DR typing. 3000 donors were used as controls for
the HLA-A and -B typing.

RESULTS

The results of HLA-A and -B typing in patients and controls are shown in table 1. The HLA-DR results are shown in
table 2. The only significant difference between patients
and controls was the reduction in the frequency of DR2 in the
patient group. Allowing for the number of antigens tested
[eight], this difference was significant statistically
[$\chi^2 = 8.23$, p[corrected] = 0.03].

Table 1. Numbers of HLA-A and -B antigens in 142 patients
with inflammatory bowel disease and 3000 normal
controls [Percentage phenotype frequencies in
brackets].

	ulcerative colitis	Crohn's disease	I.B.D.	controls
	n = 75	n = 67	n = 142	n = 3000
A				
1	19 (25.3)	21 (31.3)	40 (28.2)	1092 (36.4)
2	42 (56.0)	38 (56.7)	80 (56.3)	1438 (47.9)
3	17 (22.7)	23 (34.3)	40 (28.2)	816 (27.2)
9	8 (10.7)	11 (16.4)	19 (13.4)	517 (17.2)
11	9 (12.0)	3 (4.5)	12 (8.5)	362 (12.1)
25	1 (1.3)	0	1 (0.7)	112 (3.7)
26	5 (6.7)	3 (4.5)	8 (5.6)	146 (4.9)
28	6 (8.0)	3 (4.5)	9 (6.3)	205 (6.8)
29	5 (6.7)	10 (14.9)	15 (10.6)	218 (7.3)
w30/w31	11 (14.7)	3 (4.5)	14 (9.9)	156 (5.2)
W32	5 (6.7)	4 (6.0)	9 (6.3)	233 (7.8)

Table 1 continued

B

5	6 (8.0)	5 (7.5)	11 (7.8)	277 (9.2)
7	21 (28.0)	13 (19.4)	34 (23.9)	813 (27.1)
8	17 (27.7)	13 (19.4)	30 (21.1)	860 (28.7)
12	26 (34.7)	29 (43.3)	55 (38.7)	863 (28.8)
13	4 (5.3)	2 (3.0)	6 (4.2)	124 (4.1)
14	5 (6.7)	6 (9.0)	11 (7.8)	198 (6.6)
15	13 (17.3)	10 (14.9)	23 (16.2)	456 (15.2)
w16	0	0	0	88 (2.9)
17	3 (4.0)	9 (13.4)	12 (8.5)	280 (9.3)
18	6 (8.0)	4 (6.0)	10 (7.0)	247 (8.2)
w21	2 (2.7)	2 (3.0)	4 (2.8)	112 (3.7)
w22	1 (1.3)	4 (6.0)	5 (3.5)	113 (3.8)
27	5 (6.7)	2 (3.0)	7 (4.9)	232 (7.7)
w35	9 (12.0)	13 (19.4)	22 (15.5)	358 (11.9)
37	1 (1.3)	1 (1.5)	2 (1.4)	85 (2.8)
40	9 (12.0)	8 (11.9)	17 (12.0)	404 (13.5)
w47	0	0	0	25 (0.8)

Table 2. Numbers of HLA-DR[w] antigens in 142 patients with inflammatory bowel disease and 500 normal controls [percentage values in brackets].

antigen	ulcerative colitis	Crohn's disease	I.B.D.	controls
n = 8	n = 75	n = 67	n = 142	n = 500
DR1	17 (22.7)	11 (16.4)	28 (19.7)	95 (19.0)
DR2	18 (24.0)	14 (20.9)	*32 (22.5)	179 (35.8)
DR3	18 (24.0)	12 (17.9)	30 (21.1)	143 (28.6)
DR4	29 (38.7)	24 (35.8)	53 (37.3)	166 (33.2)
DR5	9 (12.0)	9 (13.4)	18 (12.7)	79 (15.8)
DRw6	16 (21.3)	19 (28.4)	35 (24.6)	109 (21.8)
DR7	17 (22.7)	20 (29.9)	37 (26.1)	119 (23.8)
DRw4x5	5 (6.7)	4 (6.0)	9 (6.3)	13 (2.6)

*Statistically different from controls p(corrected) =0.03.

Calculation of the relative risk of developing inflammatory bowel disease for those individuals possessing DR2 was performed using the formula

$$\frac{P_1 [P_2 + P_4]}{P_2 [P_1 + P_3]}$$

Where P_1 and P_2 are the numbers of positive and negative patients respectively and P_3 and P_4 the corresponding values in the controls. The relative risk was 0.59 : 1 for IBD. For Crohn's disease alone, this was 0.51 : 1 and for ulcerative colitis alone, it was 0.61 :1. The reduction in the frequency of HLA-DR2 did not achieve statistical significance when each disease was considered separately, although the trends are clearly the same. One of the patients with a family history of ulcerative colitis possessed DR2.

The elevation of the frequency of HLA-B12 in the patients was not quite statistically significant [χ^2=6.04; p[corrected for 17 antigens]= 0.24].

DISCUSSION

The reduction of DR2 among patients with inflammatory bowel disease was seen in both ulcerative colitis and Crohn's disease. Individuals possessing DR2 had a 40% less chance of developing inflammatory bowel disease. However, in each disease considered separately, the reduction in HLA-DR2 was not statistically significant. Work carried out in Leiden [Holland] in patients with Crohn's disease shows a similar reduction in HLA-DR2, but no difference in HLA-B12 between patients and controls (7). This confirms the HLA-DR2 results, but indicates that those for HLA-B12 in this study may represent a sampling error.

Many diseases have been found to be positively correlated with HLA antigens (5). However, a negative association with a disease is less commonly seen. In juvenile onset diabetes mellitus, there is a relative lack of HLA-DR2, but an increase in HLA-DR3 and -DR4. Clearly, one of these changes may be compensating for the other in order to maintain a genetic balance. However, if the reduction in HLA-DR2 is the primary one, then it may be that this gene [or associated genes] has a "protective" effect in normal individuals. In diabetes mellitus, it has been proposed that HLA linked genes control the immune responsiveness to environmental agents, such as viruses (6); these may have a potential cytopathic effect on the βcells in the pancreas. It is possible that a similar mechanism operates in inflammatory bowel disease. An environmental agent is thought to be involved in the aetiology and susceptibility to this agent may be genetically mediated.

The fact that between a fifth and a quarter of patients with inflammatory bowel disease [including one with a family history] possess HLA-DR2 indicates that this gene is not itself absolutely protective. However, HLA-DR2 may be in linkage disequilibrium with another gene, as yet unidentified, which does have this role. This postulated gene may be found once the many other loci in the major histocompatibility region have been investigated. An alternative possibility is that HLA-DR2 may be found to be a composite of several determinants and one of these may be more closely correlated with resistance to inflammatory bowel disease.

REFERENCES
1. Lewkonia RM, McConnell RB. (1976) Familial Inflammatory Bowel Disease - heredity or environments. Gut 17:235-243
2. Stastny P. (1978) Association of the B cell alloantigen DRw4 with rheumatoid arthritis. New Eng.J.Med. 298:869871
3. Bodmer JG. (1978) Ia antigens. Definition of the HLA-DRw specificities. Br.Med.Bull. 34:233-240
4. Gelsthorpe K. (1980) Serological determination of Ia like determinants (HLA-DR) on human B lymphocytes. Ph.D. thesis Univ. of Sheffield
5. Dick HM. (1978) HLA and disease. Br.Med.Bull. 34:271-274
6. Cudworth AG, Festenstein H. (1978) HLA genetic heterogeneity in diabetes mellitus Br.Med.Bull. 34:285-289
7. Pena AS, Biemond I, Kuiper G, Weterman IT. Leeuwen van A, Schreuder I, Rood van JJ. (1980) HLA antigen distribution and HLA haplotype segregation in Crohn's disease. Tissue Antigens 16:56-61.

SEARCH FOR GENETIC MARKERS ASSOCIATED WITH CROHN'S DISEASE IN
THE NETHERLANDS

I. BIEMOND, IRENE T. WETERMAN, J.J. VAN ROOD, E.C. KLASEN, P.
MEERA KHAN and A.S. PEÑA

INTRODUCTION

It is now well established that Crohn's disease [CD]
occurs significantly more frequently in the relatives of the
patients than in the general population (1). More over, several families have been reported with more than one sibling
affected with CD, and the majority of the affected monozygous
twins so far reported are concordant for the disease (2).
Ankylosing spondylitis, a disease with a well known genetic
background was found to be associated with CD more than was
expected by chance alone (2). All these arguments suggest a
genetic predisposition for CD. Parameters to define susceptibility should bring an enormous advance in understanding
familial CD. Therefore, we started a systematic search for
genetic markers in CD.

The following well defined genetic polymorphisms have
been studied: the ABO and Rhesus blood groups, the HLA-A,-B,
and -DR antigens, both in unrelated patients and in selected
families with more than one member affected with CD, and the
electrophoretic variants of α_1-antitrypsin and of nine red
cell enzymes.

PROCEDURE

Materials and Methods

All the patients included have been attending the in-
and/or out-patient clinic of the Department of Gastroenterology of the Leiden University Hospital. In about 90% of the
patients the diagnosis was confirmed by the histological
criteria of Morson (3).

Typing of the ABO and Rhesus blood groups and HLA-A,-B,-C

and -DR antigens was performed according to the standard techniques in the Department of Immunohaematology (4).

α_1-Antitrypsin electrophoretic variants were typed according to the methods mentioned earlier (5).

Red cell enzyme markers were typed by enzyme electrophoresis on cellulose acetate gel (6).

RESULTS

ABO Blood groups.

In table 1 the ABO phenotype distribution in 145 patients with Crohn's disease is compared with 3194 Dutch healthy blood donors (7). The ABO and Rhesus blood group distributions were in Hardy-Weinberg equilibrium and none of the phenotypes were significantly different from the controls.

Table 1. Distribution of ABO and Rhesus blood group phenotypes in unrelated patients affected with Crohn's disease and unrelated controls.

	Phenotype	Patients No.	%	Controls No.	%	χ^2	p
ABO	0	55	37.9	1464	45.8	3.4953	0.062
	A	68	46.9	1306	40.9	2.0670	0.151
	B	14	9.7	299	9.4	0.0141	0.905
	AB	8	5.5	125	3.9	0.9334	0.334
Rhesus	D+	127	88.2	668	84.0		
	D-	27	11.8	127	16.0	1.632	0.201

HLA-A,-B,-C and -DR antigens.

In our population study of the HLA-A and -B antigens we found a weak positive association with HLA-B18. No significant deviation was observed in the distribution of HLA-DR antigens (4). A segregation analysis of parental HLA haplotypes in families with more than one affected sibling did not reveal any major influence of the HLA haplotype in Crohn's disease.

α_1-Antitrypsin electrophoretic [α_1-AT] variants.

The distribution of α_1-AT variants in a group of 310 unrelated patients showed no significant deviation from the controls (5).

Red cell enzyme markers.

The results of typing of 321 unrelated patients with CD for nine Red cell enzymes is shown in table 2. All nine polymorphisms were in Hardy-Weinberg equilibrium. The phenotypic distribution of GPT showed a significant deviation from the controls. The phenotype 4-1 of Diaphorase 2 [DIA2] exhibited a weak but significant association with Crohn's disease.

Table 2. Distribution of electrophoretic variants of different red cell enzymes in patients affected with CD compared to controls (8,9,10).

Enzyme	Pheno-type	Patients no	%	Controls no.	%	χ^2	p
Acid Phosphatase-1	CB	13	4.1	44	5.6	1.1326	0.287
(ACP1)	CA	12	3.8	30	3.8	0.0046	0.946
	BA	151	47.2	343	43.9	1.0154	0.314
	A	32	10.0	99	12.7	1.5338	0.215
	B	112	34.9	266	34.0	0.0977	0.755
Adenosine deaminase	2-1	30	9.3	102	12.8	2.5977	0.107
(ADA)	1	289	90.0	696	87.2	1.7186	0.190
	2	2	0.7	0	0.0	2.1008*	0.147
Adenylate Kinase-1	2-1	24	7.5	54	6.7	0.2153	0.643
(AK1)	1	294	92.2	747	93.3	0.4176*	0.518
	2	1	0.3	0	0.0	0.2275	0.633
Glutamic pyruvic	2-1	144	45.4	402	51.6	3.4408	0.064
transaminase(GPT)	2	86	27.2	162	20.8	5.1623	0.023
	1	87	27.4	214	27.5	0.0001	0.992
6-phosphogluconate	CA	11	3.4	33	4.1	0.2921	0.584
dehydrogenase(PGD)	A	310	96.6	768	95.9	0.2921	0.584
Phosphoglucomutase$_1$	2-1	90	28.8	225	31.8	1.5522	0.213
(PGM1)	2	16	5.0	45	5.6	0.1789	0.672
	1	215	67.0	501	62.5	1.9488	0.163
Diaphorase-2	2-1	7	2.2	20	2.5	0.0976*	0.755
(DIA2)	3-1	0	0.0	1	0.1	0.2242	0.634
	4-1	9	2.8	7	0.9	6.0715	0.014
	1	305	95.0	773	96.5	1.3481	0.246
Esterase D	1	249	77.8	748	73.5	2.4094	0.121
(ESD)	2-1	65	20.3	252	24.8	2.6571	0.103
	2	6	1.9	18	1.8	0.158	0.900
Glyoxalase I	1	62	19.3	158	20.8	0.3365	0.562
(GLO1)	2-1	154	48.0	372	49.1	0.1227	0.726
	2	105	32.7	227	29.9	0.7845	0.376

* Yates corrected

DISCUSSION

The present study on ABO blood groups confirms the results of an earlier study of Atwell et al. (11) which showed that there is no relationship between CD and any of the ABO blood group phenotypes and implicitly the antigens.

It is interesting to note that there exists a remarkable geographic variation of the association of HLA-B18 with Crohn's disease. [See table 3].

Table 3. HLA-B18 and Crohn's disease in different parts of the world

Country	City	Patients no. +	Patients no. −	Controls no. +	Controls no. −	RR Haldane	Ref.
England	Birmingham	1	99	17	266	0.23	(15)
England	Liverpool	1	42	19	356	0.65	(12)
England	Nottingham	4	63	247	2753	0.79	(17)
Holland	Amsterdam	14	43	33	445	4.43	(12)
Holland	Leiden	18	131	258	3742	2.04	(4)
Norway	Oslo	2	17	6	137	3.02	(18)
Sweden	Uppsala	7	55	23	312	1.80	(16)
Canada	Toronto	6	42	30	531	2.67	(13)
Israel	Tel-Aviv	1	17	47	584	1.05	(14)
U.S.	Vermont	3	61	5	95	0.99	(19)

The question arises as to the relevance of these findings to Crohn's disease. An explanation can be sought in the genetic heterogeneity in the causation of this disease. Possibly we are dealing with a subgroup of patients in whom HLA-B18 does have some influence and this subgroup varies in its size in different geographical areas.

The distribution of other HLA antigens in the patient population and in a limited number of families studied so far failed to implicate any major influence of genes in the MHC region in determining the predisposition to Crohn's disease.

Further critical investigations are necessary, in order to explain the significance of deviation of the phenotypic distribution of GPT in CD patients from that in controls. Nevertheless, the occurence of a "null" allele for GPT at a higher frequency in the CD population may be considered as the basis for this deviation. The existence of a "null" allele occuring rarely in the European populations has been well documented (23).

Considering the possible occurence of the "null" allele in the patient and control populations and using the maximum likelihood method of Yasuda (21), we recalculated the frequencies of the GPT alleles 1,2 and the "null" We found the frequency of the "null" allele to be 0.031 in the CD patients and 0.000 in the controls. The expected number of the patients heterozygous for the null allele was estimated to be 19 while that of the controls to be 0: the p-value was calculated to be 2×10^{-7} using Fisher's exact test. It is interesting to note that the locus for epidermolysis bullosa is known to be linked to the GPT locus (21), while a gene for predisposition to breast cancer has been shown to be weakly linked to the same locus in man (21).

The variant 4 of DIA2 is another proven "null" allele in man. The hypothesis that HLA-B18 might have some influence in a subgroup of CD patients [see above] can be extended also to the apparent association of CD with the allele 4 of DIA2 and the "null" allele of GPT.

SUMMARY

1. The antigen B18 of the HLA system was found to be weakly associated with CD in certain populations only.

2. Similar weak association was found between the electrophoretic variant 4-1 of DIA2 and CD during the present study in the Dutch patients.

3. It is postulated that a "null" allele of GPT is significantly associated with CD.

4. No associations were found between the genetic variants of α_1 AT, ABO, Rh, ACP1, ADA, AK1, PGD, PGM1, ESD and GLO1.

ACKNOWLEDGEMENTS

The red cell enzyme phenotyping was performed by Mr. Herbert Rijken, Mrs. Ada Ebeli-Struijk and Mrs. L.M.M. Blankestein-Wijnen with the financial support from FUNGO and Preventie Fonds (Netherlands).

REFERENCES
1. Singer HC, Anderson JGD, Frischer H, Kirsner JB. (1971) Familial aspects of inflammatory bowel disease. Gastroenterology 61:423-430
2. Lewkonia RM, McConnell RB. (1976) Familial inflammatory bowel disease-heredity or environment? Gut 17:235-243
3. Morson BC. (1972) Pathology of Crohn's disease. Clin. Gastroenterol. 1:265-277
4. Peña AS, Biemond I, Kuiper G, Weterman IT, Leeuwen van A, Schreuder I, Rood van JJ. (1980) HLA antigen distribution and HLA haplotype segregation in Crohn's disease. Tissue Antigens 16:56-61
5. Klasen EC, Biemond I, Weterman IT. (1980) α_1-Antitrypsin levels and phenotypes in Crohn's disease in the Netherlands. Gut, in press.
6. Meera Khan P. (1971) Enzyme electrophoresis on cellulose acetate. Gel.Arch.Biochem.Biophys. 145:470-483
7. D'Amaro J. (1978) HLA polymorphisms in the Netherlands. M.D. Thesis Leiden
8. Fraser GR, Volkers WS, Bernini LF, Loghum van E, Meera Khan P, Nijenhuis LE. (1974) Gene frequencies in a Dutch population. Human.Hered. 24:435-448
9. Ebeli-Struijk AC, Wurzer-Figurelli EM, Ajam F, Meera Khan P. (1976) The distribution of Esterase D variants in different ethnic groups. Hum.Genet. 34:299-306
10. Meera Khan P, Doppert BA. (1976) Rapid detection of Glyoxalase I (GLO) on cellulose acetate gel and the distribution of GLO variants in a Dutch population. Hum.Genet. 34:53-56
11. Atwell JD, Duthie HL, Goligher JC. (1965) The outcome of Crohn's disease. Brit.J.Surg. 52:966-972
12. Woodrow JC, Lewkonia RM, McConnell RB, Berg van den-Loonen EM, Johnson NM, Meuwissen SGM, Dekker-Saeys BJ, Nijenhuis LE, Mowbray YF. (1978) HLA antigens in Inflammatory Bowel Disease. Tissue Antigens 11:147-152
13. Cohen Z, McCullock P, Leung MK, Mervart H. (1980) Histocompatibility antigens in patients with Crohn's disease. Second International Workshop on Crohn's disease, Noordwijk, The Netherlands
14. Delpre G, Kadish U, Gazit E, Joshua H, Zamir R. (1980) HLA antigens in Ulcerative Colitis and Crohn's Disease in Israel. Gastroenterology 78:1452-1457
15. Mallas EG, MacKintosh P, Asquith P, Cooke WT. (1976) Histocompatibility antigens in inflammatory bowel disease Gut 17:906-910

Bergman L, Lindblom JB, Safwenberg J, Krause U. (1976) HL-A frequencies in Crohn's disease and Ulcerative Colitis. Tissue antigens 7:145-150

17. Burnham WR, Gelsthorpe K, Langman MJS. (1980) HLA-DR Antigens in Inflammatory Bowel Disease. Second International Workshop on Crohn's Disease, Noordwijk, The Netherlands.

18. Thorsby E, Lie SO. (1971) Relationship between the HL-A system and susceptibility to diseases. Trans.Proc. 3: 1305-1307

19. Eade OE, Moulton C, MacPherson BR, Andre-Ukena SSt, Albertini RJ, Beeken WL. (1980) Discordant HLA haplotype Segregation in familial Crohn's disease. Gastroenterology 79:271-275

20. Yasuda N, Kimura M. (1968) A gene-counting method of maximum likelihood for estimating gene frequencies in ABO and ABO-like systems. Ann.Hum.Genet. 31:409-420

21. Olaisen B, Gedde-Dahl T. (1973) GPT-Epidermolysis bullosa simplex (EBS-Ogna) linkage in man. Hum.Hered. 23:189-196

22. King MC, Rodney LPG, Eslton RC, Lynch HT, Petrakis NL. (1980) Allele increasing susceptibility to human breast cancer may be linked to the Glutamate-Pyruvate Transaminase locus. Science 208:406-408

23. Olaisen B. (1975) Genetic studies on the GPT system of human red cells. MD Thesis, Oslo, Norway

D4 Summary of Discussions relating to topics D1 to D3

Strober: The HLA system in man has been shown to consist of a number of sub-loci. In addition to the HLA-A, B, C and DR loci there is a locus governing the B-cell antigen system which is detected with antisera derived from inbred multiparous women. It is still possible that some of these other loci will prove to have positive associations with this disease.

Peña: We have made a preliminary screening of maternal antisera. We have found three out of 20 maternal sera which appear to recognize some specifities on B-lymphocytes more frequently in patients with CD than in controls. The degree of cytotoxicity is not very high and we will have to use better techniques of B-cell isolation to establish that there is indeed an association with this other B-cell system and CD.

Asquith: If you look at particular clinical subgroups, there may be an association, such as the people with Crohn's disease, who have associated eye complications having an excess of B5. Has the Leiden group clinical study determined if there is any particular type of disease associated with a particular HLA antigen?

Biemond: Most of the patients with ankylosing spondylitis and Crohn's disease have the well known marker HLA-B27. We have not yet looked into other subgroups.

Meuwissen: In 1978 we published a study in the Annals of
              Rheumatic Diseases on the HLA types in 50 IBD cases
              of whom all had rheumatologically established anky-
              losing spondylitis. You would expect if they all
              had classical ankylosing spondylitis [AS], the
              percentage with HLA-B27 would be 80 to 90%; in
              certain subgroups however, this did not prove to be
              the case.

	All patients n = 50		UC n = 12		CD n = 38	
HLA-B27	+	−	+	−	+	−
Precedence of AS symptoms [mean age at onset]	12 20.9	5 33.4	2	0	10	5
Simultaneous AS + IBD-symptoms [mean age at onset]	13 24.2	7 27.1	3	3	10	4
Precedence of IBD symptoms [mean age at onset]	3 32.0	10 32.6	3	1	0	9

As shown in the table, of these CD patients who
started with spondylitic complaints only 10 of 15
were B-27 positive. Of those patients with simultaneous occurrence of spondylitis and bowel disease,
10 of 14 were positive, while of those patients with
preceding bowel symptoms a striking zero of 9 cases
were positive. The HLA-B27 positive cases almost
always had a positive family history of ankylosing
spondylitis but not of inflammatory bowel disease
and in addition nearly all had a history of iridocy-
clitis. These data therefore indicate that the ankylosing spondylitis appearing after the onset of
Crohn's disease is genetically different from ordinary ankylosing spondylitis.

McConnell: Are you quite confident that all these patients had ankylosing spondylitis, or had some of them merely radiological evidence of sacro-iliitis?

Meuwissen: At the time of this study, we followed the New York criteria for the diagnosis of ankylosing spondylitis. However, I think it would be very worthwhile to look at these patients again and see if five years later there is any definite involvement of the sacro-iliac joint or possibly regression.

McConnell: This is one field in which HLA typing is potentially useful clinically. It is possible by HLA typing to identify patients with CD who may develop ankylosing spondylitis. What is the risk of a B27 positive CD patients developing spondylitis? In my very small series in Liverpool, out of six male patients who were B27 positive, four had already developed ankylosing spondylitis.

Strober: Recently there has been a series of publications from Geczy in Australia, that an antigen derived from klebsiella had the capacity to bind to lymphocytes bearing HLA-B27 and that antisera raised against klebsiella had the capacity in the presence of complement to kill these lymphocytes with the bound klebsiella antigen. This opens the possibility that in CD you harbour organisms that can produce materials which will bind to lymphocytes or other structures in the body, and thereby set up a situation in which you will develop AS. So in a sense the development of CD may be due to an environmental factor which in turn changes the environment of the host in such a way as to bring out an underlying genetic disease. Against this theory is the information from Meuwissen that those patients who developed AS after the onset of CD did not in fact have

B27. Perhaps in CD patients, there was another antigen which can function in the way that B27 ordina-
rily functions.

Biemond: Burnham has found a negative association with
DR2. Does he think that there will be found a positive association with DR antigens not yet established? When we counted all the antigens found at the DR
locus in our study and subtracted them from the
double of the total of patients, [a measure for the
number of "blanks" in the series] we detected a significant positive association with Crohn's disease
with these "blanks". Is there any comment on that?

Burnham: It is hard to sort out what these "blanks" mean
although some are due to patients who are homozygous
for particular genes. I do not think they necessarily mean that there is something else which we have
not found at the DR locus although that is of course
a possibility that cannot be absolutely excluded.

EPIDEMIOLOGICAL EVIDENCE FOR A HEREDITARY COMPONENT IN
CROHN'S DISEASE

B.I. KORELITZ

INTRODUCTION

Evidence for a significant familial incidence of Crohn's
disease has been presented from many sources (1-5). Despite
this, geneticists have not yet concluded that this familial
association has a hereditary basis. The traditional lines of
investigation of the past into the etiology of Crohn's disease such as dietary and psychosomatic have lost their en-
thusiasts, immunological factors seem to have a supplementary
role and even the recently promising microbiological transmission studies warrant less hope than earlier (6). It is
therefore understandable for the gastroenterologist to turn
once again to his patients to find whether the strong familial association observed clinically is statistically significant and whether any new direction for further investigation might be forthcoming through this route.

MATERIAL AND METHODS

The incidence of Crohn's disease in New York City has
increased during the past decade just as it has elsewhere in
many parts of the world (7). Between 1960 and 1979, 350
patients with documented Crohn's disease were seen in the
author's private practice. Each patient had been specifically
asked to identify blood relatives who also had Crohn's disease, an illness suggestive of Crohn's disease, or ulcerative
colitis, in order to achieve a reasonable accurate appraisal
of the incidence and specific relationships of Crohn's disease in families.

Seventy-two patients [20%] had one or more blood relatives who also suffered with Crohn's disease or ulcerative colitis. When the name of the relative's disease was disclosed

by the patient as ulcerative colitis [UC], but not necessarily documented, it was listed as Crohn's disease vs. ulcerative colitis. Symptomatology suggestive of Crohn's disease
[CD] without verification was listed as possible Crohn's
disease.

The relationships are listed in table 1. The discrepancy
in the total is accounted for by more than one member of a
family being a patient.

Table 1. Family relationships in 72 patients with Crohn's
disease.

	CD	CD vs UC	Possible CD
Father-Daughter	13	3	1
Father-Son*	8	3	1
Mother-Daughter	5	2	2
Mother-Son*	3	3	-
Brother-Sister	14	1	-
Brother-Brother	6	2	-
Sister-Sister *	4	2	-
Grandparents-Grandchild	3	1	1
First Cousin	14	6	-
Second Cousin	2	1	-
Paternal Aunt	7	3	-
Paternal Uncle	6	2	-
Maternal Aunt	-	4	-
Maternal Uncle	3	2	-
Total	88	35	5

* 3 generations of Crohn's disease in 2 families

Table 2 shows the number of family relationships for each
patient with Crohn's disease who had one or more relatives
with the same disease.

Table 2. Number of family relationships in 353 patients with
Crohn's disease

No. Relatives	No. Families
0	281
2	36
3	15
4	3
8	1

Familial Crohn's disease occurred most commonly among Jews, in whom inbreeding is prevalent. Nevertheless, the 56 family relationships included 14 [19%] gentile families. In eight of these 14, the relatives of the patient probably had ulcerative colitis rather than Crohn's disease, while in 25 of 42 Jewish families, the relative was more likely to have Crohn's disease. The two families with three generations of Crohn's disease were both Jewish. Five patients belonged to one family with eight members suffering with Crohn's disease, including a father with four children, his sister, his brother and his brother's son. This family was also Jewish. Two patients had twin siblings, neither of whom had any indication of the disease.

Table 3 shows other relationships of interest among the Crohn's disease patients. These include a woman whose husband developed the disease after they were married, but this is rare. [Subsequently the older of two sons has also developed Crohn's disease.] The infrequent occurrence of such cases provides evidence against exposure to a common organism as an etiologic factor in contrast with genetic predisposition.

Table 3. Other family relationships in patients with Crohn's disease

Husband and wife with IBD	2
Mother with carcinoma of colon	4
Father with carcinoma of colon	4
Mother with carcinoma of small bowel	1
Father with Hodgkin's disease	1
Brother with Hodgkin's disease	1

The incidence of carcinoma of the colon occurring in parents of patients with Crohn's disease is remarkably high and raises consideration of increased risk of malignancy in bowel involved with Crohn's disease.

DISCUSSION

It is very difficult for the gastroenterologist who sees large numbers of patients with Crohn's disease to be dissuaded from a genetic factor in the etiology when in his own practice there is a 20% incidence of the same disease in blood relatives. If this is not convincing, then caring for a family of eight members suffering from the same disease should eliminate all doubt.

If an estimated 100 people have a disease in a population of 1,000,000, then the prevalence of the disease is 1/10,000 and the probability of any two members of one family suffering with the disease by chance would be 1/100,000,000. Crohn's disease must then have a hereditary component. The relationships in a family of eight suggest a peculiar kind of autosomal dominant, probably homozygous. The four sibling children must be heterozygous. The father's parents must both have been carriers. Though there was no clinical evidence of the disease in either, they were most likely vulnerable to the missing component necessary to create the disease.

The most common specific family relationships in this study were, in order: 1] first cousins; 2] father-daughter; and 3] brother-sister. These suggest a polygenic type of inheritance, those at greatest risk being those who share the most genes with the patient (8-10).

Patients with Crohn's disease have many relatives with ulcerative colitis as well as Crohn's disease, and patients with ulcerative colitis have many relatives with ulcerative colitis but few with Crohns's disease. It may be postulated that Crohn's disease results from a larger concentration or summation of genes and ulcerative colitis from a lesser (4). This pattern too is consistent with a polygenic type of inheritance (8-10).

In further support of a genetic factor and/or a polygenic type of inheritance, Kirsner has shown concordance for inflammatory bowel disease in monozygotic twins but no concordance in dizygotic twins: the concordance is higher for Crohn's disease than for ulcerative colitis (4).

In both patients with Crohn's disease and ulcerative colitis who also have ankylosing spondylitis, there is a high frequency [over 90%] of the histocompatibility antigen HLA-B27 (11). Ankylosing spondylitis, however, is an infrequent complication of inflammatory bowel disease in the United States and studies of 15 sibling pairs without this complication showed no support for a gene locus close to HLA-A and -B predisposing to a familial form of either disease (12).

The evidence for a genetic component in the etiology of Crohn's disease thus remains strongly suggestive but lacking final conviction. Better genetic markers are being sought. Meanwhile, promising immunological or microbiological experiments regarding etiology and pathogenesis would seemingly show more hope of success in the study of families than study of sporadic familial occurrences.

REFERENCES
1. Kirsner JB, Spencer JA. (1973) Familial occurrences of ulcerative colitis, regional enteritis and ileocolitis. Ann.Int.Med. 59:133-144
2. Almy TP, Sherlock P. (1966) Genetic aspects of ulcerative colitis and regional enteritis. Gastroenterology 51:757-763
3. Singer HC, Anderson JGD, Frischer H, Kirsner JB. (1971) Familial aspects of inflammatory bowel disease. Gastroenterology 61:423-430
4. Kirsner JB. (1973) Genetic aspects of inflammatory bowel disease. In: Clinics in Gastroenterology. Ed. McConnell RB, WB Saunders, Philadelphia Vol 2: pp 557-575
5. Farmer RG, Michener WM, Mortimer EA. (1980) Studies of family history among patients with inflammatory bowel disease. In: Clinics in Gastroenterology. Ed. Farmer RG, WB Saunders, Philadelphia Vol 9: pp 271-278
6. Gitnick GL. (1979) Etiology of inflammatory bowel disease. Are we making progress? Gastroenterology 78:1090-1102
7. Korelitz BI. (1979) From Crohn to Crohn's disease:1979. An epidemiological study in New York City. Mt.Sinai J.Med. 46:533-540
8. Falconer DS. (1965) The inheritance of liability to certain diseases estimated from the incidence among relatives. Ann.Hum.Genet. 29:51-76
9. Lewkonia RM, McConnell RB. (1976) Familial IBD-heredity or environment? Gut 17:235-243
10. McConnell RB. (1966) Crohn's disease and Ulcerative Colitis. In: The Genetics of Gastrointestinal Disorders. Ed. McConnell RB, Oxford Univ. Press, London. pp 128-142
11. Emery AEH, Lawrence JS. (1974) Genetics of ankylosing spondylitis. J.Med.Genet. 4:239-244
12. Kemler BJ, Glass D, Alpert E. (1980) HLA studies of families with multiple cases of inflammatory bowel disease [IBD]. Gastroenterology 78:1194

STUDIES OF FAMILY HISTORY IN INFLAMMATORY BOWEL DISEASE

R.G. FARMER, W.M. MICHENER and D.S. SIVAK

INTRODUCTION

Although it has been known for many years that inflammatory bowel disease [IBD] can occur in family clusters (1,2), in recent years there has been an increasing number of reports of familial occurrences of IBD. A study from the University of Chicago described a familial occurrence rate of 17.5% with 113 of 646 patients reporting a positive family history (3). Other studies have emphasized occurrence of IBD in multiple family members and the predilection for familial aggregation of patients with ankylosing spondylitis in Crohn's disease [CD] (4,5). In a progress report in 1976, Lewkonia and McConnell (6), stated that "study of the families of patients with IBD leaves no doubt that ulcerative colitis and Crohn's disease are closely associated. This association within families may be due to a common environmental aetiology, but more probably it is due to a shared genetic background."

MATERIALS

During a study of 838 patients with onset of IBD under age 21, special attention was paid to presence of IBD in additional family members (7). Information concerning their family histories was obtained from all patients. Each patient was specifically interviewed in regard to family history, and questions were posed concerning a definite diagnosis of IBD among their relatives, including parents, siblings, grandparents, and blood relatives - aunts, uncles and first cousins. Follow-up information was obtained from 826 patients [98.4%]. All patients had the diagnosis of IBD established at the Cleveland Clinic prior to attaining the age of 21 years, and diagnosis was established between the years

1955 and 1975. There were 280 patients [34%] with a positive family history for IBD with at least one other family member afflicted.

As shown in table 1, there were 316 patients with UC, and a positive family history was obtained for IBD for 93 patients [29%]. Among 552 patients with CD, 187 [35%] had a positive family history for IBD. The table also shows the occurrence of disease in different types of relatives.

Table 1. Association of IBD in families

	UC n = 316		CD n = 522	
Family history for IBD	93 [	29%]	187 [	35%]
Parents	31 [	9.8%]	48 [	9%]
Siblings	19 [	6%]	39 [	7.5%]
Relatives	48 [	15%]	101 [	19%]
Grandparents	13 [	4%]	29 [	5.5%]

Multiple members of families were found to have IBD in 21 instances of patients with UC [6.6%] and 46 instances [8.8%] of patients with CD. Two families each had 8 members afflicted while 3 - 5 members were involved 18 times. Both families with 8 members involved were patients with CD. There were five instances in which patients with UC had more than two family members afflicted; 13 families with Crohn's disease had more than 2 members afflicted in addition to the two families with 8 members involved.

Familial incidence of IBD was reported by patients with ulcerative colitis more frequently in the second decade covered by this study than in the first. In the first decade, 29 of 138 patients [21%] gave a positive family history; this increased to 64 to 178 patients [35%] in the second decade. For patients with CD, there were 42 patients [35%] with a positive family history reported in the first decade, and 145 of 404 patients [35%] with a positive history reported in the second decade.

Particular attention was paid to IBD in immediate family members. These are shown in table 2.

Table 2. Inflammatory bowel disease among immediate family
         members

Affected members	UC		CD	
Father-Son	4	[1.3%]	14	[2.7%]
Father-Daughter	8	[2.5%]	6	[1.1%]
Mother-Son	10	[3.2%]	14	[2.7%]
Mother-Daughter	9	[2.8%]	14	[2.7%]
Sibling-Sibling	19	[6.0%]	39	[7.5%]
Total	50	[15.8%]	87	[16.6%]

137/83 8=16.3%

There was a mean of 2.4 siblings in these families [680
siblings in 280 families]. Among 558 patients without a positive family history, 1,205 siblings were present [mean 2.2
siblings per family].

A more detailed study has now been undertaken. During the
period 1970 to 1975 there were 302 patients under the age of
21 for whom the diagnosis of IBD was established at the
Cleveland Clinic - 92 with UC and 210 with CD. Among these
were 95 [31.5%] with a positive family history for IBD. Of
these, 62 cases were CD and 33 cases were UC. Those patients
who had affected siblings and cousins, a horizontal family
history, were designated as having a positive recessive family history. Those patients who had affected parents, grandparents, uncles or aunts with affected offspring, a vertical
family history, were designated as having a dominant family
history. Of the 62 Crohn's disease patients, 17 had what
appeared to be a recessive family history as compared with 45
who appeared to have a dominant family history. With respect
to the ulcerative colitis patients, there were 10 who appeared to have a recessive family history and 23 who appeared to
have a dominant family history.

Because of the dichotomy of this data, it was decided
that some of these histories should be thoroughly scrutini-
zed. Four such kindreds have been evaluated. Although the
primary pattern is that of an autosomal dominant gene of
incomplete penetrance, other inheritance patterns cannot be
eliminated from consideration.

216

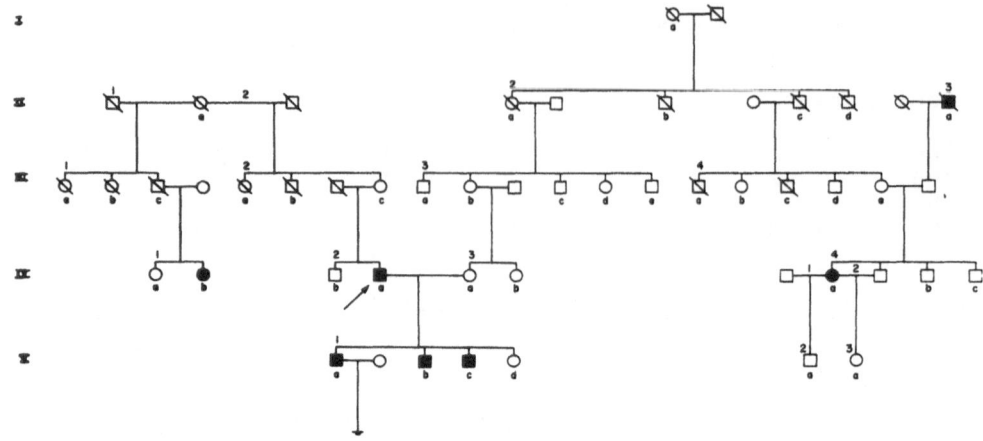

Kindred 1: This is a Jewish kindred which immigrated from Poland and Russia. The proband [IV 2a] and his three
sons [V 1a, V 1b, V 1c] have UC as does IV 2a's
first cousin [IV 1b]. On the proband spouse's side
of the family, a first cousin [IV 4a], has CD.
However, IV 4a has a deceased grandfather who
married into this kindred who had UC. This history
presents as a possible incomplete penetrant autosomal dominant syndrome, transmission being from
II 1a to the half-siblings III 1c and III 2c.

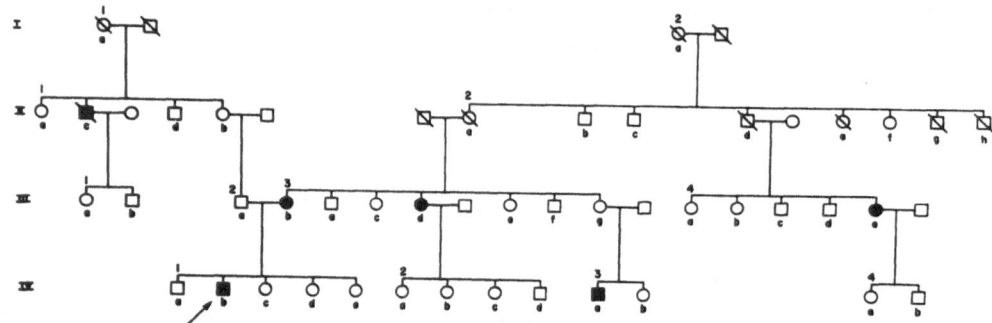

Kindred 2: This is a Jewish kindred with immigrants from Russia and Poland. The proband [IV 1b] has UC. On the
paternal side of the family, there was a great uncle [II 1c] who had UC and died of cancer of the
colon. On the maternal side of the family, the
proband's mother [III 4e] and also his own first
cousin [IV 3a] had UC. This kindred presents a
confused genetic picture. The maternal side appears to be either an autosomal or X-linked dominant gene of incomplete penetrance. It is difficult to assess the effect of the paternal history;
perhaps several genes are involved in this
kindred.

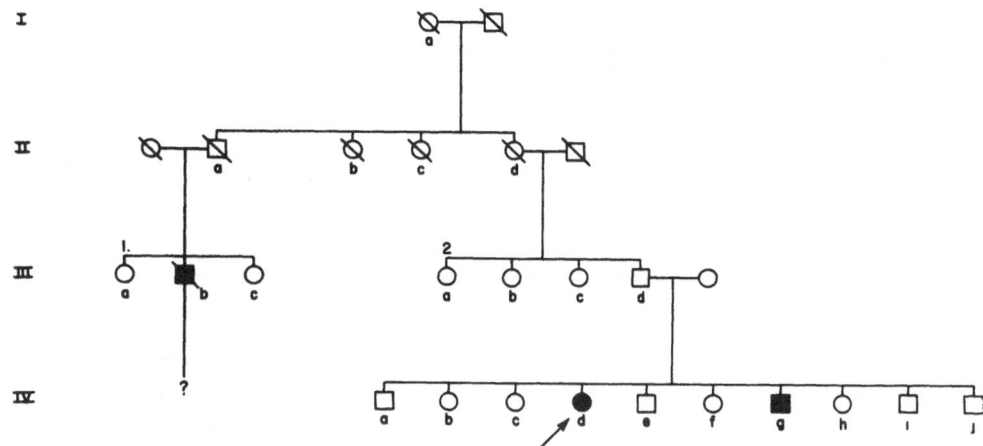

Kindred 3: This gentile kindred immigrated from Germany. The proband [IV d] has UC, while her sibling [IV g] has CD. There was a paternal first cousin [III lb] who also has UC. This history suggests an autosomal dominant gene of incomplete penetrance; however, a recessive form cannot be discounted.

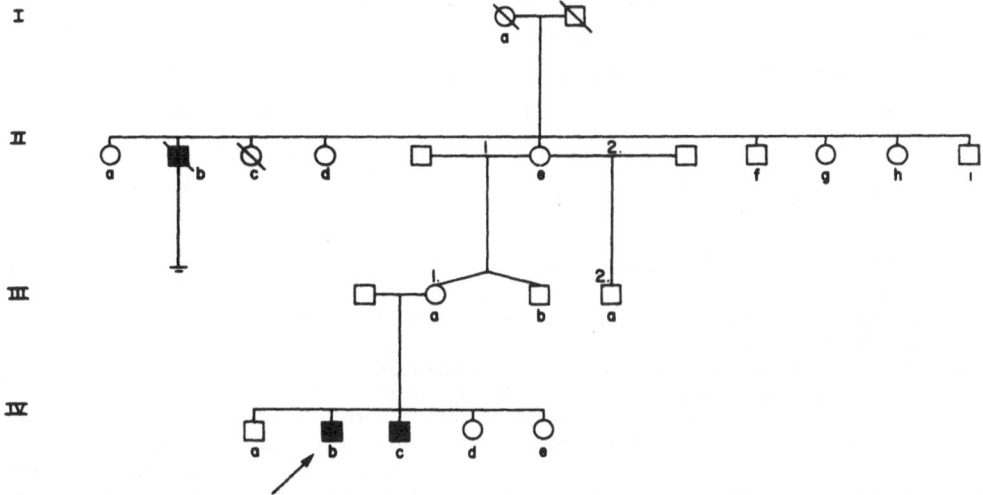

Kindred 4: This gentile kindred came originally from Poland and Sicily. The proband [IV b] has UC and his sibling [IV c] has CD. The maternal great uncle [II b] of the proband had UC also. This kindred again suggests an autosomal dominant gene with incomplete penetrance. However, it should be noted that an X-linked dominant or X-linked recessive form of inheritance is also possible.

DISCUSSION

The most significant problem in a genetic study of this type is that of reduced penetrance and failure to diagnose subclinical disease. Because of this, a prospective study could be utilized to define a range of genotypes which would be assigned after the correct designation of phenotypes in a kindred. These genotypes then would be statistically compared with various models of inheritance. Such a study is being formulated by our group with special emphasis on the criteria to be utilized for phenotypic designation.

CONCLUSIONS

Our study of family history of 838 patients with IBD diagnosed under the age of 21 disclosed a positive family history of approximately one-third of all patients; in addition 15% of all patients had relatives in their immediate families afflicted. Four kindres are described. Although the primary pattern may be that of an autosomal dominant gene with incomplete penetrance, other inheritance patterns cannot be eliminated from consideration. Although no conclusions can be drawn, it is our opinion that a large number of kindreds taken in this manner may provide enough data for a statistical evaluation from a genetic point of view.

REFERENCES
1. Kirsner JB, Spencer JA. (1963) Family occurrences of UC, RE and ileocolitis. Ann.Intern.Med. 59:133-144
2. Almy TP, Sherlock P. (1966) Genetic aspects of UC and RE. Gastroenterology 51:757-763
3. Singer HC, Anderson JGD, Frischer H, Kirsner JB. (1971) Familial aspects of IBD. Gastroenterology 61:423-430
4. Kuspira J, Bhambhani R, Singh SM, et al. (1972) Familial occurrence of Crohn's disease. Hum.Hered. 22:239-242
5. Macrae I, Wright V. (1973) A family study of ulcerative colitis with particular reference to ankylosing spondylitis and sacroiliitis. Ann.Rheum.Dis. 32:16-20
6. Lewkonia RM, McConnell RB. (1976) Familial inflammatory bowel disease-heredity or environment? Gut 17:235-243
7. Farmer RG, Michener WM, Mortimer EA. (1980) Studies of family history among patients with IBD. In: Clinics in Gastroenterology. WB Saunders, Philadelphia Vol 9: pp 271-278.

D7 Summary of Discussions relating to topics D5 to D6

Meera-Khan: Some observations presented earlier indicate that we are probably dealing with a degree of heterogeneity, whether genetic or non-genetic. The family aggregations suggest that there is a genetic component although it is possible that the environmental factors are more important in the causation of CD.

Fielding: How do the speakers calculate their figures when they have more than one member of a family attending their clinic? In what proportion of their UC-relatives, their Crohn's-relatives, and in Korelitz' case, the carcinoma-patients, are the diagnosis based on histological grounds?

Korelitz: As far as the carcinoma relatives are concerned, they were not identified histologically because they were not patients of mine. The evidence was rather solid in that it was the child telling me that his parent had died of carcinoma of the colon.

Farmer: Only one patient was registered as the proband and the relatives were considered to be supplementary. We attempted to verify the diagnosis at least by communication with the physician in most of the cases. I would say the only area which I fell uncertain about are the grandparents. I believe that we were able to identify with reasonable clinical accuracy the diagnosis in the other relatives.

D8 General Discussion and Conclusions

Reported by R.B. McConnell

The genetic contributions made to this workshop have given strong support to the results of research done previously.

HLA Testing

The search for associations between CD and HLA types reported from Nottingham, Toronto and Leiden have confirmed the previous impression given by smaller studies that there is not likely to be any strong association with a particular DR1 antigen and that there is probably no association with A or B locus antigens.

The DR typing from Nottingham showed a nearly significant negative association with DR 2. Our discussions resulted in a consensus view that this possible association should be born in mind in the future if subdivision of DR2 takes place or when other developments in DR typing are made, but that there is no strong indication for the DR typing of another CD series in the immediate future.

Other Genetic Markers

The testing in Leiden of genetic markers other than HLA has not yet uncovered any definite association, but this is a potentially fruitful line of research which should be pursued. Though the highest priority should be given to testing for associations with genetic polymorphisms which are likely to be concerned in gut physiology, genes often have pleotropic effects and therefore no polymorphism need be excluded from this work.

Family Data

We had 3 papers presenting data on the familial distribution of CD, Korelitz's, Farmer's and Mayberry's data which was presented in the Epidemiological Section. Taken with previously published data there is a remarkable unanimity in the findings. It would seem that the following facts can be regarded as firmly established:-

1. There is more CD in the relatives of CD patients than would be expected from knowledge of population frequencies.

2. There is more UC in the relatives of CD patients than would be expected by chance.

3. The percentage of CD patients with a first-degree relative affected by IBD has varied from 9 to 20 percent, the proportions of relatives being about 6 CD to 4 UC.

4. There is a lesser incidence of IBD in more distant relatives.

5. Parallel studies of UC patients have shown a lesser frequency with a positive family history than that found with CD patients (though this difference was much less marked with early onset patients studied by Farmer).

6. Both types of IBD are found in the relatives of UC patients, the proportions being about 3 CD to 7 UC.

Interpretations

This repeated demonstration of the occurrence of CD and UC within the same family is probably the most striking feature of the family studies. The reason for this intra-familial association is open to a variety of interpretations ranging from both conditions having the same environmental cause to both having the same genetic basis. Both extreme interpretations seem highly unlikely and they cannot explain all the known facts. It seems very probable that the aetiology of CD is similar to that of many other relatively common diseases - that is one or more environmental factors operating widely on a population of varying susceptibility which is largely genetically determined. The disease will develop when the environmental factor strikes a genetically susceptible individual or perhaps when the environmental dose received by an individual is high enough to overcome the genetic resistance. What is the likely nature or mechanism of the genetic basis of CD? We have considered many genetic mechanisms to see if they can fit the facts.

Is CD a single distinct entity? Meera Khan has pointed out that several genetic defects can result in the same phenotype or disease. Many rather uncommon diseases have been shown in different families to be due to several different mutant genes. Examples of this splitting of a clinical entity into several genetic entities are xeroderma pigmentosa and glycogen storage disease. Genetic studies are good for splitting a disease into several types and it is curious that so far our family studies are tending to bring CD and UC closer together rather than separating them.

It is highly unlikely that the genetic basis of CD is one gene. The pattern of inheritance does not indicate anything Mendelian and a polygenic inheritance is likely. Individual families with a particular aggregation of cases can be attributed to a chance high concentration of genes which one would expect to occur in a large population. Within the polygenic system however, the possibility is not ruled out of a major gene which need a number of genes at other loci on other chromosomes to express itself but which is not an essential component of the genotype. This may be the situation in ankylosing spondylitis which develops in less than 1 % of the men in the population who have HLA-B27 and in a few men without B27, and yet the B27 gene is obviously of major importance in the ankylosing spondylitis genotype.

Whether the genetic relationship of CD and UC is due to overlapping genotypes or to a quantitative difference within a shared polygenic system is uncertain. The latter explanation fits the known facts but so might overlapping genotypes if the non-overlapping part of the CD genotype contained a major gene.

SECTION E

CYTOGENETICS

Section Editor: P. Meera Khan

CHROMOSOMAL BREAKAGE IN CROHN'S DISEASE

INGRID EMERIT and A.M. MICHELSON

INTRODUCTION

Chromosomal instability or chromosomal breakage are terms employed for a situation characterized by an increased number of disrupted and rearranged chromosomes. This acquired chromosome damage is variable from one cell to the other and can be due to the influences of various physical, chemical and biological factors. Previous work of our laboratory has shown that increased chromosome breakage is observed in lymphocyte cultures from patients with so-called autoimmune diseases (1,2). The high risk of cancer and leukemia in patients with the hereditary diseases Fanconi's anemia, Bloom's syndrome and ataxia telangiectasia, suggests the role of chromosomal instability as the origin of cancer, since these disorders are characterized by an increase in chromosome breakage and rearrangement (3). New Zealand black[NZB] mice are also characterized by a high incidence of lymphoreticular malignancies and autoimmune reactions with chromosomal instability (4). Selective matings of NZB mice, according to chromosome breakage frequencies, leads to two NZB substrains, a high and a low breakage strain (5). Both are significantly different for the incidence of autoimmune hemolytic anemia and malignant lymphomas. This breeding experiment thus confirms the correlation between chromosome breakage, autoimmunity and malignancy and suggests that the study of the causes of chromosomal instability will lead to the elucidation of the origin of autoimmune diseases and cancer.

The present study reports the results of chromosome studies in 50 patients with Crohn's disease, a disorder associated with autoimmune phenomena and a 20-fold increase in the incidence of colorectal cancer compared to the general population.

PROCEDURE

In each patient, the diagnosis was established on the basis of typical proctoscopic and colon X-ray examinations with classic histological findings on biopsy or surgical specimens. In the majority of patients the cytogenetic analysis was done before diagnostic X-ray procedures and before treatment.

Either whole blood or lymphocytes separated by standard Ficoll-Hypaque gradient centrifugation were incubated for 72 hours in TCM 199 from the Pasteur Institute or from Flow laboratories supplemented with 20% human AB serum. Cell division was obtained by phytohemagglutinin M and P. Chromosomes were counted and scored for aberrations by means of coded photographic prints. The aberration frequencies were calculated on a minimum of 50 mitoses.

In certain experiments, lymphocytes from patients and from healthy volunteers were cocultivated and the breakage rate in the two cell populations was compared to that of simultaneous lymphocyte cultures from the donor and the control. Usually the control was a male subject and only mitoses in which the Y chromosome was clearly identifiable were scored for aberrations.

Whole blood or lymphocytes from healthy subjects were incubated in presence of patients' serum or ultrafiltrates of serum for which Diaflo filters of different pore size were used. The aberration rate in these cultures was compared to that of simultaneous cultures supplemented with serum from a healthy subject.

Simultaneous cultures were set up in 12 patients with culture media differing in their L-cysteine content [TCM 199 0.1 mg/l and RPMI 1629 30 mg/l respectively].

The influence of the drug D-penicillamine [DPcA] and of the enzyme superoxide dismutase [SOD] on the breakage rate in vitro and in vivo was studied in another series of patients.

RESULTS

The incidence of chromosome breaks was found to be increased in all 50 patients compared to that of the 50 controls. The number of aberrations per 100 mitoses was 28.5 and 9.9 respectively [P<0.001], if TCM 199 from the Pasteur Institute was used. Besides gaps and breaks of one or of both chromatids, there were single and double minute fragments as well as long acentrics. Rings, dicentrics and morphologically abnormal chromosomes were observed in 0.7% of mitoses compared to 0.1% in controls. Individual incidences varied between 11 and 64% of abnormal mitoses. A low breakage rate was observed in mild, limited or resolved disease (6).

Highly significant differences in the chromosome breakage rate were observed, if the patient's blood was incubated in RPMI 1629 instead of TCM 199 Pasteur : 10.2 aberrations per 100 mitoses compared to 44.7, mean of 12 cultures from 12 patients [P<0.001].

DPcA added to the culture medium [TCM 199 Pasteur] at a final concentration of 100 g/ml reduced the aberration rate in blood cultures from 10 patients from 35.1 to 14.0%. In three patients studied before and during treatment with DPcA, the breakage figures returned to normal values after 2 months.

Bovine Cu-SOD added to the culture medium at a final concentration of 50 g/ml reduced the aberration rate regularly in 5 other patients, mean 26.6 and 10.4 respectively.

In 2 of the 3 cocultivations of patients' lymphocytes with normal lymphocytes, a high aberration rate was induced in the normal lymphocytes [45.5 and 23.4 respectively], while the aberration rate of the patients' lymphocytes remained unchanged. If SOD was added to the cocultivations, the normal lymphocytes showed no increase in the incidence of aberrations. Cocultivation of two populations of lymphocytes from normal subjects does not result in aberration induction.

In 4 of the 5 experiments designed to detect a clastogenic agent in the serum or in ultrafiltrates from patients' serum, an increase of chromosome aberrations was observed in the lymphocytes of the healthy volunteer, cultured with patients' serum or ultrafiltrate of serum but not control materials. The "chromosome breaking agent" present in the ultrafiltrates has a molecular weight between 1000 and 10,000 daltons. Unconcentrated ultrafiltrates of serum did not produce breakage except for the experiment with the highest aberration induction [48.6%]. The action of the chromosome breaking agent was inhibited by SOD.

DISCUSSION

As in other autoimmune diseases (7,8,9) the increased chromosome breakage rate observed in lymphocyte cultures from patients with Crohn's disease is correlated with a chromosome damaging agent of low molecular weight, that produces also chromosome breaks in cells from healthy subjects. The fact that contact with patients' lymphocytes also produces chromosome breaks in normal lymphocytes suggests that the chromosome damaging agent is released from the cells into the serum. Since radioprotectors such as L-cysteine and free radical scavenging enzymes such as superoxide dismutase inhibit the production of chromosome breaks as well in lymphocytes from patients as in normal lymphocytes exposed to the breakage factor from patients, it is probable that activated oxygen species such as the superoxide anion radical $O_2^{-\cdot}$ or secondarily formed hydroxyl radicals $OH^{\cdot}$ are involved in the breakage phenomenon. D-penicillamine and dimethylcysteine may act similarly to L-cysteine due to their SH-groups or may mimic the enzyme superoxide dismutase in the destruction of $O_2^{-\cdot}$ as suggested by Younes and Weser (10). The role of free radicals at the origin of chromosome damage is well-known from radiation induced chromosome damage. In living organisms they are produced in a variety of processes and are able to alter the structure of DNA (11). Furthermore some of the changes seen during inflammation are related to the $O_2^{-\cdot}$ release from inflammatory cells (12). The extracellular space is poor in SOD and damage may occur as a consequence of incomplete dismutation.

The reason for the increased flux of $O_2^{-\cdot}$ and of other active oxygen species remains to be determined. Theoretically there may be an increased production of free radicals or a decreased capacity of radical scavenging. For this reason, the levels of copper and manganese SOD in the plasma of Crohn's patients are currently under study.

As in other autoimmune diseases, the role of viruses has been suggested as the origin of Crohn's disease (13). Both DNA and RNA viruses are capable of producing chromosome damage (14), their influence on the 0_2^- production of infected cells is not known at present.

REFERENCES
1. Emerit I. (1979) Chromosomal abnormalities in progressive systemic sclerosis. Clin.Rheum.Dis. 5:201-214
2. Emerit I, Michelson AM. (1980) Chromosome instability in human and murine autoimmune disease. Acta Physiol.Scand., in press
3. German J. (1972) Genes which increase chromosomal instability in somatic cells and predispose to cancer. Prog. Med.Genet. 8:61-101
4. Emerit I, Halpern B, Feingold J. (1975) Chromosomal breakage in NZB mice. Biochem.Exp.Biol. 11:365-369
5. Emerit I, Feingold J, Levy A, Martin E, Housset E. (1980) Tumor incidence and development of autoimmune hemolytic anemia in two breeding lines of the NZB mouse strain that differ in chromosome breakage. J.Nat.Cancer Inst. 64:513-517
6. Emerit I, Emerit J, Levy A, Keck M. (1979) Chromosomal breakage in Crohn's disease. Hum.Genet. 50:51-57
7. Emerit I, Levy A, Housset E. (1974) Breakage factor in systemic sclerosis and protector effect of L-cysteine. Hum.Genet. 25:221
8. Emerit I, Michelson AM, Levy A, Camus JP, Emerit J.(1980) Chromosome breaking agent of low molecular weight in human systemic lupus erythematosus.Hum.Genet., in press
9. Emerit I, Levy A, de Vaux Saint Cyr C. (1980) Chromosome damaging agent of low molecular weight in the serum of New Zealand black mice. Cytogenet.Cell Genet. 26:41-48
10. Younes M, Weser U. (1977) Superoxide dismutase activity of copper penicillamine. Biophys.Res.Commun. 78:1247-1251
11. White JR, Vaughan TO, Shiang Yeh W. (1971) Superoxide radical in the mechanism of action of streptonigrin. Fed.Proc. 30:1145-1147
12. Babior BM. (1979) Oxygen dependent microbial killing by phagocytes. New.Engl.J.Med. 298:659-668
13. Riemann JF. (1977) Viral agent in Crohn's disease. Acta Hepatogastroenterol. 24:403-406
14. Nichols WM. (1974) Viruses and chromosomes. In: The Cell Nucleus. Acad. Press, New York Vol.II: p 43

SIGNIFICANCE OF CHROMOSOMAL ABERRATIONS OBSERVED IN HUMAN PERIPHERAL BLOOD LYMPHOCYTES

A.T. NATARAYAN and J.L.S. VAN RIJN

Human peripheral blood lymphocytes offer unique possibilities to study dividing somatic cells in vitro and have been utilized for diverse purposes including the detection of structural and numerical chromosomal aberrations in man. Chromosomal aberrations are indicative of some damage to genetic material. The type of chromosomal aberrations observed - such as chromosome type or chromatid type, stable or unstable type - can give an indication to the time and origin of these aberrations. In many inherited human recessive diseases such as ataxia telangiectasia, Bloom's syndrome, Fanconi's anemia, etc., stimulated blood lymphocytes as well as cells from bone marrow exhibit a high frequency of spontaneous chromosomal aberrations when compared to control subjects. In addition, several of such disorders are sensitive to specific physical or chemical mutagenic carcinogens e.g., xeroderma pigmentosum cells are sensitive to UV and other agents which induce dimer like lesions in DNA, ataxia telangiectasia cells are sensitive to all types of ionizing radiations and bleomycin and Fanconi's anemia cells are sensitive to cross linking agents. This increased sensitivity is related to some defect in repairing different classes of lesions in the DNA. These specific types of responses allow one to characterise these diseases as well as help in diagnosis of suspected cases. Possible utilization of such techniques for identifying heterozygotes for these diseases, which should be in order of 1 to 2% in human population, is being explored in several laboratories. If found valid, these will be of great value in genetic counseling as well as regulating occupational exposure to physical and chemical mutagens for this specific group.

Chromosomal aberrations observed in diseases such as Crohn's disease appear to be different in nature from those of the above mentioned disorders. In Crohn's disease, the chromosomal aberrations can be observed only in cells which are grown in very specific culture medium, maximum effect being observed in a medium devoid of L-cysteine, and containing Tween 80 (2), whereas in the other diseases mentioned above, the chromosomal aberrations can be observed in any type of medium.

Chromosomal aberrations can originate due to damage in the nucleoprotein, but the main target appears to be DNA itself. The types of chromosomal aberrations observed will depend on the type of lesions induced in the DNA and the cell cycle stage in which these lesions are induced. In the case of ionizing radiations, in which case the primary lesions responsible for chromosomal aberrations appear to be DNA double strand breaks, the lesions are repaired or misrepaired immediately after induction, thus giving rise to chromosome type [dicentrics, rings and chromosome breaks] of aberrations when irradiated in G_0 or G_1 cell stage and chromatid type [chromatid breaks and exchanges] when irradiated in G_2 cell stage. On the other hand, most chemical mutagens and UV light-induced lesions, need a S dependent DNA repair to be developed into an aberration, mainly due to errors in replications process. Thus, these agents induce chromatid type of aberrations even when the cells are treated in G_1 cell stage. When treated in G_2 stage, the aberrations which are of chromatid type do not appear immediately in the next oncoming mitosis, but in the second mitosis, i.e., after a S phase.

The human peripheral blood lymphocytes represent a heterogenous population of cells and most of them are in G_0 stage while circulating in the body. On stimulation in vitro, with a mitogen, RNA and protein synthesis start within a few hours and DNA synthesis starts around 24 hours. First mitotic cells appear around 36 hours, reaching a peak at about 48 hours. At 72 hours, a time period which is generally employed by many clinical workers, the lymphocytes are mostly in their second or third mitotic divisions. In general, about 90% of cells are in first mitosis at 48 hours, whereas 50 to 90% of cells are in 3rd division at 72 hours. The latter is true for patients of Crohn's disease as well [Table 1].

Table 1. Frequencies of chromosomal aberrations and sister chromatid exchanges [SCEs]

	48 hrs.		72 hrs.	
	MEM	F 10	MEM	F 10
Patient 1				
Gaps + breaks [%]	10.3[32][a]	0[25][a]	0[100][a]	17.0[100][a]
I,II,III division cells (5)			3,6,91	6,16,78
SCEs/cells[b]			9.1	4.8
Patient 2				
Gaps + breaks [%]	14.2[24][a]	14.0[100][a]	2.0[100][a]	9.0[100][a]
I,II,III division cells (5)			8,20,72	12,33,55
SCEs/cells[b]			7.8	7.2

a] number of cells scored
b] 25 cells were scored for SCEs. For scoring SCEs the lymphocytes were grown for 72 hours in the presence of 10 M BrdUrd, and the preparations were stained with H.33258 and Giemsa. The same slides were used for the determination of 1st, 2nd and 3rd division cells. Culture media were from Flow, and 15% fetal calf serum was added to the medium.

If the chromosomal aberrations arise due to lesions induced in vivo, one would expect chromosome or chromatid type of aberrations during the first mitosis and at 72 hours [mainly containing 2nd and 3rd mitoses] the aberrations observed should be chromosomal type, representing derived aberrations. In our preliminary study of two patients with Crohn's disease [Table 1], we found mainly chromatid type of aberrations irrespective of the time of fixation. Two different culture media were employed, namely Ham's F 10 and Eagles MEM. MEM does not contain L cysteine, whereas F 10 contains this amino acid. We found more aberrations in cells grown in F 10 medium than those in MEM.

The two patients responded differently. One had fewer aberrations at 48 hours fixation [only 25 to 32 cells scored] and many aberrations at 72 hours fixation. The other had higher frequencies of aberrations at both fixation times. Though these results are preliminary and are based on only two patients, the frequencies are higher than those observed in control population, based on several thousands of cells (5). We also estimated the frequencies of sister chromatid exchanges [SCEs] in these two patients, in the lymphocytes grown in both types of media. The frequencies varied between 4.8 to 9.1 per cell, a range which is well within the control values observed in normal population (4).

From our preliminary results as well as the extensive results from Emerit et al. (2) one can speculate on the nature of lesions that lead to chromosomal aberrations in the cultured blood lymphocytes of patients of Crohn's disease. The lesions are induced in vitro as [1] the frequencies of chromosomal aberrations depend on the type of medium employed for culturing and [2] chromatid type of aberrations are induced in 2nd and 3rd divisions. These lesions give rise to mainly chromatid breaks and gaps and a few exchanges. The increased frequencies of aberrations are not accompanied by an increased frequency of SCEs. Agents such as alkylating agents and UV light, which are S dependent agents, efficiently induce both chromosomal aberrations and SCEs, whereas S independent agents such as X-rays and bleomycin induce chromosomal aberrations efficiently but not SCEs. Among the lesions induced in DNA by ionizing radiations, strand breaks are important for production of aberrations and these lesions are repaired in an S independent manner. Such a repair is not accompanied with an increase in the frequencies of SCEs. Thus, one can postulate that the increase in the frequencies of aberrations without concomitant increase in SCEs in the lymphocytes of Crohn's disease patients points toward DNA strand breaks in these cells induced during culture. Possible role of several factors, such as free radicals, absence of radical scavengers - cysteine, superoxide dismutase, Tween 80 in the medium [making cells specially permeable] as well as involvement of DNA/RNA viruses, have been considered by

Emerit et al. (2). Though the types of aberrations produced, namely chromatid breaks and gaps are similar to those observed in virus infected cells, the dependency of their occurrence on the type of culture medium used in the case of Crohn's disease makes a viral origin of these aberrations difficult to justify. However, medium dependent effect observed in Crohn's disease as well as detection of fragile sites in human chromosomes in cells grown in starvation medium (7) have opened up a new field of research in clinical cytogenetics.

Since this phenomenon of chromosome breakage is heavily dependent on the culture media employed, inter laboratory comparisons are difficult to make. Secondly, the predominant types of aberrations are chromatid breaks and gaps and the scoring criteria of these types of aberrations, especially gaps, vary from laboratory to laboratory. In population monitoring studies for industrial exposure, we have successfully employed an additional method of scoring aberrations in interphase cells, namely micronuclei. These micronuclei are formed by lagging chromosomal breaks and their frequencies are positively correlated with the frequencies of other types of aberrations (1,3). This technique may prove to be a relatively easy one to generate quantitatively comparable data between laboratories. In several chromosomally unstable syndromes we have noticed an increased frequency of HGPRT$^-$ variant cells in peripheral blood lymphocytes. These variants can be considered as point mutations occuring in vivo (6). It will be interesting to investigate whether an increase in these variants occurs also in the case of Crohn's disease. These investigations are underway in our laboratory. Since majority of agents which induce chromosomal aberrations and point mutations are carcinogenic as well, increased frequencies of these biological events in lymphocytes may indicate a higher cancer proneness of the individual.

ACKNOWLEDGEMENTS

We are thankful to Dr. Meera Khan for discussions, Dr. Peña for blood samples and Prof. F.H. Sobels for encouragement. This research is partially supported by the Koningin Wilhelmina Fonds [S.G.74], and the Association of Euratom and the University of Leiden, contract no. 052-64-1 BIAN.

REFERENCES
1. Countryman PI, Heddle JA. (1976) The production of micronuclei from chromosome aberrations in irradiated cultures of human lymphocytes. Mutat.Res. 41:321-332
2. Emerit I, Emerit J, Levi A, Keck M. (1979) Chromosomal breakage in Crohn's disease. Anticlastogenic effect of D-penicillamine and L-cysteine. Hum.Genet. 50:51-57
3. Iskander O, Jager MJ, Williemze R, Natarajan AT. (1980) A case of pure red cell aplasia with a high incidence of spontaneous chromosome breakage. A possible X ray sensitive syndrome. Hum.Genet. (in press)
4. Morgan WF, Crossen PC. (1977) The incidence of sister chromatid exchanges in cultured human lymphocytes. Mutat.Res. 42:305-312
5. Natarayan AT, Obe G. (1980) Screening of human populations for mutations induced by environmental pollutants: Use of human blood lymphocyte system. Ecotoxicology and Environmental Safety (in press)
6. Strauss GH, Albertini RJ. (1979) Enumeration of 6 thioguanine resistant peripheral blood lymphocytes in man as a potential test for somatic mutations arising in vivo. Mutat.Res. 61:353-379
7. Sutherland GR. (1979) Heritable fragile sites on human chromosomes. I. Factors affecting expression in lymphocyte culture. Am.J.Hum.Genet. 31:121-135

E3 Summary of Discussions relating to topics E1 to E2

Das: Do you have any other information as to the nature of the agent? Have you examined diseased tissue extracts?

Emerit: This agent is present in CD, and in connective tissue diseases and has a molecular weight below 10,000 daltons. This excludes a virus. The lupus factor loses its activity when exposed to ribonucleases, but not after exposure to proteolytic enzymes. As in lupus patients the agent photosensitizes; it could be similar to flavin mononucleotides.

Riis: Have you read your preparations blindly? Is it important that the controls were not exposed to X-rays in contrast to the patients with CD and UC?

Emerit: We worked with coded slides or coded photographs. Twenty among the 50 patients studied had had no X-ray studies or treatment at the time the blood samples were taken.

Elson: I do not recall any increased incidence of abnormal births in patients with CD. You would expect this from the high level of chromosome damage. Phytohemagglutinin is a very potent stimulator of human monocytes, a cell which produces superoxide radicals. Therefore it might be better to deplete your cells of adherent cells before you culture them with phytohemagglutinin so as to eliminate this source of materials capable of producing chromosome breakage.

Booth: Has Emerit studied patients with cancer? And
              what is Bloom's syndrome?

Emerit: Cancer patients have no increased chromosome
              instability except when treated with cytostatic
              drugs. Bloom's syndrome is a congenital hereditary
              breakage syndrome described by Bloom and then by
              James German in New york. These patients have a
              high frequency of chromosome breaks and of sister
              chromatid exchanges. They also have a high risk of
              cancer and leukemia.

Fiocchi: Have you measured the level of superoxide dis-
              mutase in patients with Crohn's disease.

Emerit: This is in progress.

Jarnerot: Mittelman and his group studied chromosome
              aberrations in patients with Crohn's disease who
              were treated with metronidazole or sulphasalazine.
              He could not find any increase of chromosome aber-
              rations in the metronidazole treated group, but he
              did find a slight increase in the sulphasalazine
              treated group. Does treatment with corticosteroids,
              azathioprine or 6-mercaptopurine influence the rate
              of chromosome aberrations?

Emerit: Cortisone treatment may reduce breakage, and
              this could be explained by the fact that the O_2^-
              production of cells is diminished by cortisone.
              Mercaptopurine produces chromosome breaks.

E4 General Discussion and Conclusions
Reported by P. Meera Khan

The findings of Natarajan did, in principle, agree with those of Emerit whose pioneering work showed an increase in the incidence of chromosomal aberrations in the cultured lymphocytes of CD patients. Moreover, certain in vitro conditions appear to influence this observed instability of the chromosomes. Since added superoxide dismutase [SOD] or D-penicillamine or a related thiol compound prevents the damage, Emerit suggested that an accumulation of highly reactive superoxide radicals, known to be clastogenic, might play a role in the pathogenesis of CD. It is plausible that in CD the gut directly exposed to various extraneous agents, is susceptible to the intracellular storage of free radicals as a result of part interaction between CD gene[s] and the triggering environment. In this connection it is interesting to note that the number of macrophages, which are producers of superoxide radicals were found to be increased in the lamina propria of CD patients (Sommers and Ginsel).

As McConnell pointed out, the hereditary component of CD, appears to be polygenic, a fraction of which might be "dominant". The target cells, which carry the same genetic information and are exposed to the same environment, are equally predisposed. But the typical lesions appear to be initiated in an occasional cell [e.g., "focal necrosis" observed in electron microscopy by Dourmashkin and Gebbers], and spread around. It may be put forth, as a working hypothesis, that an onset of "focal necrosis" at a single cell level primarily requires homozygotization or hemizygotization of the gene[s] in the "dominant" component which may be achieved by the occurrence of chromosomal rearrangements. As a result "focal necrosis" as well as "neoantigens" generation may initiate the characteristic local lesions which eventually merge to manifest extensive devastating pathological changes. Further critical exploration of the involvement of free radicals in CD may be rewarding and help developing a rational therapy.

SECTION F

Environmental Factors

Section Editor: J.E. Lennard-Jones

240

INFECTIOUS AGENTS IN INFLAMMATORY BOWEL DISEASES

G.L. GITNICK

INTRODUCTION

Cytopathic agents have been reported in bowel filtrates from patients with Crohn's disease [CD] and ulcerative colitis [UC] (1-4). Recently, this has been confirmed in three separate independent laboratories with a high degree of concordance (5). Even though the cytopathic effects [CPE] is similar to that produced by viruses, may be subpassaged for up to twenty-five passages and is produced by filtrates which have been passed through 0.2 micron filters, controversy has arisen as to whether this CPE is produced by a virus, a cell wall-defective bacteria, or a toxic chemical product. Unfortunately, the CPE is often ephemeral, titers are low, and insufficient for complete biophysical characterization, antigen analysis, or formal neutralization studies. We have attempted to characterize the agents responsible for this CPE.

METHODS

Surgical specimens were obtained from UC patients, CD patients or patients with other bowel diseases. Surgical specimens were washed ten times in Hank's Balanced Salt Solution, minced and homogenized at 4°C in a rotary homogenizer which did not utilize glass of silica parts. The preparation was suspended in 0.9% saline solution and was centrifuged at 1800 rpm for 30 minutes at 4°C. The supernatant was then passed through coarse filter paper and then through a 0.2 micron filter and this filtrate was used for subsequent assessment. This methodology differs from that reported by Aronson et al. (1) in that whole biopsy specimens are not layered on monolayer cultures and the tissues and conditions of incubation and maintenance employed differed. Some of the specimens processed using the technique of Aronson et al. (1)

have been shown to harbor mycoplasma contamination (5). The
filtering process was used to exclude possible luminal contaminants such as bacteria and mycoplasma to the greatest
degree feasible. Mycoplasma testing was performed on all
specimens and included utilization of the Hoechst stain,
electron microscopy, immunofluorescent studies, and cultivation in agar and broth culture with multiple subcultures.

Whereas we initially reported the ability of rabbit ileum
[RI] tissue culture to support the growth of these agents
(2), we subsequently learned that commercially available Riff
free chick embryo tissue and duck embryo tissue culture were
also sensitive to the CPE produced (4). The utilization of
these tissues provided advantages in terms of convenience and
time although the CPE which resulted was not as dramatic as
with RI tissue culture. The studies reported here were performed utilizing Riff free chick embryo tissue culture plant-
ed in tubes and commercially obtained. Maintenance medium
consisted of Eagle's Minimum Essential Medium with 2% streptomycin and penicillin [250 μ g/l and 250 U, respectively] per
ml, 1% nonessential amino acids, 1% L-glutamine, and 2% Reha-
tuin prefiltered and preselected fetal calf serum [Reheis
Chemical Company, Phoenix-Arizona]. Preselected calf serum
was necessary because many lots of fetal calf serum contain
inhibitors preventing the development of CPE. The media was
changed at 5 to 7 day intervals depending on the degree of
acidity present. For each isolation or inhibition assay,
groups of 5 tubes were used. Standard viral neutralization
[inhibition] testing was employed, but where titers did not
exceed 2 logs, inhibition was determined to be positive if
all tubes at a given dilution were prevented from producing
CPE even though a two log reduction in titer could not be
obtained because of initial low titer. Isolation were considered positive only if the CPE could be subpassaged for at
least three subpassages.

RESULTS
CPE was observed in tissue specimens obtained from 51 of

54 CD patients and from 36 of 40 UC patients. CPE was observed in specimens from the bowel wall of 22 of 24 colon carcinoma patients. A specimen from a child with necrotizing enterocolitis, from 1 of 22 diverticulitis patients, 1 of 2 radiation enteritis patients and each of 2 familial polyposis patients were also positive. In order to determine if each of the positive cytopathic isolates represented the same agent, inhibition studies were undertaken. Antisera were prepared in guinea pigs hyperimmunized with a CD isolate or a prototype UC isolate. We also used a human serum rich in antibody to the Crohn's disease associated isolate.

Each of the isolated agents were resistant to heat at $56^{\circ}C$ for 15 minutes, ether and acid pH. Antisera against the CD associated agent did not inhibit the UC associated agent, the agents found in colon carcinoma or that from necrotizing enterocolitis. Similarly, the antisera directed against the UC associated agent, although it inhibited each of the UC isolates, failed to inhibit the CD, colon carcinoma, or necrotizing enterocolitis isolates. Recently, we assessed the isolates obtained in other bowel diseases and found that antisera directed against the herpes group of viruses reproducibly inhibits the agents isolated from colon carcinoma patients but not those isolated from CD or UC patients.

The utilization of methotrexate was found to significantly enhance titer. Methotrexate, $10^{-5}M$, was added to the maintenance media of each of the tissue culture systems. Twenty inflammatory bowel disease [IBD] specimens were tested at the first passage level and at the fourth passage level. Initial isolations were performed in methotrexate-containing media and these same specimens were simultaneously inoculated into cultures with media lacking methotrexate. Serial specimens were then obtained in order to yield a growth curve and these were titered in tissue culture with media with and without the addition of methotrexate. In each instance the utilization of methotrexate enhanced titer by approximately one log. These data were found to be statistically significant with a p value of less than 0.05. Electron microscopic studies of the tissue cultures so treated revealed that methotrexate produced electron microscopic evidence of cell membrance damage even in control specimens which were not inoculated with IBD tissues. Thus, methotrexate may permit virus to enter the cell and enhance titer, but since there is an electron microscopic CPE in control tissues we may be enhancing the expression of CPE rather than actually increasing the number of viral particles. Under direct light microscopy the CPE of methotrexate on control tissues not inoculated with IBD specimens was not evident.

CONCLUSIONS

The current literature now reveals a number of infectious agents having been identified in bowel preparations from CD and UC patients as well as from occasional patients with other bowel diseases. We and others have described virus-like agents (1-4). Others have described cell wall-defective bacteria (6) and mycoplasma in Crohn's disease (5). We have described cytomegalovirus (7) and a small RNA virus in specimens obtained from UC patients (4) and thus far other agents have not been identified in ulcerative colitis. About 20% of control specimens tested have been shown to produce CPE. We have now shown that methotrexate enhances the CPE produced. Thus, IBD tissues have been shown to contain a variety of infectious agents. These agents singly or in combination may be operative in the development of the complications of these diseases such as diarrhoea or other manifestations of disease such as the development of malignancies. Alternatively, they may singly or in combination initiate an immune process which leads to the development of disease. It is equally likely that these agents play no role in disease causation or symptom development. Nevertheless, it is encumbent on the scientific community to explain the presence of these agents and determine what role, if any, they play in disease. In order to characterize the virus-like agents, the titer must first be increased to levels allowing further characterization. Although these studies serve to assess the flora of the gastrointestinal tract during IBD, there is no evidence that infectious agents cause IBD, diarrhoea or the cancer of IBD.

REFERENCES
1. Aronson MD, Phillips CA, Beeken WL. (1974) Isolation of a viral agent form intestinal tissue of patients with Crohn's disease and other intestinal disorders. Gastroenterology 66:661
2. Gitnick GL, Arthur MH, Shibata I. (1976) Cultivation of viral agents from Crohn's disease. A new sensitive system. Lancet 2:215-217
3. Gitnick GL, Rosen VJ. (1976) Electron microscopic studies of viral agents in Crohn's disease. Lancet 2:217-219
4. Gitnick GL, Rosen VJ, Arthur MH, Hertweck SA. (1979) Evidence for the isolation of a new virus from ulcerative colitis patients: comparison with virus derived form Crohn's disease. Dig.Dis.Sci. 24:609-619
5. Cave D, Kirsner JB, Gitnick GL, et al. [IBD Research Group]. (1980) Infectious agents in inflammatory bowel disease [IBD]: A status report. Gastroenterology 78:1185
6. Parent K. Mitchell PD. (1976) Bacterial variants: Etiologic agent in Crohn's disease. Gastroenterology 71:365-368
7. Farmer GW, Vincent MM, Fuccillo DA, Barbosa LH, Ritman S, Sever JL, Gitnick GL. (1973) Viral investigations in ulcerative colitis and regional enteritis. Gastroenterology 65:8-15

STUDIES OF THE IN VITRO CYTOPATHIC EFFECT OF INFLAMMATORY
BOWEL DISEASE TISSUE PREPARATIONS

R.G. STRICKLAND and L.C. McLAREN

INTRODUCTION

Two laboratories, using different inocula, cell lines and
tissue culture systems recently reported that inflammatory
bowel disease [IBD] tissues produce transmissible cytopathic
effects [CPE] in cell culture (1-4). Both groups described
virus-like particles in cell cultures undergoing CPE (3,4)
and limited characterization suggests these to be RNA-viru-
ses. Gitnick et al. (4) presented evidence for antigenic
differences between the agents isolated from Crohn's disease
[CD], ulcerative colitis [UC] and control intestine and Whorwell et al. (3) reported that the CD-associated agent may be
a reovirus. The positive culture results obtained at the
University of Vermont and UCLA have been tempered by a report
of mycoplasma contamination of cell culture passage material
in some of these systems (5) and by a negative report of
virus isolation from IBD tissues (6). We report here our
experience with the isolation and characterization of cytopathic agents in IBD. These studies have been in progress
since 1978.

PROCEDURE

Tissue sources

Colonic or small intestinal tissue obtained at surgery
included 38 samples from 20 CD patients, 12 samples from 8 UC
patients and 27 samples from 25 patients with non-IBD intestinal disorders. The latter included colonic cancer [8],
diverticular disease [7], vascular disease [3], bowel trauma
[3], colostomy closure [2], colonic polyposis [1] and colonic
pseudo-obstruction [1]. Endoscopic colorectal biopsies were
obtained from 13 patients with IBD [6 CD, 7 UC] and 13 con-

trols [3 radiation proctitis, 3 colon cancer, 5 irritable colon, 1 sigmoid volvulus, 1 ischemic bowel disease].

Preparation of Inocula and Cell Culture Procedures

Homogenates and 0.2μ filtrates were prepared by the method of Gitnick et al. from fresh or frozen surgical bowel samples and directly inoculated into cell culture (2,4). Fresh colorectal biopsies were finely minced and cell suspensions used for modified co-cultivation experiments as described by Aronson et al. (1). Cultures were accepted as showing CPE if inoculated as compared to uninoculated monolayers showed 25% or greater cell destruction and this effect was transmissible for at least two passages. Susceptible cell cultures using direct filtrate inoculation included mammalian fibroblast lines established in our laboratory from adult or fetal rabbit or human intestine, rabbit kidney and human skin, as well as commercially obtained fibroblast lines IMR-90, MRC-7 and two avian lines, Peking duck embryo and chick embryo [SPAFAS]. The co-cultivation experiments were carried out using WI-38 [Pass 14][*]. Homogenates, filtrates and minced biopsies, as well as cell culture passage material were routinely cultured for mycoplasma (7). Inoculated and uninoculated cell cultures were selectively tested for non-culturable mycoplasma by fluorochrome staining (8).

Characterization Experiments

The following properties of the isolates have been examined - sedimentability by homogenate ultracentrifugation, filterability through membrane filters of various mean pore size, fluorocarbon extractability, and stability of filtrates to treatment with diethylether, heating to $56^{O}C$ for 30 minutes, or IUdR. Filtrates were also treated with polyvalent anti-clostridial globulin and the effect on CPE production observed.

Augmentation of Infectivity

Attempts to augment the rate of appearance of CPE and virus yield have included alteration of incubation tempera-

[*]American Type Culture Collection

ture [33°C to 39°C] or pH [6.8 to 7.8] treatment, of inoculated cells with inhibitors of cell function such as actinomycin D or cyclohexamide, supplementation of medium with proteolytic enzymes such as trypsin and use of serum free medium and roller tube culture.

Serum Neutralization

Equal volumes of 14 normal, 14 IBD sera [final dilutions 1:2 to 1:40] and intestinal filtrate were incubated for one hour at 37°C. The mixture was then inoculated into cell culture and the tubes followed for appearance of CPE in parallel with untreated filtrate-inoculated and uninoculated cells.

RESULTS AND DISCUSSION

Cytopathic Effects [CPE] of Filtered Intestinal Specimens

Thirty-five of 38 [92%] CD filtrates, 10 of 12 [83%] UC filtrates and 7 of 27 [26%] control filtrates produced transmissible CPE in cell culture. The latter included cancer [3], diverticular disease [3] and ischemic bowel [1]. CPE commenced focally at day 7 and was slowly progressive reaching a maximum [50-75% destruction of monolayers] at day 14-21. CPE was transmissible with either infected cells or 0.2_μ filtrates of sonicated infected cells and up to six serial passages have been accomplished. This observation suggests that the CPE is due to a replicating agent(s) and not to a tissue-associated toxin. CPE production was independent of disease site, degree of gross involvement of the tissue by disease or whether the starting material was fresh or frozen. No differences in quality or extent or CPE were observed between filtrates from the three patient groups studied. However, in preliminary experiments, it appears that the range of cell line susceptibility to CPE is broad with IBD filtrates and more restricted with control filtrates. PPLO cultures of filtered bowel wall samples and cell culture passage material were uniformly negative and selective fluorochrome staining of both inoculated and uninoculated cell cultures have also been negative for mycoplasma.

Cytopathic Effects [CPE] of Unfiltered Intestinal Biopsies

The modified co-cultivation technique using WI-38 [Pass 14] yielded transmissible CPE with 12 of 13 biopsies from patients with IBD and 4 of 13 biopsies from disease controls [2 radiation colitis, 1 volvulus, 1 irritable bowel]. PPLO cultures were positive in 6 of the 13 IBD biopsies and 3 of the 13 control biopsies. There was, however, no correlation with CPE positivity. Moreover, gentamycin treatment of two IBD biopsies which were positive for both mycoplasma and CPE 'cured' the mycoplasma but these biopsies still yielded CPE following such treatment.

Characterization of Cytopathic Effect

CPE was produced by untreated and fluorocarbon extracted homogenates and by 100,000 x G sonicated homogenates. The CPE was not affected by treatment of the filtrates with IUdR, ether or heating to 56°C for 30 minutes. Filterability experiments indicated that CPE was produced by 100 nm filtered material but not by 50 or 10 nm filtrates. Treatment of active filtrates with anticlostridial globulin did not inhibit the rate of appearance or extent of CPE, indicating that the effect is unlikely to be due to tissue-associated clostridial toxin. These results suggest that the CPE is produced by a particulate agent, 50-100 nm in size, with physico-chemical properties consistent with RNA virus[es].

Augmentation of Infectivity

TCD_{50} titrations have indicated infectivity titers which averaged 10^4 per ml. Serial passage, incubation temperature or pH, and treatment with actinomycin D or cyclohexamide had no enhancing effect. The use of serum-free medium, 2 µg per ml Trypsin, and culture in roller tubes modestly augmented the appearance and extent of CPE. This difficulty in achieving high titer virus growth in tissue culture has been reported by others (1-4) and may indicate that the agents being isolated are highly defective.

Serum Inhibition of CPE

Ten of the 14 IBD sera [all from patients whose bowel wall filtrates had yielded CPE in culture] inhibited CPE at dilutions of 1:2 or greater. However, 11 of the 14 control sera also inhibited CPE at similar dilutions. These results offer no support for specificity of the cytopathic agents isolated to IBD tissues or significant differences in immune responses to the agents between patients with IBD and controls. However, it is equally possible that the method used lacks the sensitivity and specificity needed to demonstrate such differences.

CONCLUSIONS

Our results confirm the observations of Gitnick et al. (2,4) and Aronson et al. (1) that intestinal tissues from patients with Crohn's disease or ulcerative colitis consistently produce a transmissible cytopathic effect in mammalian fibroblast or avian cell cultures using either direct inoculation of tissue filtrates or unfiltered tissues and modified co-cultivation. Non-IBD control tissues produce similar CPE but with significantly lower frequency and more restricted cell line susceptibility than do IBD tissues. Mycoplasma contamination does not account for the CPE induced in these cell culture systems. Characterization of the CPE is consistent with its production by intestinally-derived RNA virus-[es]. Confirmation and extension of this work will depend on the results of studies in progress aimed at virus isolation in liquid phase along with further characterization and immunologic studies.

ACKNOWLEGEMENTS

Supported by grants from the National Foundation for Ileitis and Colitis, Inc. and the US Public Health Service No: AM-19497.

REFERENCES
1. Aronson MD, Phillips CA, Beeken WL, Forsyth BR. (1975) Isolation and characterization of a viral agent from intestinal tissue of patients with Crohn's disease and other intestinal disorders. Progr.Med.Virol. 21:165-176
2. Gitnick GL, Arthur MH, Shibata I. (1976) Cultivation of viral agents from Crohn's disease. A new sensitive system. Lancet 2:215-217

3. Whorwell PJ, Phillips CA, Beeken WL, Little PK, Roessner KD. (1977) Isolation of reovirus-like agents from patients with Crohn's disease. Lancet 1:1169-1171
4. Gitnick GL, Rosen VJ, Arthur MH, Hertweck SA. (1979) Evidence for the isolation of a new virus from ulcerative colitis patients. Comparison with virus derived from Crohn's disease. Dig.Dis.Sci. 24:609-619
5. Kapikian AZ, Barile MF, Wyatt RG, Yolken RH, Tully JG, Greenberg HB, Kalica AR, Chanock RM. (1979) Mycoplasma contamination in cell culture of Crohn's disease material. Lancet 2:466-467
6. Phillpotts RJ, Hermon-Taylor J, Brooke BN. (1979) Virus isolation studies in Crohn's disease: A negative report. Gut 20:1057-1062
7. Hayflick L. (1965) Tissue culture and mycoplasmas. Tex.Rep.Biol.Med. 23:285-303
8. Chen TR.(1977) In situ detection of mycoplasma contamination in cell cultures by fluorescent Hoechst 33258 Stain. Exp.Cell Res. 104:255-262

EVIDENCE AGAINST THE INVOLVEMENT OF CONVENTIONAL VIRUSES IN CROHN'S DISEASE

R.J. PHILLPOTTS, J. HERMON-TAYLOR and B.N. BROOKE

INTRODUCTION

Research into the aetiology of Crohn's disease [CD] was revitalized by the demonstration of Mitchell and Rees in 1970 of a putative transmissible agent in CD tissues (1). Investigations into the physico-chemical characteristics of this putative agent suggested that it may be a virus, or a cell wall-deficient microorganism (2). Because of these findings, and the promising preliminary results of virus isolation studies conducted in other laboratories (3,4,5), we undertook an extensive series of experiments designed to demonstrate the presence of conventional viruses in CD tissues (6,7).

PROCEDURES

Gut and lymphoid tissue removed at surgery from CD, ulcerative colitis [UC] and control patients with other gastrointestinal diseases was snap-frozen in liquid nitrogen, and stored at $-70^{\circ}C$ prior to washing and homogenization in the Biotec X-press, or washed and homogenized immediately in an MSE blender. All homogenates were centrifuged to remove coarse debris. Fresh homogenates were filtered through a 220 nm Millipore membrane, before inoculation into cell cultures; frozen tissue homogenates were used without filtration. Each homogenate was stored in separate 1 ml aliquots at $-70^{\circ}C$ for future use. A variety of cell cultures were inoculated, and incubated at $33^{\circ}C$ or $37^{\circ}C$, stationary or rolling, and with or without 5% CO_2 in the atmosphere.

Evidence of virus growth was sought by observation for cytopathic effect [CPE], and indirect immunofluorescence using human CD serum, and calf anti-rotavirus serum.

In a parallel series of experiments cell cultures from CD and control tissues were established in vitro, and examined by the following tests for persistent virus infection.

[i]   Thin section electron microscopy
[ii]   Indirect immunofluorescence using CD serum
[iii]   Fluorescent lectin binding
[iv]   Spontaneous and poly I:poly C induced interferon induction
[v]   Challenge with Semliki forest virus
[vi]   Co-cultivation with human and animal cell lines with and without the nucleic acid inhibitor iododeoxyuridine, followed by assay of the cell culture fluid for reverse transcriptive activity [in collaboration with Dr. N.M. Teich, of the Imperial Cancer Research Fund, Lincoln's Inn Fields, London, England]

RESULTS

Six CD, 2 UC and 5 control frozen tissue homogenates were inoculated into vero- [continuous African Green Monkey Kidney] and BCL-D1 cells [human embryo lung fibroblasts, Flow Laboratories, Scotland]. Six CD, 2 UC and 2 control tissue homogenates were inoculated into MRC_5 human embryo lung fibroblasts and 13 CD, 3 UC and 12 controls homogenates into human foetal ileal fibroblasts. None of the tissue homogenates produced any CPE after incubation times of up to 6 weeks, and one blind passage. There was no specific fluorescence detected in the cell cultures using serum from 5 CD patients.

Seven CD, 3 UC and 6 control homogenates prepared from fresh tissues were inoculated into rabbit ileal cells. All these cultures showed spontaneous degeneration, but all were restored to normal appearance by the substitution of growth medium for maintenance medium at any time up to 14 days of incubation. Twelve CD, 6 UC and 16 control homogenates were inoculated into WI38 human embryo lung fibroblasts. Six CD, 6 UC and 6 acute appendicitis homogenates produced a CPE.

CPE was usually visible in 2-4 days, but occasionally took up to 10 days to appear. Cytopathogenic activity had the following characteristics:

[i]   It could be passaged up to three times

[ii]   The severity was reduced by regular changes of cell cultured fluid

[iii]   The severity was increased by doubling the inoculum size

[iv]   It was not prevented by arcton 113 extraction of the homogenate

[v]   It was not destroyed by a dose of UV irradiation shown to kill $10^{6.25}$ plaque forming units of Rhinovirus No.2.

[vi]   It was not inhibited by serum from 4 CD patients

[vii]   There was no positive correlation with acid phosphatase levels [lysosomal enzyme marker] in the tissue homogenates

[viii] It was abolished by dilution of the inoculum 1:5

[ix]   It was destroyed by proteolytic digestion

[x]   Activity was present in gel filtration fractions corresponding to molecular weights in the range >100,000, 40-60,000, 25-35,000 and <25,000

No specific fluorescence was detected in WI38 cells using calf anti-rotavirus serum.

Eight CD [4 ileum, 2 colon, 2 lymph node] and 7 controls [3 ileum, 3 colon, 1 lymph node] cell cultures were established in vitro. During 11 passages, non of these showed any sign of degeneration or CPE, which could be attributed to a virus. None of the tests previously described gave any indication of persistent virus infection of any of the cell lines, and no differences were apparent between the CD and control cultures.

DISCUSSION

Although tissue from a total of 16 CD patients was examined by inoculation into cell cultures which were incubated for various times, and under a variety of conditions, no viruses were detected. A CPE produced in WI38 cells by fresh CD tissue homogenates was also produced by an equal number of controls. This activity appeared to be due to proteins with a range of molecular weights, although no evidence was found to suggest that these were lysosomal enzymes.

Persistent virus infection was not detected in any of the CD-derived cell cultures. However, this result must be evaluated recognising the possibility of the cell selecting effects of trypsinization during the establishment of these cultures. Consequently it does not enable persistent virus infection of CD tissues to be completely excluded.

CONCLUSIONS

Non-confirmation was provided for earlier reports of virus isolations from CD tissues (3,4,5). While not completely excluding any involvement of conventional viruses in the aetiology of CD, these results contribute greatly towards the weight of evidence against such a possibility.

REFERENCES
1. Mitchell DN, Rees RJW. (1970) Agent transmissible from Crohn's disease tissue. Lancet 2:168-171
2. Cave DR, Mitchell DN, Brooke BN. (1975) Experimental animal studies on the aetiology and pathogenesis of Crohn's disease. Gastroenterology 69:618-624
3. Aronson MD, Phillips CA, Beeken WL, Forsyth BR. (1975) Isolation and characterisation of a viral agent from intestinal tissue of patients with Crohn's disease and other intestinal disorders. Progr.Med.Virol. 21:165-176
4. Gitnick GL, Arthur MH, Shibata I. (1976) Cultivation of viral agents from Crohn's disease. Lancet 2:215-217
5. Whorwell PJ, Phillips CA, Beeken WL, Little PK, Roessner KD. (1977) Isolation of reovirus-like agents from patients with Crohn's disease. Lancet 1:1169-1171
6. Phillpotts RJ, Hermon-Taylor J, Brooke BN. (1979) Virus isolation studies in Crohn's disease: A negative report. Gut 20:1057-1062
7. Phillpotts RJ, Hermon-Taylor J, Teich NM, Brooke BN. (1980) A search for persistent virus infection in Crohn's disease. Gut 21:202-207

F4 Summary of Discussions relating to topics F1 to F3

Gitnick: I would like to congratulate Phillpotts on his
interesting work and I do not think our disagreement is great. We have all tested IBD filtrates in
African Green Monkey tissue and a variety of other
tissue culture systems and have not found any cytopathic change. It is only a very narrow range of
tissue culture systems that CPE is found. With the
human diploid lung cell studies the difference in
the data is easily explained. Phillpotts of necessity used high-passage WI-38 but our laboratory,
Phillips and Dolan's laboratory, and McLaren and
Strickland's laboratory have all used high-passage
WI-38 and got nothing. It is very hard to get low-
passage WI-38 but that is the material McLaren and
Strickland used. With rabbit ileum you also need to
use low-passage material. You found a toxic protein
and we all should strive now to confirm its presence and identify it. In the work published in Gut
on rabbit ileum cultures I could not see that Eagles medium was used; each of us have used Eagles
minimum essential medium with 2% streptomycin and
penicillin, 1% glutamine and pre-selected foetal
calf serum. Many foetal calf sera are insensitive
culture systems and are in themselves cytotoxic. We
should exchange reagents, just as we have done in
the USA.

Phillpotts: The difference between us is in interpretation.
To my mind you have not presented hard evidence
that your CPE is due to a virus; I was unable to
show that the CPE I observed was due to a virus.

Versteeg: Did you do any electron microscopy on your viruses?

Strickland: We were able to get one sample of Crohn's colitis colon into explant culture and after a period of about 6 weeks in culture that explant underwent spontaneous cytopathic change. A thin section EM of that tissue did reveal virus-like particles of fairly uniform size many of which were without a central core.

Gitnick: We are dealing with an agent in a liquid phase of too low a titre to see on EM. In a thin section we see virus-like material, 60 nanometres in diameter in the tissue cultures. We need to get very concentrated material and try liquid phase electronmicroscopy and immunoelectronmicroscopy.

Jewell: Could you tell us to what agent the antisera were made which neutralize your CPE?

Gitnick: At best we proved inhibition, that is, we completely prevented the development of cytopathic change using guinea pig antisera and human antisera to partially purified tissue culture agents.

Strober: If you raise an antiserum from Crohn's patients specifically with materials obtained from the small intestine or from the large intestine do you find that the antisera obtained are different in their pattern of blocking?

Gitnick: We have not compared ileal to colonic Crohn's disease.

Strickland: We have tried to use classical immuno-fluores-
               cent techniques to detect antibodies within IBD or
               control sera using the infected versus the non-in-
               fected cell lines but have not been able to show
               any clear specificity reactions.

Tijtgat: Were the inocula studied by negative staining
               at the EM level before inoculation?

Gitnick: We have never seen evidence of a virus particle
               in the tissue specimen only in tissue culture
               cells.

TRANSMISSION OF IBD HOMOGENATES IN INBRED MICE AND RABBITS

Z. COHEN, M.K. LEUNG, D. JIRSCH, S. ARCHIBALD, J. CULLEN and J. GARDNER

INTRODUCTION

In 1970, research into inflammatory bowel disease advanced with a new investigation of an old concept, namely that the cause of Crohn's disease was due to an infectious agent. Mitchell and Rees (1) injected Crohn's disease tissue homogenates into the footpads of normal and thymectomized CBA mice. They reported the appearance of classic focal epithelioid granulomas in several mouse footpads upon injection of ileal or mesenteric lymph node homogenates from one patient with Crohn's disease. They postulated that a transmissible agent from human Crohn's disease tissue must be responsible. In 1973, Cave and Mitchell (2) reported successful reproduction of lesions similar to Crohn's disease by injection of Crohn's tissue homogenates from two patients into the ileal wall of rabbits. They were also able to successfully passage this positive rabbit tissue into a second group of rabbits. Control tissue identically injected produced no reaction in rabbits. In contradiction to this, Bolton et al. (3) reported a consistent failure to produce granulomas in various animal models using techniques similar to Cave and Mitchell. Heatley et al. (4) then reported that inoculation of tissue homogenates from 24 patients with Crohn's disease into more than 400 experimental animals of four species showed no evidence of granuloma formation at the inoculation site. Taub et al. (5) were able to transmit focal granulomas into less than 10% of A2G strain mice inoculated with both Crohn's and ulcerative colitis tissue homogenates. In addition, these same authors noted the appearance of granulomas in CBA mice inoculated with Crohn's disease, ulcerative colitis, and control tissue homogenates (6). In this paper, we report the results of inoculating IBD tissue homogenates into inbred mouse strains and NZW rabbits.

PROCEDURE

Materials and Methods

Animals:

Experiment no 1. Twenty mice each of the following strains were used: CBA/J [H-2^k], AKR [H-2^k], C57BL/10 [H-2^b], AJAX [H-2^a], and BALB/C [H-2^d]. Each group was equally divided between Crohn's disease and control tissue inoculations.

Experiment no 2. One hundred and forty-four mice each of C57BL/10 and BALB/C were equally inoculated with Crohn's, ulcerative colitis, and control tissue.

Experiment no 3. Forty-two NZW rabbits were used. These were divided into controls [13], Crohn's inoculated [20], and ulcerative colitis [UC] inoculated [9]. In 32 of these, a laparotomy was performed and a Thiry-Vella [T-V] loop created using an isolated 25 cm segment of distal ileum.

Tissue samples: Tissue was obtained following surgical resection after confirmation of histological diagnosis. Ileal tissue from right hemicolectomy specimens for carcinoma was used as control tissue.

Experiment no 1: 2 Crohn's patients and 2 controls.

Experiment no 2: 8 Crohn's patients, 5 ulcerative colitis patients and 6 controls.

Experiment no 3: 6 Crohn's patients, 3 ulcerative colitis patients and 4 controls.

Homogenates: Full thickness bowel was cut, snap frozen, and stored at -70° and then processed in a Biotec X-press homogenizer. Twenty per cent homogenates were used in all experiments. In rabbit experiments, 40% homogenates were also used. The homogenates were centrifuged and filtered through a 0.22 μ millipore filter prior to inoculation.

Injection of homogenates: All mice received 0.03 ml of homogenate into each hind footpad and 0.5 ml intraperitoneally. Rabbits received multiple intramural 0.2 ml injections of both 20% and 40% homogenates. Four rabbits received 1.0

ml of 20% homogenate intravenously.

Harvesting tissue

Mouse tissues - A full thickness biopsy specimen initially of the same and later of the contralateral footpad was obtained 3 - 12 months after inoculation. Samples of ileum, spleen, and liver were taken at autopsy.

Rabbit tissues - All were sacrificed at 1 year. The incontinuity bowel as well as the T-V loop were examined histologically. Samples of liver and spleen were also taken.

Histologic assessment. Histologic assessment was made from coded specimens of mouse footpads and mouse and rabbit viscera by two independent pathologists. In addition, representative samples from each experiment were sent to Prof. J. Yardley for further assessment. The presence of granulomatous infiltration was considered a positive response.

RESULTS

Mice. No macroscopic or microscopic abnormalities were seen in ileum, liver or spleen. No granulomas were seen in any of the footpad biopsies taken from CBA/J, AKR, and AJAX mice in Experiment no 1. Three of 25 biopsies [12%] from BALB/C mice inoculated with control tissue and 6 of 25 [24%] inoculated with Crohn's disease homogenates showed granulomas [Table 1]. Three of 27 biopsies [11%] from C57BL/10 mice ino-

Table 1. Experiment no 1: Results of all footpad biopsies taken to 1 year

| | Control tissue homogenates | | | Crohn's disease tissue homogenates [CR] | | |
	+ve	equiv.	-ve	+ve	equiv.	-ve
CBA/J	0	1	26	0	0	29
AKR	0	1	25	0	0	23
AJAX	0	0	27	0	0	27
BALB/C	3	1	21	6	3	16
C57BL/10	3	0	24	11	0	10

culated with control tissue and 11 of 21 [52%] inoculated with Crohn's homogenates showed granulomas microscopically. The granulomas which were seen following control tissue inoculation at the 3 and 6 month biopsies were not seen at 12 months.

In experiment no 2 [Table 2], footpad biopsies were taken only at 1 year. In C57BL/10 mice, 18 of 46 [39%] Crohn's di-

Table 2. Experiment no 2: Results of footpad biopsies taken at 1 year.

	Control tissue homogenates			Crohn's disease tissue homogenates			UC tissue homogenates		
	+ve	equiv.	-ve	+ve	equiv.	-ve	+ve	equiv.	-ve
C57BL/10	3	2	38	18	3	25	14	5	27
BALB/C	1	3	44	10	2	35	8	3	34

sease tissue homogenates inoculated and 14 of 46 [30%] ulcerative colitis tissue homogenates inoculated mice developed granulomas. However, 3 of 43 [7%] control inoculated mice also developed granulomas. After further histologic assessment by Dr. J. Yardley, it was found that approximately 25% of all positive granulomatous reactions were associated with keratin or hair. These findings were equally distributed within the test groups.

Rabbits. No significant macroscopic changes occurred in any of the rabbits. From Table 3, it can be seen that none of the control animals showed any significant microscopic changes. One of 9 rabbits inoculated with ulcerative colitis tissue developed granulomas. Of the 20 Crohn's tissue inoculated animals - 3 of 16 inoculated intramurally and 1 of 4 inoculated IV developed granulomas. No granulomas were seen in any of the Thiry-Vella loops. There was no difference in the frequency of positive microscopic results with differences in homogenate concentration used. The granulomas found in the Crohn's tissue inoculated rabbits were confirmed by Dr. Yardley. However, that found in the ulcerative colitis tissue inoculated rabbit was assessed as a "non caseating granuloma containing small refractile particles" and was considered to be a normal finding in rabbits.

Table 3. Experiment no 3: Histology of rabbit viscera taken
at autopsy at 12 months.

Tissue	Rabbits (n)	Granulomas (n)
Control tissue (13)		
1. T-V loop (not injected)	3	0
2. Saline injected (no T-V loop)	3	0
3. Tissue injected (no T-V loop)	4	0
4. Bowel + T-V loop	3	0
Crohn's disease tissue		
1. Intravenous [IV]	4	1
2. Bowel (no T-V loop)	4	2
3. Bowel + T-V loop	12	1
Ulcerative colitis tissue		
1. Bowel + T-V loop	9	1

DISCUSSION

The overwhelming feature of animal transmission studies
related to inflammatory bowel disease research is the lack of
agreement and reproducibility of reported results (1-6). We
have attempted to develop a more reliable and consistent
mouse model for the transmission of inflammatory bowel disease homogenates. We based this work on the fact that different mouse strains having different genetic histocompatibility complexes might also have different susceptibility rates
to the formation of granulomas following inoculation with
Crohn's tissue homogenates. In two experiments, granulomas
were produced in C57BL/10 mice to a greater extent than in
other strains. The reported results of 52% and 39% granuloma
formation however must be viewed with some scepticism because
of the presence of foreign material in 25% of positive responses. We were not able to produce granulomas in any of our
CBA mice. This again is contrary to other reports (1,2,5).
The C57BL/10 mouse appears to give the best reported results.
However, we still are not certain if this response is directed towards a specific etiologic agent or if it is a mouse
lesion which occurs in response to a foreign material inoculation, and is completely irrelevant to the underlying human
disorder.

The reports regarding a viral or infectious etiology to

Crohn's disease and ulcerative colitis are equally conflicting and confusing. Gitnick (7), following earlier work by
Beeken et al. (8), has isolated "viral agents" from ileal
homogenates of patients with Crohn's disease. Exact characterization of these agents was not possible because of the
extremely low titres of the agents grown in tissue culture.
Gitnick (9) has also reported the isolation of a new virus
from ulcerative colitis tissue homogenates differing from
that described as being isolated from Crohn's disease tissue
homogenates. However, to this date, no "viral agents" have
been isolated from any of the positive granulomatous responses seen in experimental animal transmission studies. In
addition, the inoculation of these "viral agents" into animals has not as yet yielded positive granulomatous reactions.

We have been able to produce granulomas in mice following
inoculation with ulcerative colitis tissue. Others have
produced similar results (6,10). This observation does not
necessarily mean that ulcerative colitis is a transmissible
disease caused by a viable agent. It, in fact, reinforces
the concept that other inflammatory non-Crohn's disease tissue homogenates must be used as controls to distinguish specific from more general animal responses.

A granulomatous response was seen in rabbit ileum following inoculation with Crohn's disease tissue homogenates.
However, the gross lesions reported by Cave (2) and the more
non-specific lesions reported by Simonowitz (11) have not
been confirmed. It is of interest that in one animal, the
intravenous inoculation of Crohn's disease homogenates produced a granulomatous reaction in the distal ileum. It is
also noted that no positive reaction was seen in any of the
Thiry-Vella loops. This might indicate that lumenal factors
are necessary to either initiate or propagate the responses
seen.

Our studies confirm that it is possible to produce granulomas in experimental animals following inoculation of IBD
tissue. The C57BL/10 mouse appears to offer the highest
response rate. However, this response rate is still relati-

vely low. The response does become more specific after prolonged incubation, but in some cases it is still seen following inoculation of control tissue. Confirmation of these and
other studies must await an ongoing National Co-operative
Trial.

ACKNOWLEDGEMENT

This work was supported by a grant from the Canadian
Foundation for Ileitis and Colitis.

REFERENCES
 1. Mitchell DN, Rees RJW. (1970) Agent transmissible from
    Crohn's disease tissue. Lancet 2:168-171
 2. Cave DR, Mitchell DN, Kane SP, Brook BN. (1973) Further
    animal evidence of a transmissible agent in Crohn's dis-
    ease. Lancet 2:1120-1122
 3. Bolton PM, Owen E, Heatley RV, Jones Williams W, Hughes
    LE. (1973) Negative findings in laboratory animals for a
    transmissible agent in Crohn's disease. Lancet 2:1122-
    1124
 4. Heatley RV, Bolton PM, Owen E, Williams W, Jones Williams
    W, Hughes LE. (1975) The search for a transmissible agent
    in Crohn's disease. Gut 16:528-532
 5. Taub RN, Sachar D, Siltzbach LE et al. (1974) Transmis-
    sion of ileitis and sarcoid granulomas to mice. Trans.As-
    soc.Am.Physicians. 87:219-224
 6. Taub RN, Sachar D, Janowitz H, Siltzbach LE. (1975) In-
    duction of granulomas in mice by inoculation of tissue
    homogenates from patients with inflammatory bowel disease
    and sarcoidosis Ann.N.Y.Acad.Sci. 278:560-564
 7. Gitnick GL, Rosen VJ. (1976) Electron microscopic studies
    of viral agents in Crohn's disease. Lancet 2:217-219
 8. Beeken WL, Acharya Goswami KK, Mitchell DN. (1975) Stu-
    dies of a viral agent isolated from patients with Crohn's
    disease and other intestinal disorders. Gut 16:401
 9. Gitnick GL, Rosen VJ, Arthur MH, Hertweck SA. (1979) Evi-
    dence for the isolation of a new virus from ulcerative
    colitis patients. Comparison with virus derived from
    Crohn's disease. Dig.Dis.Sci. 24(8):609-619
10. Cave DR, Mitchell DN, Brook BN. (1975) Observations on
    the transmissibility of Crohn's disease and ulcerative
    colitis. Gastroenterology 68:871
11. Simonowitz D, Block GE, Riddell RH, Sumner C, Kraft SC,
    Kirsner JB. (1977) The production of an unusual tissue
    reaction in rabbit bowel injected with Crohn's disease
    homogenates. Surgery 82:211-218

INDUCTION OF LYMPHOMA IN ATHYMIC [NU/NU] MICE BY CROHN'S DISEASE TISSUE FILTRATES: A MODEL FOR THE STUDY OF CROHN'S DISEASE

K.M. DAS, SUSAN E. WILLIAMS, ISABEL VALENZUELA and S. BAUM

INTRODUCTION

Crohn's disease [CD] is a chronic inflammation of unknown etiology, usually involving the small and large intestine. Different infectious agents such as L-forms of bacteria, mycobacteria and viruses have been isolated from tissues of patients with CD at different times in various laboratories (1-3). Similar conflicting results have been encountered in attempts to transfer the disease to normal animals (4-5). Athymic, T-cell deficient, nude mice have been found to be unique suited to studies of various infectious agents including bacteria, parasites and viruses (6). The agents express their phenotype and grow better in nude mice. In a search for a disease specific transmissible agent(s) of CD, we used homozygous nude mice [nu/nu] on a BALB/C background and reported production of lymphoma by CD lymph node filtrates (7). Here we update this work and examine the possibility of using nude mice as an experimental model of CD.

PROCEDURE

Injection of nu/nu mice with tissue filtrates: 0.45μ m filtrates of intestinal mucosa or lymph node homogenates from 5 patients with CD were injected intraperitoneally into groups of 8-12 nu/nu totaling 50 mice. Twenty four mice received filtrates from 3 patients with ulcerative colitis [UC] and another 24 mice were injected with control filtrates of normal mesenteric lymph nodes and colonic mucosa from 5 patients with cholecystitis or colon carcinoma. Mice were examined regularly and sacrificed after 12 months.

Immunofluorescent studies: Sera were obtained from 21

patients with CD [8 active, 13 in remission], 23 with UC [11 symptomatic, 12 asymptomatic], 11 with other gastrointestinal diseases and 10 normal subjects. The sera were coded, decomplemented and absorbed sequentially with nude mouse normal spleen cells and mouse serum proteins bound to Sepharose 4B. Cryostat sections of lymphoma or other tissues [liver, spleen, kidney, ileum and colon] of nu/nu mice were incubated with serum for 45 min., washed, and incubated again with fluorescein isothiocyanate [FITC] conjugated antihuman IgG [Fab'$_2$ fragments] for 45 min. Coded slides were examined under an immunofluorescent microscope independently by 3 investigators and scored as negative, weakly positive or strongly positive. Lymphomas and other tissues were also incubated directly with FITC conjugated anti-mouse serum against IgG, IgM or Thy 1-2 antigen and examined under the microscope.

RESULTS

Table 1 summarizes the clinicopathological findings in 98 mice. To date, approximately 80% of the mice have been killed or died and more than 90% of them were histologically examined. Nine mice which received CD filtrates developed generalized lymphadenopathy due to lymphoma [Fig.1]. In 3 additional mice, lymphadenopathy was due to plasma cell hyperplasia. Tissue from each patient with CD produced at least one lymphoma. Two additional mice developed ascites without lymphadenopathy. Filtrates from patients with UC or control subjects did not produce lymphadenopathy or ascites.

Table 1. Clinicopathological findings of nu/nu mice injected with filtrates

Source of tissue	no.of patients	Nu/nu mice	Lymphoma	Plasma cell hyperplasia	Ascites
Crohn's disease	5	50	9*	3	2
Ulcerative colitis	3	24	0	0	0
Control	5	24	0	0	0

*Each tissue from patients with CD produced at least one lymphoma.

268

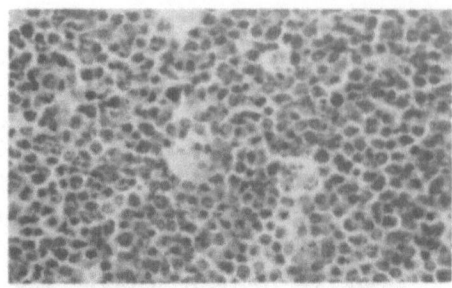

Figure 1. Histology of the enlarged lymph node showing lymphoma.

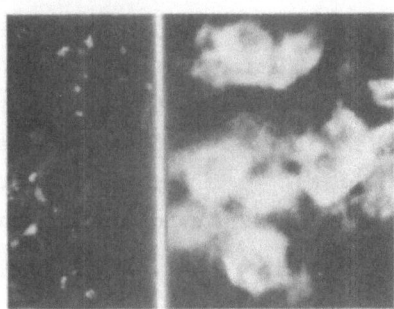

Figure 2. Indirect immuno-fluorescent stai-ning of lymphoma with serum from a patient with CD [right] and UC [left]. Cytoplasmic staining was present with CD serum only.

Sera obtained from 8 patients with active CD showed strongly positive cytoplasmic immunofluorescence in clusters of lymphoma cells [Fig.2]. However, none of the 32 sera from 11 patients with symptomatic UC, 11 with asymptomatic UC and 10 normal subjects showed any fluorescence. Sera from all 13 patients with asymptomatic CD showed weakly positive immuno-fluorescence or did not stain at all. Specificity of immuno-logic recognition of mouse lymphoma by CD serum was demon-strated by retesting for immuno-fluorescent staining follow-ing absorption of serum with homogenates of CD intestinal mucosa or of the lymphoma. Sera from 4 patients with CD were absorbed with homogenates of CD mucosa or normal colonic mucosa. Following absorption with CD mucosa, immunofluor-escent staining of the lymphoma by CD serum disappeared. Staining did not decrease on absorption with mucosal homoge-nates of normal colon. Immunofluorescent reactivity disap-peared following similar absorption of CD sera with homoge-nates of the lymphoma but not of a mouse myeloma cell line. These results suggest presence of a common antigen both in CD intestinal mucosa and the lymphoma recognized by CD sera.

Sera from 5 patients with active CD were restudied 3 wks to 1 yr later when they were completely asymptomatic. The immunofluorescent staining of the lymphoma significantly decreased and was weakly positive or negative. Lymphomas fluoresced with anti-mouse IgG and IgM but not with the anti-serum against Thy 1-2 antigen suggesting that they are B cell lymphomas.

Using sera from 2 patients with active CD, 2 with active UC and 1 normal subject, other nu/nu tissues were examined for any antigenic recognition. No staining was noted in any organ except kidney. Five of the 13 mice injected with CD filtrates showed 3+ glomerular staining, while 10 nu/nu mice injected with UC or control filtrates were negative. Glomeruli of the kidneys which were positive with CD serum also showed positive staining with FITC conjugated anti-mouse IgG and IgM, suggesting deposition of immune complexes of an antigen derived from CD tissue and mouse Ig.

Transmission studies: Mouse to mouse: [i] 0.45μm filtrates of 2 lymphomas were injected intraperitoneally into 5 nu/nu mice. Within three months, 2 mice developed lymphoma. [ii] 0.45μm filtrate of ascitic fluid was also injected into 4 nu/nu mice. Within 4 months, one mouse developed lymphoma. Another developed ascites.

Electron microscopic studies: Electron microscopic examination of 3 lymphomas produced by CD tissue filtrates were performed. As a control, lymph nodes from 3 mice which received filtrates of UC or normal tissue were also examined. No viral particles were found in the control lymph nodes. However, each lymphoma produced by CD tissue filtrate contained cytoplasmic particles which look like C type murine virus. In addition budding from the surface of the lymphoma cells was observed [Fig.3].

270

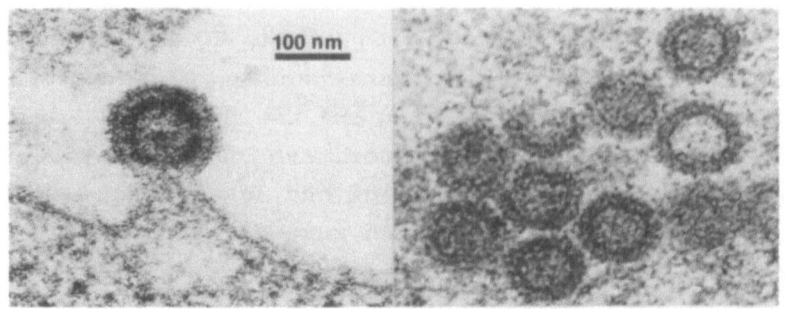

Figure 3. C type murine virus like particles fludding from
the surface of a lymphoma cell

SUMMARY AND CONCLUSIONS

Filtrates of intestinal lymph nodes and mucosa from patients with CD produce lymphoma and immune complex glomerulonephritis in athymic nu/nu mice. These effects are not seen
when similar filtrates are prepared from tissues obtained
from patients with UC or from normal subjects.

Sera from patients with active CD recognize the lymphoma
and the glomeruli. Antigenic recognition of the lymphoma by
CD serum was abolished by absorption with CD mucosa or the
lymphoma.

"C" type virus particles were found in 3 lymphomas.
These results suggests that 0.45μm filtrates of tissues from
patients with CD contained an agent(s) which induced lymphomas in athymic mice directly or by activation of an oncogenic
murine "C" type virus. The antigen persists in the lymphoma.
If the phenomenon of multiplication of the agent(s) in the
nu/nu mice is due to enhanced growth and expression of the
agent, nude mice may serve as an exciting model for further
studies of the putative agent related to Crohn's disease.

ACKNOWLEDGEMENTS

This work is supported by grants NIAMDD-RO1 AM26403 and
N.C.I. - CA 10945-10 from the National Institutes of Health,
Bethesda, Maryland, U.S.A.

REFERENCES
1. Gitnick GL, Arthur MH, Shibata I. Cultivation of viral
    agents from Crohn's Disease. (1976) Lancet 2:215-217

2. Parent K, Mitchell PD. (1978) Cell wall-defective vari-
    ants of Pseudomonas-like (Group Va) bacteria in Crohn's
    disease. Gastroenterology 75:368-372
3. Burnham WR, Lennard-Jones JE, Stanford JL, Bind RG.(1978)
    Mycobacteria as a possible cause of inflammatory bowel
    disease. Lancet 2:693-696
4. Cave DR, Mitchell DN, Brooke BN. (1978) Induction of
    Granulomas in mice by Crohn's Disease Tissues. Gastroen-
    terology 75:632-637
5. Heatley RV, Bolton PM, Owen E, Williams W, Jones WW,
    Hughes LE. (1975) A search for a transmisseble agent in
    Crohn's disease. Gut 16:528-532
6. Armstrong D, Walzer P. (1978) Experimental infections in
    the nude mouse. In: The nude mouse in experimental and
    clinical research. Eds. Fogh J, Giovanella BC. Academic.
    Press, New York. pp 477-491
7. Das KM, Valenzuela I, Morecki R. (1980) Crohn's disease
    lymph node homogenates produce murine lymphoma in athymic
    mice. Proc.Natl.Acad.Sci. 77:588-592

F7 Summary of Discussions relating to topics F5 to F6

Yardley: I wish to confirm Cohen's statement that we have seen material from some of the experimental work done on mouse footpads. There was a recurrent appearance of foreign material in these specimens and frequently foreign body giant cells could be found that had refractive or other intracytoplasmic substance in them. Sometimes hairs had entered the tissue, either with the needle or because of the local injury. I have seen the specimens from Cohen's experiments with injection of the mouse cheek pad. There are large masses of histiocytic cells with numerous giant cells, some of them of the Langhans type. This is unlike any lesion that I have seen in any of the previous material, though there were possible particles in some of these cells which will have to be checked with polarization and other techniques.

One of the problems in working with human tissues, looking for an infectious agent, is what to use as the control. I would suggest that investigators particularly try to obtain tissue from bacterial infections and from other disorders of known cause such as ischaemic colitis.

Diverticulitis is not really a mucosal disease. It is a localized disease where the diverticula have become inflamed, and I do not think it is an appropriate control.

Strober: Das has apparently ruled out the possibility that he is transferring material which induces murine virus to produce a tumour. He finds something in the patients that reacts with the tumour cell surface and potentially this becomes a diagnostic test for CD.

Das: We have now initiated a double blind study of diagnosis and correlation with disease activity using sera collected during the National Co-operative Crohn's Disease Study.

Emerit: Does Das know the paper of Watta and Schwartz about the induction of lymphomas in mice by lymph node and spleen cell extract from dogs with lupus?

Das: They used different animal systems whereas we used nude mice because of their unique immune system defect. There are a number of agents that have been shown to activate the oncogenic viruses. Something is activating the virus particles which we have seen or they happen to be present in the rapidly proliferating cell system. We do not know whether the antigen in the tumour recognised by the CD serum is incorporated in the virus or is incorporated somewhere in the cell.

Hermon-Taylor: I should like to suggest that Das grows his lymphoma in the immune competent relatives of his nu/nu mice, because he may find that they will develop antibodies in their serum to the human component, and this will give him a reciprocal reagent to use on CD tissues.

Das: I think that is an excellent suggestion. We recently injected heterozygous animals but we have not got any results yet.

ACID FAST ORGANISMS IN CROHN'S DISEASE AND ULCERATIVE COLITIS

J.L. STANFORD

INTRODUCTION

The similarities between Crohn's disease and intestinal tuberculosis have made many workers consider the possibility of a relationship although it has never been possible to demonstrate mycobacteria reproducibly in tissues from Crohn's disease. Nevertheless progress in mycobacteriology and the observations being made in sarcoidosis indicated that the time had come for reinvestigating the possibility.

MATERIAL AND METHODS

To avoid the necessity for decontamination procedures lymph nodes draining intestinal lesions were selected for study rather than the gut lesions themselves. Nodes were collected from cases of Crohn's disease, ulcerative colitis and other intestinal lesions. As far as possible no clinical details accompanied the specimens, so that to some extent at least, the study could be considered "blind".

Within a few hours of operative removal, the nodes were ground up with sand in nutrient broth or saline and this inoculum was applied to many different bacteriological media which were incubated for an indefinitely long time at 32°C. When changes were observed in the media subcultures were made and smears of the growth were stained by Gram's and the Ziehl-Neelsen[ZN] method.

To demonstrate that microscopic appearances similar to those found in our cultures could be obtained from a typical mycobacterium an experiment was set up as illustrated in the flow diagram [Table 1]. Organisms were produced that were visually identical to those isolated from the cases of inflammatory bowel disease.

Table 1. In vitro transformation of M. Kansasii into acid fast forms indistinguishable from forms obtainable from culture of Crohn's disease materials.

M. kansasii from L-J medium
↓
glycine and sucrose enriched
liquid medium
↓
abnormal forms
↓
add very dilute human serum
lysozyme [egg lysozyme won't do]
↓
E.M. evidence of cell wall-
defective forms
↓
0.45μ membrane filtration
↓
ZN: abnormal acid fast forms
↓
0.22μ membrane filtration
↓
ZN: negative filtrate
↓
incubate filtrate at 32° for
ten days
↓
ZN: abnormal acid fast forms ⟶ Try to recover typical
indistinguishable from our   culturable mycobacterium
Crohn's cultures   ↓
                              Impossible so far

As a special blind study 15 samples were supplied and coded by Dr. D.N Mitchell and examined in our system. For this series which was known to include mouse passage tissues, very heavy inocula were used on the primary cultures and subcultures onto Löwenstein-Jensen and Robertson's cooked meat media were made after 4 months incubation. These subcultures were examined intermittently by eye and by smear after 3 years. The results were sent to Dr. Mitchell who then broke the code [Table 2].

RESULTS

From 6-18 months after cultures commenced macroscopic changes in some media occurred. Notably on Löwenstein-Jensen slopes a thin iridescent sheen appeared and in Robertson's cooked meat medium a deposit formed at the meniscus; in both cases smears made of the material showed irregular acid fast masses, 2-5 microns in diameter some of which were also Gram positive. This only occurred in some cases and was not present in uninoculated media incubated in the same manner. The material can be subcultured on the same media and the appearance of growth again takes several months. Growth of this kind has been obtained from 42 of 76 nodes from Crohn's disease, 14 of 27 nodes from ulcerative colitis and from 3 of 41 nodes from control patients with other diseases.

The results of the special blind study are shown in table 2. It can be seen that there were 3 [3, 7 and 10] control tissues and one centrifuged supernate [2] that would be expected to yield negative cultures. Of them only the Robertson's culture of specimen 7 was inappropriately positive. Of the remaining 11 samples many of which were mouse passage material, 9 produced positive cultures. One of these cultures [11], produced typical growth of a mycobacterium on Lowenstein-Jensen medium.

Table 2. Results of subcultures onto Löwenstein-Jensen[L/J]- and Robertson's cooked meat medium. Double blind trial.

Code	Specimen	L/J	Robertson's		Result
			Meniscus	Deep	
		ZN	ZN	Gram	Gram	
1	Crohn's [H]	-ve	+ve	-ve	+ve	+ve
2	Supernate from 1	-ve	-ve	-ve	-ve	-ve
3	Control tissue	-ve	-ve	-ve	-ve	-ve
4	Crohn's [M]	-ve	+ve	-ve	+ve	-ve
5	Crohn's [M]	-ve	+ve	-ve	-ve	+ve
6	Crohn's [M]	+ve	+ve	+ve	+ve	+ve
7	1-autoclaved	-ve	+ve	+ve	+ve	+ve
8	Crohn's [M]	+ve	+ve	-ve	-ve	+ve
9	Crohn's [M]	-ve	-ve	-ve	-ve	-ve
10	Sarcoid [H]	-ve	-ve	-ve	-ve	-ve
11	Crohn's [M]	+ve*	-ve	+ve	+ve	+ve
12	Crohn's [M]	+ve	-ve	+ve	+ve	+ve
13	Crohn's [M[	-ve	+ve	+ve	+ve	+ve
14	Crohn's [M]	+ve	-ve	+ve	+ve	+ve
15	Crohn's [M]	+ve	-ve	+ve	+ve	+ve

* Typical mycobacterium grown from this sample
M = murine origin
H = human origin

DISCUSSION

There can be little doubt that an unusual organism producing acid-fast material, if not itself acid-fast, can be isolated with difficulty from a preponderance of mesenteric lymph nodes of patients with IBD. The organism is exceedingly slow growing under the conditions described and its true identity remains uncertain. Early in this work a single isolate of <u>Mycobacterium kansasii</u> was obtained from one of the cultures showing acid-fast material from a case of CD (1). Despite many attempts it has not been possible to obtain any further culturally "normal" mycobacteria except for the strain which has not yet been identified from tissue of mouse origin in the special blind study.

The nature of the acid fast material found in our cultures has not been fully established. It is either made up of sphaeroplastic organisms themselves or is aggregated acid fast matter, perhaps a wax containing mycolic acids which has been released from the organisms.

Certainly the organisms we have isolated are associated with IBD, but whether they are present casually or as the aetiological agent of CD, UC or both, we are still far from proving. However, in the case of CD at least, the association of a potentially granulomagenic organism with a granulomatous disease suggests an aetiological relationship.

CONCLUSION

An abnormal form of acid-fast organism is present in the lymph nodes of many cases of IBD. The identity of this organism remains obscure but there is some collateral evidence that mycobacteria can be made to produce these appearances. It is quite within the theoretical capabilities of such an organism to induce the basic pathological changes of CD.

REFERENCE
1. Burnham WR, Lennard-Jones JE, Stanford JL, Bird RG. (1978) Mycobacteria as a possible cause of inflammatory bowel disease. Lancet 2:693-696

INVESTIGATION INTO THE IDENTITY OF ACID FAST ORGANISMS ISO-
LATED FROM CROHN'S DISEASE AND ULCERATIVE COLITIS

SUSAN A. WHITE

INTRODUCTION

The identity of the acid fast organisms described in the
previous paper remains obscure. Various studies have been
carried out to investigate their relation to Mycobacteria and
inflammatory bowel disease.

Skin tests were performed using the strain of M.kansasii
1129 to test the significance of the isolation. In the first
trial (1), using reagents prepared from 17 Mycobacterial
species and Candida, there was a significantly lower proportion of positive reactions to tuberculin in the patient group
[44%] compared to the control group [71%]. However, there was
a greater proportion of positive reactions to kansasin [1129]
in the patient group [46%] as compared to controls [20%]. No
difference was apparent between the groups with kansasin 8.
When this skin test trial was repeated these results were not
confirmed, an increased proportion of positive reactions to
kansasin was found in control subjects [51%]. However, the
actual number of positive responses separating the two studies was very small.

Serological studies have also been carried out using the
sensitive ELISA technique. Firstly, levels of the different
antibody classes were measured in Crohn's disease, ulcerative
colitis patients and controls against antigens prepared from
M. kansasii 1129 and from the pleomorphic acid fast organisms.

When measured against M.kansasii 1129 antigen, only a
significant increase in IgA class antibodies between Crohn's
disease [CD] patients and controls, as well as between ulcerative colitis [UC] patients and controls was found.

Similarly, when measured against an antigen prepared from

a Crohn's disease mesenteric lymph node culture, there is a significant increase in the levels of IgA class antibodies in CD patients as compared to controls. However, in this case, UC patients do not give a significantly increased value. Although these results would appear to implicate these organisms in the aetiology of Crohn's disease and ulcerative colitis it has been found (2) that inflammatory bowel disease [IBD] patients do tend to have generally raised IgA levels. This may also be an example of the 'leaky gut phenomenon'.

The ELISA technique was also used to help identify the possible cell-wall deficient [CWD] organisms by reacting antigens prepared from some of the cultures against a panel of antisera to various bacterial species. In most cases the highest responses were to M.kansasii related Mycobacteria and Corynebacteria antisera. Other bacterial antisera such as against Klebsiella sp. gave very low responses. This helps confirm that the acid fast organisms belong to the Mycobacterium/Corynebacterium group.

In the present study we cultured the acid fast organisms obtained from Crohn's disease tissue in simple media under different conditions of aeration. In this way, gram positive Coryneform organisms became cultivable.

PROCEDURE

Material from cultures prepared from mesenteric lymph nodes in which gram positive rods were seen and some from those in which they were absent were cultivated into various media including blood agar plates. In each case they were incubated aerobically, anaerobically and under microaerophilic conditions [approximately 6% O_2]. In preliminary attempts to identify the organisms isolated, cell wall amino acids and neutral sugars were determined by thin layer chromatography of acid hydrolysates. The presence of mycolic acids was also detected in a similar manner.

RESULTS

Gram positive Coryneform organisms were seen as follows in table 1 and the results of the cell wall amino acid analysis of the isolates is shown in table 2.

Table 1. Gram positive Coryneform organisms in different cultures

	Acid fast material present	Gram positive Coryneforms present	Gram positive Coryneforms isolated
CD cultures	42 / 76 55%	27 / 76 32%	12 / 76 16%
UC cultures	14 / 27 52%	3 / 27 11%	2 / 27 7%
C cultures	3 / 41 7%	3 / 41 7%	3 / 41 7%

Table 2. Cell wall amino acid analysis of different cultures isolates

Patient No.	Disease	Acid fast material	Mycolic acids	Cell wall amino acids	Cell wall sugars
1	CD	+	+	meso DAP	gal,man ara
2	CD	+	+		
3	CD	+	+		
4	CD	+	+		
5	C	+	+		
6	UC	++	+		
7	CD	++	+		
8	CD	+			
9	CD	+	+		
10	CD	+		L DAP	gal,glu
11	CD	+			
12	CD	+			
13	CD	+			
14	CD	+/-			
15	C	+/-			
16	C	-			
17	UC	+			

When cell wall amino acid analysis was carried out the isolates were as follows in table 2.

One group have L DAP, galactose and glucose in their cell wall which suggests Propionibacterium spp. The other group have also meso DAP and mycolic acids. The structure of these mycolic acids in 7 out of 8 is suggestive of Corynebacterium and the other of a Mycobacterium species. The meso DAP group are still from cultures which contained acid fast material and include one control culture from a patient with Hirschsprung's disease. These organisms have been sub-cultured into Robertson's Cooked Meat medium, [RCM]. There was no acid fast material after three months incubation but after six months incubation some cultures show partially acid fast organisms and also acid fast amorphous material.

DISCUSSION

The ability of the Coryneform organisms to produce acid fast material in RCM medium indicates a direct association between the two. It is known that all the Coryneform genera share some antigens with the Mycobacteria (3) and these shared antigens could account for our serological and skin test findings. O'Grady and his colleagues in 1969 (4), found that patients with Crohn's disease had greatly depressed numbers of diphtheroids at all levels of the gut, as compared to normal subjects. This suggests that IBD patients may have some immunological mechanism, such as IgA, directed specifically against Coryneform organisms.

CONCLUSIONS

Acid fast pleomorphic organisms are found in a large percentage of IBD patients lymph node cultures. Out of a proportion of these cultures, gram positive Coryneform organisms can be isolated which might be of the Corynebacterium or Propionibacterium genera. Much more work is necessary on all these organisms to completely identify and characterise them.

Our observations of these organisms suggest that Inflammatory Bowel Disease may be associated with or caused by an organism from the Mycobacterium-Corynebacterium axis. This organism may assume an unusual [possibly cell-wall deficient] form in the lymph nodes or other tissues: Under these circumstances become cultivable generating acid fast material at the surface of the medium and at a late stage in culture developing into a gram positive Coryneform organism.

REFERENCES
1. Burnham WR, Lennard-Jones JE, Stanford JL, Bird RG. (1978) Mycobacteria as a possible cause of Inflammatory bowel disease. Lancet 2:693-696
2. Asquith P, Thompson RA, Cooke WT. (1971) Quantitation of serum secretory IgA in gastrointestinal disease. Clin. Res. 19:562
3. Stanford JL, Rook GAW, Convit J, Gondal T, Kronvall G, Rees RJW, Walsh AP. (1975) Preliminary taxonomic studies on the Leprosy bacillus. Br.J.Exp.Pathol. 56:579-585
4. O'Grady F, Dawson AM, Dyer NH, Hamilton JD, Vince A. (1970) Patterns of disturbance of the gut microflora in gastrointestinal disease. In: Nutrition. Proc.VIIIth Int. Cong. Nutrition Prague 1969. Eds. Masek J, Osancova K, Cuthbertson DP. Excerpta Medica, Amsterdam pp 438-441

F10 Summary of Discussions relating to topics F8 to F9

Hodgson: Angela Vince, University College Hospital, London, grew out a Corynebacterium which was eventually identified as Corynebacterium bovis from a patient with Whipple's disease. I had hoped we had identified the Whipple's bacillus, but I now wonder whether a leaky gut allowing Corynebacteria into the body accounts for this finding.

Booth: Corynebacteria were described in Whipple's disease by Caroli's group in Paris with Prevot at the Institute Pasteur about fifteen years ago.

Stanford: We are not claiming that these organisms are necessarily aetiological to the disease and it is quite possible that they get in through leaky walls. My interest is primarily in leprosy and when a colleague of mine saw our cultures and slides he could not tell them from organisms cultured from leprosy patients. So both in leprosy and in Crohn's disease we are growing an organism which doesn't follow any of the rules, even for L-forms.

v.d. Waay: The diversity of micro-organisms that are isolated suggests that CD patients do not respond normally to the different micro-organisms. Could one of the immunologists comment on this?

Strober: The probable answer is that you have one or more organisms involved in the pathogenesis of CD, but that organism does not cause disease in every individual. One might postulate that an immunologic deficiency relative to that organism must be present for disease to result.

Phillpotts: I would like to ask Stanford what was present in his cooked meat cultures when he assessed them for contaminants.

Stanford: We started using Robertson's cooked meat as a contamination control. A few of the cultures were obviously contaminated when they were examined after about a week in that they were cloudy and showed all the signs of normal growth and were discarded. We subcultured them on to blood medium and they all contained Coliforms of various varieties. In other samples the medium remains looking precisely like uninoculated medium put up in parallel with it for at least six months and then changes begin to appear. So far we have been unable to grow Corynebacteria directly from biopsy samples and they have only appeared in a small number of those cultures showing acid fast material. The culture for the double blind study were in culture for three years.

Thayer: A number of years ago Manciewicz did some interesting work on mycobacteriophage infected mycobacteria and proposed that this is a mechanism of sarcoidosis. She was able to reproduce a sarcoid-like lesion and noticed that these mycobacteriophage infected organisms did not stain very well and did not grow very well in tissue culture. Could some of your results be due to a mycobacteriophage infected organism?

Stanford: The one strain of Mycobacterium kansasii that we grew out was examined by a colleague of mine who works specifically on mycobacteriophage and he was unable to find any in it.

Peña: I wonder whether Stanford has some information on the world distribution of these organisms and whether this correlates with the high incidence of Crohn's disease in certain areas?

Stanford: Mycobacteria are very unevenly distributed throughout the world. Factors which control their frequency in the environment are temperature, amount of ultra-violet light, water vapour, and very particularly, the pH value of the soil. In Sweden and Norway, mycobacteria are exceedingly common in the sphagnum swamps from which much more of the drinking water is derived. The richest known source of environmental mycobacteria is the grey layer of the sphagnum bog.

PRELIMINARY STUDY OF THE FAECAL FLORA IN FAMILIES OF PATIENTS WITH CROHN'S DISEASE

F. WENSINCK and A.M. SCHRÖDER

INTRODUCTION

It is likely that both genetic and environmental factors are involved in the aetiology of Crohn's disease [CD]. Inheritance appears to be polygenic and, as far as the environment is concerned, it can only be said that the disease is not contagious. In many cases, intestinal infections [by Campylobacter, Yersinia, viral infections, 'ulcerative colitis'] appear to trigger the onset of CD. In a previous investigation (1) we found that the faecal flora of patients with CD localized in the terminal ileum differs from the flora of apparently healthy subjects by higher numbers of anaerobic gram-negative rods [Bacteroides, Fusobacterium] and of anaerobic coccoid rods [species of Eubacterium and Peptostreptococcus]. Neither duration of illness nor ileocaecal resection had an effect on flora composition and it appears that the Crohn flora is permanently abnormal. To investigate whether prolonged intimate contact with a CD patient has an effect on the flora of familial household contacts we analysed the flora of married patients, their spouses and children and of unmarried patients, their parents and siblings. The preliminary results are presented in this paper.

PROCEDURE

The relevant data on patients and contacts are given in table 1. Faeces were cultured within 2 h after passage according to the methods described by Wensinck et al. (1). The median number of samples cultured from patients was 6 [3-10] and from the other subjects 3 [2-5]. The floras were characterized by ^{10}log median numbers of anaerobic gram-negative and coccoid rods.

Table 1. Composition of the families of Crohn's patients

	Patients	Spouses	Children	Parents*	Siblings*
Number	10	8	20	4	3
Age **	41 [22-59]	44 [25-52]	16 [5-34]	52 [48-56]	20 [11-28]
Duration of illness**	15 [3-20]				
Married [children]	7				
No. of children	20				
- median [range]	3 [1- 6]				
Married [no children]	1				
Unmarried	2			4	3
Total period of contact**		16 [5-25]	16 [5-25]	23 [11-25]	13 [11-21]
-after onset of disease		15 [5-25]	14 [4-22]	10 [0-16]	3 [0- 8]
Faecal flora determined	10	8	20	4	3

* Data refer to family members of two unmarried patients.
** Median; range in parentheses [years].

RESULTS

Fig. 1 shows the results of a previous investigation of the faecal flora of CD patients (1). The floras of the patients form a cluster which is well separated from the normal cluster. The line of demarcation is used in Figs. 2,3 and 4. As shown in Fig. 2, the floras of the married patients – except the flora of a patient using salazopyrin for years – are within the Crohn's cluster and those of the spouses in the normal cluster.

288

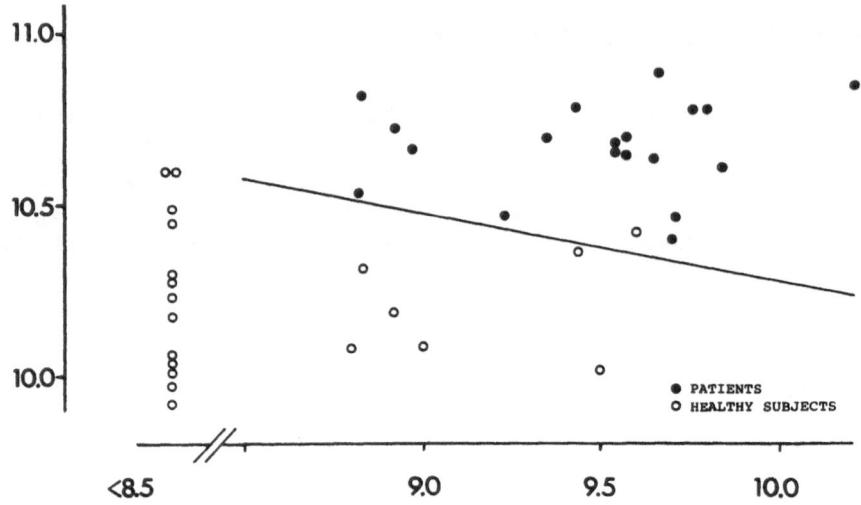

Figure 1. ^{10}Log median numbers of gram-negative rods [abscissa] and coccoid rods [ordinate] in Crohn's disease and controls(1).

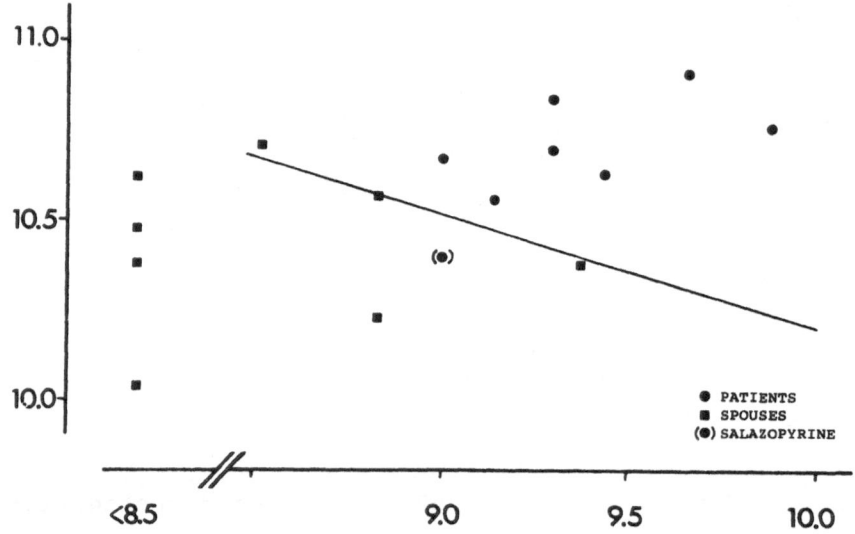

Figure 2. ^{10}Log median numbers of gram-negative rods [abscissa] and coccoid rods [ordinate] in married Crohn's patients and their spouses.

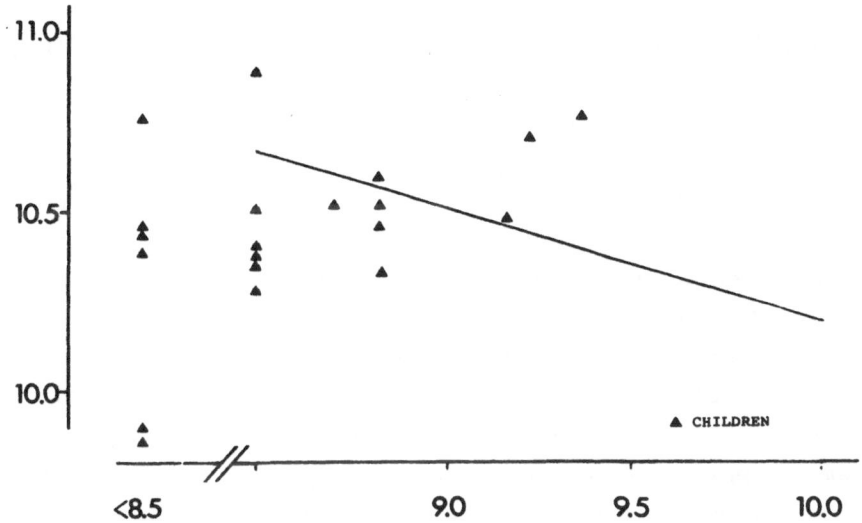

Figure 3. ^{10}Log median numbers of gram-negative rods [abscissa] and coccoid rods [ordinate] in children of patients affected with Crohn's disease.

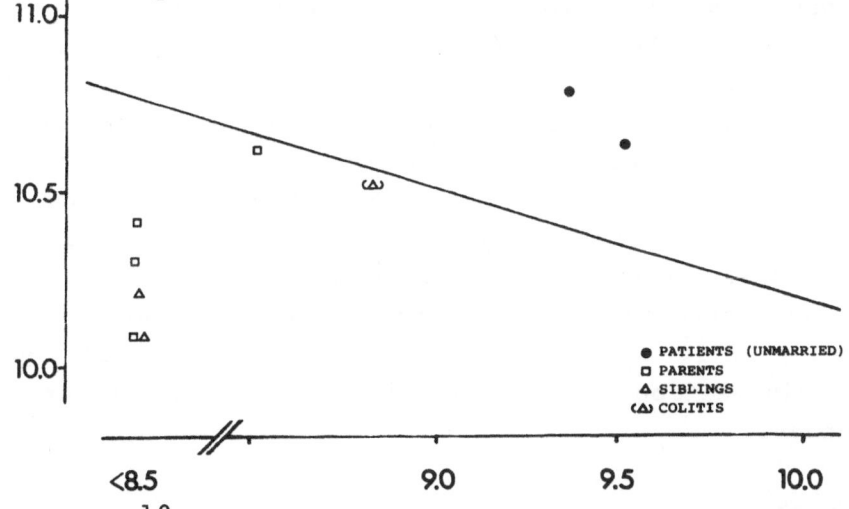

Figure 4. ^{10}Log median numbers of gram-negative rods [abscissa] and coccoid rods [ordinate] in two un-married Crohn's patients, their parents and their siblings.

From the children [Fig. 3], 17 have a normal flora, 2 a Crohn flora and the position of one flora is uncertain [high numbers of anaerobic gram-negative rods but low numbers of coccoid rods].

Two unmarried patients have a Crohn flora, their parents

and siblings a normal flora [Fig. 4]. Thus, from 35 familial household contacts 32 have a normal flora, 2 a Crohn flora and 1 an intermediate flora.

DISCUSSION AND CONCLUSIONS

This preliminary study of the faecal flora of contacts of CD patients shows that an intimate contact for years does not result in the installation of a Crohn flora in most of the 35 familial contacts. This holds for contacts already exposed in early childhood as well as for adults. The two children with a Crohn flora are daughters [12 and 14 years of age] of two female patients and both have been under medical treatment for chronic diarrhoea and atypical appendicitis respectively. In our opinion the Crohn flora is a necessary determinant of the disease and may be an expression of the genetic predisposition. The two girls with the Crohn flora may thus be considered to be predisposed to the disease. As far as we know the intestinal flora of families has only been studied in connection with methane production, due to the presence of relatively high numbers of metabolically active methane bacteria in the intestinal tract (2,3). When both parents produce methane [expired in quantities of 20 p.p.m. or more] their children nearly always do as well. Early colonization by methane bacteria seems to be due to environmental and not to genetic influences. In the case of the Crohn flora, genetic predisposition appears to be much more important than environment.

REFERENCES
1. Wensinck F, Custers-Lieshout van LMC, Poppelaars-Kustermans PAJ, Schroder AM. The faecal flora of patients with Crohn's disease. J. of Hygiene 1981 in press
2. Bond JH jr., Engel RR, Levitt MD. (1971) Factors influencing pulmonary methane excretion in man: an indirect method of studying the in situ metabolism of the methane-producing colonic bacteria. J.Exp.Med. 133:572-588
3. Levitt MD. (1974) Methane production in the gut. New Engl.J.Med. 291:528-529

A POSSIBLE ROLE OF EUBACTERIUM AND PEPTOSTREPTOCOCCUS SPECIES IN THE AETIOLOGY OF CROHN'S DISEASE

J.P. VAN DE MERWE

INTRODUCTION

The faecal flora of patients with Crohn's disease [CD] has been found to contain higher numbers of anaerobic gram-negative rods [Bacteroides and Fusobacterium] and anaerobic gram-positive coccoid rods [Eubacterium and Peptostreptoccus] than the flora of healthy subjects (1,2). Ileocaecal resection and duration and severity of illness had no effect on flora composition which suggests that the "abnormal" flora not merely results from the inflammatory process (3) but is likely to be the resident intestinal flora of subjects predisposed to CD.

To four strains of the coccoid rods, identified as Peptostreptococcus [strain C_{18}], Eubacterium contortum [strain Me_{44} and Me_{47}] and Eubacterium rectale [strain Me_{46}], agglutinating antibodies were found in a considerable percentage of sera from patients with CD (4). In patients with ulcerative colitis, other diseases and in healthy subjects, these antibodies were found less frequently, allowing them to be used as a diagnostic test (4,5).

The agglutinins to the coccoid rods are predominantly IgG and IgM antibodies (6). To investigate a possible role of the coccoid rods and the specific antibodies in the pathogenesis of CD, activation of complement by the bacteria and biological effects of antibodies such as activation of complement and opsonization were studied.

MATERIALS AND METHODS

Sera were obtained from patients with CD and selected for the presence of antibodies to the coccoid rods. Antibodies were demonstrated as described elsewhere (4).

Bacteria were sensitized with test samples as described previously (6). Unless mentioned otherwise, test samples were heated for 30 min at 56°C to inactivate complement.

Bacteria and sensitized bacteria were tested for complement fixation (7) by incubation during 16h at 4°C with guinea-pig complement. Residual complement was measured by the degree of lysis of the haemolytic system. The anticomplementary titre of samples is given by the highest dilution which produces 50% lysis of the red cells. Test samples were undiluted and diluted CD sera. Control experiments showed that three unsensitized strains inhibited red cell lysis. To see whether this occurred by activation of the alternative pathway, the classical pathway was prevented with Mg EGTA (8,9). Before addition to the haemolytic system, 0.1 ml of 100 mM $CaCl_2$ per ml of sample was added.

Opsonization was studied with neutrophils from healthy subjects. Test samples were whole CD sera, IgG and IgM fractions obtained by gel filtration, specifically absorbed fractions and IgG fractions with anti-Me_{46} antibodies from patients with colonic carcinoma. Neutrophils were suspended in concentrations of 2.10^6 cells/ml in "Hijmans" fluid (10). To 0.2 ml of cell suspension, 0.2 ml of "Hijmans" fluid and 0.2 ml of the suspension with [sensitized] bacteria were added and the mixture was incubated for 30 min at 37°C under continuous rotation. The tubes were centrifuged for 10 min at 90g, the pellet was washed and resuspended, and gram-stained slides were prepared. Ingested bacteria were seen in large puffy vacuoles, in clear contrast to those adhering onto the cell surface. The percentage of cells with ingested bacteria was calculated from duplicate counts of 200 cells. All tests were performed in duplicate and the coefficient of variation was 13%. Preliminary experiments showed that, when bacteria were ingested, phagocytosis was correlated with the amount of specific antibody. Phagocytosis of whole serum was slightly lower than with the corresponding IgG fraction if the serum contained both specific IgG and IgM antibodies, otherwise phagocytosis was similar to that induced by the IgG fraction.

Results are, therefore, given for the IgG and IgM fractions only. In addition, the opsonizing effect of complement was tested with fresh sera.

RESULTS

Complement activation: Strains C_{18}, Me_{46} and Me_{47} activated complement in contrast to Me_{44} [Table 1]. When the classical pathway was prevented, complement was still activated by the same strains, indicating alternative pathway activation.

Sensitized bacteria showed similar anticomplementary titres as unsensitized strains and anticomplementary activity could be caused, therefore, by the bacteria themselves. When bacteria were sensitized with diluted serum samples, anticomplementary activity of C_{18} diminished indicating that it was partly caused by antibodies; antibodies to the other strains lacked complement fixing properties.

Table 1. Binding of complement by coccoid rods and antibodies

Pretreatment of bacteria[a]	Anticomplementary titre with strain[b]			
	Me_{44}	C_{18}	Me_{46}	Me_{47}
Saline [n=4]	0[0-0]	8[4- 8]	32[32-64]	32[32-64]
CD serum [n=5]	0[0-0]	8[4-38]	8[4-16]	16[8-32]
CD serum				
undiluted	0	32	16	32
1/2-1/4	0	8	16	32
1/8-1/1024	0	4	16	32
CD serum and anti-Ig[n=2][c]	64	64	64	64
anti-Ig	0	8	32	16

a Pretreatment during 1h at $20^{o}C$.
b Median value and range.
c Treatment in 2 steps of 1h each at $20^{o}C$.

Opsonization: Coccoid rods sensitized with IgM were not ingested. With specific IgG antibodies, marked phagocytosis was observed of Me_{44}, C_{18} and Me_{47}; anti-Me_{46} from CD patients failed to induce phagocytosis in contrast to anti-Me_{46} from 2 patients with colonic carcinoma. Complement induced phagocytosis of all strains [Table 2].

294

Table 2. Phagocytosis of coccoid rods by neutrophils

Pretreatment of bacteria	Neutrophils containing bacteria [%][a]			
	Me_{44}	C_{18}	Me_{46}	Me_{47}
Specific IgM from CD [n=4]	1[0- 3]	15[4-20]	19[16-22]	1[0- 3]
Specific IgG from CD [n=4]	65[61-70]	80[76-83]	17[13-21]	86[84-90]
after specific absorption	11[10-13]	6[3- 7]	19[18-19]	23[20-26]
Complement [fresh serum]	95[90-99]	93[89-96]	92[87-96]	97[89-99]
Specific IgG from CC [b]	n.t.	n.t.	62[57-67]	n.t.

[a] Median value and range
[b] Two patients with colonic carcinoma

DISCUSSION

Two findings suggest a role of strain Me_{46} in the pathogenesis of CD. Firstly, like C_{18} and Me_{47}, it activates complement. Secondly, antibodies to Me_{46} from patients with CD fail to induce phagocytosis of Me_{46}, in contrast to those from two non-CD patients. These data suggest an inadequate defence against Me_{46} in patients with CD. Under physiological conditions, complement is not available in the external secretions of the bowel; when the intestinal mucosal barrier is breached from any cause however, complement can bind to strain Me_{46}. This may result in two effects (11). Firstly, strain Me_{46} initiates activation of complement by the alternative pathway. Secondly, C3b bound onto the surface of Me_{46} induces phagocytosis by neutrophils that will be attracted by chemotactic stimuli of complement cleavage products. Both effects probably occur in the mucosal area and result in comsumption of complement with release of major mediators of inflammation and an increased turnover rate of neutrophils in patients with active CD.

The absence of opsonizing and complement fixing properties of antibodies to Me_{46} in patients with CD suggests that they belong to the IgG_4 subclass. The capacity to produce antibodies of one or another subclass to particular antigens is under genetic control and shows geographic variations (12,13). The production of the non-opsonizing antibodies to strain Me_{46} in patients with CD, may thus be a reflection of the genetic predisposition for CD (14) and warrants further study of genetic determinants on immunoglobulins.

Our interpretation of the findings implies some initial intestinal damage before CD becomes manifest in predisposed subjects. This damage may result from enteritis caused by viruses, Yersinia, Salmonella, Campylobacter, clostridial toxins but also from ulcerative colitis and diverticulitis. This suggestion is in line with known associations between CD and some of these conditions (14-16).

CONCLUSIONS

Strains C_{18}, Me_{46} and Me_{47} activate complement by the alternative pathway and may thus be pathogenic. Antibodies to C_{18} and Me_{47} had opsonic properties. Antibodies to Me_{46} from CD patients failed to induce phagocytosis, in contrast to those from 2 patients with colonic carcinoma. Any inflammation of the bowel may thus initiate a chronic inflammatory process by bringing complement in contact with Me_{46} in the mucosal area. The genetic predisposition for CD is suggested to consist of the presence of strain Me_{46} in the resident intestinal flora and the property to produce non-opsonizing [IgG_4?] antibodies against strain Me_{46}.

REFERENCES
1. Wensinck F. (1975) The faecal flora of patients with Crohn's disease. Antonie van Leeuwenhoek 41:214-215
2. Wensinck F. (1976) Faecal flora of Crohn's patients. Serological differentiation between Crohn's disease and ulcerative colitis. In: The management of Crohn's disease. Eds. Weterman IT, Peña AS, Booth CC. Excerpta Medica, Amsterdam pp 103-105
3. Wensinck F, Custers-Lieshout v LMC, Poppelaars-Kustermans PAJ, Schroder AM. The faecal flora of patients with Crohn's disease. Journal of Hygiene 1981 in press
4. Wensinck F, Merwe Van de JP. Serum agglutinins to eubacterium and peptostreptococcus species in Crohn's and other diseases. Submitted for publication

296

5. Merwe van de JP, Schmitz PIM, Wensinck F. Antibodies to Eubacterium and Peptostreptococcus and the estimated probability of Crohn's disease. Submitted for publication
6. Merwe van de JP. (1980) Serum antibodies to anaerobic coccoid rods in Crohn's disease. M.D. Thesis Rotterdam
7. Verrier Jones J, Cumming RH. (1977) Tests involving the reaction of immune complexes with complement. In: Techniques in clinical immunology. Blackwell Scientific Pub., Oxford pp 138-142
8. Bryan CS. (1974) Sensitization of E.coli to the serum bactericidal system and to lysozyme by ethyleneglycolte-traacetic acid. Proc.Soc.Exp.Biol.Med. 145:1431-433
9. Fine DP. (1977) Comparison of ethyleneglycoltetraacetic acid and its magnesium salt as reagent for studying alternative complement pathway function. Infect.Immunol. 16:124-128
10. Steffelaar JW, Graaff-Reitsma de CD, Feltkamp-Vroom TM. (1976) Immune complex detection by immunofluorescence on peripheral blood polymorphonuclear leucocytes. Clin.Exp. Immunol. 23:272-278
11. Frank MM. (1979) The complement system in host defense and inflammation. Rev.Infect.Dis. 1:483-501
12. Natvig JB, Kunkel HG. (1973) Human immunoglobulins: classes, subclasses, genetic variants, and idiotypes. Adv.Immunol. 16:1-59
13. Fudenberg HH, Pink JRL, An Chuan Wang, Douglas SD. (1978) In: Basic immunogenetics. Oxford University Press, New York pp 69-74
14. McConnell RB. (1972) Genetics of Crohn's disease. In: J. Clin. Gastroenterol. Ed. Brooke BN. Vol 1, pp 321-334
15. Meyers MA, Alonso DR, Morson BC, Bartram C. (1978) Pathogenesis of diverticulitis complicating granulomatous colitis. Gastroenterology 74:24-31
16. Bolton RP, Sherriff RJ, Read AE. (1980) Clostridium difficile associated diarrhoea: a role in inflammatory bowel disease? Lancet 1:383-384

F13 Summary of Discussions relating to topics F11 to F12

Lennard-Jones: I was interested in results from Birmingham
            which suggested that metronidazole in normal sub-
            jects, affects the faecal flora very little. I
            thought it would be interesting to combine metroni-
            dazole with co-trimoxazole remembering that metro-
            nidazole affects particularly anaerobes and co-tri-
            moxazole affects aerobes. It seemed that this rela-
            tively safe antibacterial combination might perhaps
            be useful in the treatment of Crohn's disease. We
            began by organizing a small study of the effect of
            this drug combination on the faecal flora and the
            flora of rectal mucosal biopsies. The work has been
            done by M. Hudson in collaboration with M. Hill at
            the Bacterial Metabolism Research Laboratory in
            London and by Elliott and Burnham. We selected
            patients with acute active CD who were on no treat-
            ment. A faecal specimen was taken through the sig-
            moidoscope and at the same time a rectal mucosal
            biopsy was taken. Both these specimens were imme-
            diately put into a cryoprotective medium which
            protects the bacteria during freezing so that the
            specimen can be transported to the laboratory and,
            if necessary, stored aerobic and anaerobic cultures
            are performed. After the specimens had been obtain-
            ed, the patients were started on treatment with
            metronidazole 200 milligrammes 3 times a day and
            co-trimoxazole two tablets twice a day. Further
            faecal and biopsy specimens were taken 10 or 14
            days later.
                We were interested in the mucosal flora because
            we felt that this was more intimately in contact
            with the tissues. The faecal flora was quantitati-

vely greater than the mucosal flora but the proportions of the various bacteria were roughly the same in the two samples. There was no significant change in the total flora during the two weeks of treatment with this antibacterial regime. There was a marked fall in the faecal Bacteroides fragilis count (p=<0.02) but, unlike the results you have just heard, there was no obvious difference between the patients that responded and those who did not respond. There was also a fall in the B. fragilis count in the mucosal flora (p=<0.01). The total count remained approximately the same, because there was an increase in other bacterial types, in particular in the Streptococci which became the dominant flora. It is thus clear that this antibacterial combination has very large effects on both the faecal flora and the mucosal flora. What we are now interested in studying is whether or not the addition of a drug such as co-trimoxazole given in combination with metronidazole gives a clinically different effect to metronidazole alone.

Would Wensinck comments on the relative importance of anaerobic gram-negative rods and coccoid rods? I noticed from your diagram, that the total anaerobic gram negative rods are increased by about one log, if one takes the median from your diagram, whereas the anaerobic coccoid rods seem to be greatly increased over normal.

Wensinck: The total number of anaerobes is 10.65 in healthy subjects and 10.85 in the Crohn group, a very significant difference. This increase of total numbers is due to about a three-fold increase of the gram-negative anaerobic rods. The coccoid rods are also increased but that does not greatly affect the total number, because the numbers are low.

Cohen: Do you have any figures for differences in the faecal flora between CD and UC?

Wensinck: We cultured faeces of some UC patients but most patients take salazopyrine. When there is severe diarrhoea with blood, the total numbers of anaerobes decrease.

Strickland: Do you have any data on the faecal flora in other disease controls, such as radiation enteritis?

Wensinck: No.

Krook: Were the samples from CD patients without treatment and for how long?

Wensinck: The patients had not been treated with salazopyrine, corticosteroids, metronidazole or azathioprine for several months prior to the examination of the stools.

Mayberry: Does Wensinck think that altering the microbial flora of patients with CD is likely to improve their condition, or that inducing a change such as the one he describes, will induce CD in healthy subjects?

O'Morain: I noticed all of his patients had a terminal ileitis; could an element of obstruction account for some of his results?

Wensinck: In this group, no patients with colitis were included. All 22 patients we investigated with terminal ileitis have this flora and therefore we think that the flora is a necessary determinant of the disease. This does not mean that all people with this flora must get CD.

Fernandez: What is the relation between the constancy of the faecal flora, the abnormal flora and the titre of the antibodies? Is there any change with treatment?

v.d. Merwe: There is no relation between titres to the coccoid rods and parameters such as disease activity measured by the CD-activity index, α_1-acid glycoprotein or serum albumin level. There are positive correlations with other clinical parameters such as colonic CD, patients with fistulae and those with high immunoglobulin levels.

CHANGES IN THE FAECAL FLORA DURING TREATMENT WITH METRONIDA-
ZOLE OR SULFASALAZINE

AUD KROOK, D. DANIELSSON, G. JÄRNEROT and J. KJELLANDER

INTRODUCTION

In the search for etiological factors in Crohn's disease
the attention has also been directed to the possibility of a
change of the normal bowel microflora. As gut bacteria live
in close contact with the bowel mucosa, there is good reason
to believe that they play a primary or secondary role in the
pathogenesis of Crohn's disease. Observations such as increased immune response to Escherichia coli and Bacteroides
fragilis in patients with Crohn's disease (1) support this
hypothesis. The hypothesis is further supported by the fact
that metronidazole, which is highly active against anaerobic
bacteria has a good effect in some patients with Crohn's
disease (2,3) and that sulfasalazine which also has an antibacterial effect is effective in active Crohn's disease (4).
However, both these drugs have several other pharmacological
effects such as chemotactic, immunosuppressive and anti-inflammatory properties.

In an uncontrolled pilot study (5), we observed a dramatic decrease of the concentration of Bacteroides species in
the faeces of the patients with Crohn's disease who responded
to therapy, but no change was observed in controls or the
non-responders. To get more evidence of the effect on the
faecal flora during treatment with metronidazole or sulfasalazine a controlled study was performed in 20 patients with
Crohn's disease (6) and 10 healthy volunteers (7).

PROCEDURES

Eleven men and 9 women with Crohn's disease were studied
[age 12-37 years]. The duration of the disease was between 3
months and 10 years. Twelve patients had not had any medical

or surgical treatment before. No bowel resection had been performed. Fourteen patients had highly active Crohn's disease according to the criteria of the Cooperative Crohn's disease study in Sweden (CCDSS,3). Using a double dummy technique, these patients were randomized to oral treatment with metronidazole [400 mg twice daily] or sulfasalazine [1.5 g twice daily] with cross-over after 4 months of treatment. Six other patients had less active disease and were treated openly with metronidazole or sulfasalazine for 4 months.

The control subjects were treated blindly with metronidazole or sulfasalazine for two weeks with crossover for two further weeks treatment so that each control subject was given both drugs.

Faecal samples were collected before and during treatment. All samples were coded as one group and read by code. The samples were processed in the laboratory within 30 minutes after defaecation for quantitative and qualitive counts of aerobic and anaerobic bacteria. For this purpose tenfold dilutions of the samples were carried out in pre-reduced peptone yeast broth under an oxygen-free [10% hydrogen in carbon dioxide] gas flow. 0.1 ml of each dilution was inoculated into media for total counts of aerobic and anaerobic bacteria and selective media for Gram negative rods. The plates were incubated for 2 days aerobically and 6 days anaerobically after which time the number of different colonies were calculated. With the method used bacteria present in concentrations $>10^5$ colony forming units [cfu] per g could be demonstrated. Isolated anaerobic species were identified as described by Holdeman et al. (8). For fermentation tests the Minitek system [Miniaturized Micro-organism Differentation System, BBL] was used.

RESULTS

Only the evaluation of the first treatment period will be referred to. Five patients in the metronidazole and 7 in the sulfasalazine group completed 4 months of treatment. Eight patients dropped out because of treatment failure or drug intolerance. However, the faecal flora was studied in all 20 patients. Eleven control subjects started treatment. Two dropped out due to drug intolerance, one in the metronidazole and one in the sulfasalazine group. Thus faecal studies were performed in 9 subjects.

The pretreatment samples of the patients in the present study contained a higher count of E. coli than of the control subjects [p<0.02]. This count did not change significantly during treatment.

Patients

In the pretreatment samples, different Bacteroides species were the most common anaerobes isolated [9.7 $\pm$ 0.87][*]. Among the aerobic bacteria Escherichia coli [8.0 $\pm$ 1.04] and faecal streptococci [7.9 $\pm$ 1.20] dominated.

During metronidazole treatment there was a statistically significant decrease [>1 log] of the Bacteroides count [p<0.02] and an increase [> 1 log] of the streptococci count [p<0.02]. In the sulfasalazine group the bacterial count at the end of treatment was not changed significantly.

Regarding the correlation between treatment response and bacteriological chances in faeces during treatment, pronounced decrease of the Bacteroides count [> 3 log, i.e., 99.9%] was seen in five of the eight patients who responded well to therapy [S-orosomucoid value decreased > 33%] and in one non-responder.

Control subjects

In the pretreatment samples, the counts of Bacteroides were 9.2 [$\pm$ 0.85][*], E coli 6.2 [$\pm$0.99] and of faecal streptococci 6.5 [$\pm$ 0.63].

During treatment the Bacteroides count was increased [> 1 log] in one of four subjects in the metronidazole group and decreased in one of five in the sulfasalazine group. Faecal streptococci increased in two of four subjects in the metro-

[*]mean bacterial count, ^{10}log [$\pm$ 1 SD], per g wet weight

nidazole group and anaerobic Gram positive cocci and Bifido-
bacteria decreased in two of four and three of four respectively. No obvious changes were noted in the rest of the
healthy individuals. However, the number of control subjects
was too small for statistical evaluation.

DISCUSSION

The effect of metronidazole on the Bacteroides count was
significant in the patients but not in the controls. The
reason for this finding could be that microbiologically active metronidazole concentrations occurs in the large bowel
in inflammatory bowel disease but not in healthy volunteers.
We have demonstrated concentrations of metronidazole in bowel
content of treated patients with Crohn's disease but not in
control subjects (9). Such a condition could be due to a
less complete absorption of metronidazole in these patients
because of a decreased gut transit time. Another explanation
could be an exudation of metronidazole across the mucosa.

The most pronounced decrease of the Bacteroides count was
seen in patients who responded well to therapy. The one
non-responder with a decreased Bacteroides count in faeces
had a large intra-abdominal abscess which had to be drained
surgically.

It is likely that Bacteroides play a primary or secondary
role in the pathogenesis of Crohn's disease. As Bacteroides
are normally the most common bacteria in the colon, and in
these patients also in the lower ileum, a defect in the mucosa barrier could make it possible for the bowel bacteria to
initiate or modify the inflammatory process.

CONCLUSION

In patients with Crohn's disease the Bacteroides concentration in the faecal flora was generally decreased during
metronidazole treatment. Sulfasalazine did not induce the
same change. The most pronounced changes were seen in patients who responded well to treatment. The faecal flora in
control subjects was only slightly influenced by metronida

zole or sulfasalazine treatment.

REFERENCES
1. Persson S, Danielsson D. (1979) On the Occurrence of Serum Antibodies to Bacteroides fragilis and Serogroups of E. coli in Patients with Crohn's disease. Scand.J.Infect.Dis. suppl. 19: 61-67
2. Ursing B, Kamme C. (1975) Metronidazole for Crohn's disease. Lancet 1:775-777
3. Ursing B, Alm T, Bárány F, Bergelin J, Ganrot-Norlin K, Järnerot G, Krause U, Krook A, Rosén A. (1980) Cooperative Crohn's disease study in Sweden. Manuscript in preparation
4. Summers RW, Switz DM, Sessions JT Jr., Becktel JM, Best WR, Kern F Jr., Singleton JW. (1979) National Cooperative Crohn's Disease Study: Results of Drug treatment. Gastroenterol. 77:847-869
5. Krook A, Danielsson D, Kjellander J, Järnerot G. (1979) Changes in the Faecal Flora of Patients with Crohn's disease during treatment with Metronidazole. A preliminary report. Scand.J.Gastroenterol. 14:705-710
6. Krook A, Danielsson D, Kjellander J, Järnerot G. (1980) The effect of Metronidazole and Sulfasalazine on the Faecal Flora in Patients with Crohn's disease. Submitted for publication
7. Krook A. (1980) Effect of Metronidazole and Sulfasalazine on the normal human faecal flora. Submitted for publication
8. Holdeman LV, Cato EP, Moore WEC Eds. (1977) Anaerobic Laboratory Manual, 4th Ed. Virginia Polytechnic Institute and University, Blacksburg, Virginia
9. Krook A, Lindstrom B, Kjellander J, Jarneröt G, Bodin L. (1980) Concentrations of Metronidazole in Plasma and Faeces of Patients with Crohn's disease and healthy controls. Manuscript in preparation

F15 Summary of Discussions relating to topic F14

Wensinck: I see that the total number of anaerobes in
               both the studies of Krook and Lennard-Jones are
               rather low. You cultivated faeces within 15 minutes
               after passage and we always culture within two
               hours, so the difference in total numbers of anae-
               robes must lie in the anaerobic technique. What
               type of anaerobic technique do you use?

Krook: We worked on the bench not in a cabinet; when
               we compared some of these samples with the same
               samples processed in a cabinet both the total
               counts and the <u>bacteroides</u> counts were the same.
               Air was evacuated and we used 6 percent carbon
               dioxide in hydrogen.

Lennard-Jones: Samples were studied by Hudson using the
               technique originally described by Drasar with an
               anaerobic chamber.

Wensinck: Fusiform bacteria may be responsible for the
               difference in response to metronidazole between
               healthy people and Crohn's patients.

Booth: What you demonstrate are the bacterial counts
               in conditions of favourable culture in a laboratory
               which may bear no relationship to what is happening
               in the lumen of the intestine in contact with the
               mucosa.

Lennard-Jones: This is a very important point and some bio-
               chemical observations have been made on the stools
               of these patients to check it. But, as I think you

will agree, there is a change in the distribution of the bacteria before and after treatment, however we interpret it.

Strober: The period that elapsed between the production of the stools samples and the collection and culturing was up to 15 minutes. This could be considered a long time for culturing anaerobic specimens.

Lennard-Jones: Our specimens were collected by a method described by Drasar in which they are taken straight into a special medium and then deepfrozen. He has shown that this is a very good way of preserving the specimens in a form in which they can be transported until they are cultured.

Wensinck: When you follow the total numbers of bacteroides in faeces placed in the refrigerator or on the bench you get small losses within say four or five hours. Other anaerobes maintain their numbers so I do not feel that his technique gives the wrong impression on the composition of the intestinal flora. There is a great difference between the mucosal flora and the intestinal flora; the ratio between anaerobes and aerobes is about 300 to 1 in the intestine, but in the mucosa it is about one to one. This may be because the oxygen pressure is much higher in the mucosal wall than in the lumen.

Lennard-Jones: When Tabaqchali studied the mucosa of patients with CD, the ratio of aerobes to anaerobes was greater than in the normal subject.

v.d. Merwe: Did Krook observe any differences in in vitro sensitivity to metronidazole in her bacteroids species in responding and non-responding subjects?

Krook: We cannot see any difference between the res-
           ponders and non-responders.

Thompson: Super-infection with Clostridium difficile has
           been reported and we have observed cases. This
           organism will be eliminated by treatment with me-
           tronidazole. Have the patients in the Krook or
           Lennard-Jones's series, been screened with the
           faecal toxin test before treatment? Is there any
           risk of peripheral neuropathy with metronidazole
           treatment?

Krook: In our study 13 of the patients were studied
           for the toxin, 7 of them before treatment; no toxin
           was detected and we did not isolate Clostridium
           difficile from any sample.

Lennard-Jones: We did not isolate Clostridium difficile but
           the toxin was not looked for. The manufacturers
           have told me that peripheral neuropathy has been
           observed with long-courses of metronidazole. We are
           in favour of short courses of the drug.

Järnerot: In the Crohn's disease Co-operative studies in
           Sweden, we have given 400 milligrams of metronida-
           zole twice a day for four months and none of the 40
           patients has been withdrawn because of drug toxi-
           city.

SPECIFIC IMMUNOGLOBULIN E ANTIBODY TO E.COLI 0127 B8 IN SERA OF PATIENTS WITH INFLAMMATORY BOWEL DISEASE

H.F.SEWELL, M.K. BASU, R.A. THOMPSON, VICTORIA FLACK AND P.ASQUITH

INTRODUCTION

The aetiology of inflammatory bowel disease [IBD], is unknown but there is considerable evidence suggesting the participation of immunological processes. It has been speculated that a type 1 reaction may be especially involved. Employing a red cell linked antigen-antiglobulin reaction [RCLAAR] assay, a polyclonal antibody response directed to the antigen E.coli has been found in serum (1). We report here the detection of specific IgE antibodies to E.coli 0127 B8 in the sera of patients with IBD using the RCLAAR and also by an indirect immunofluorescent assay.

MATERIALS AND METHODS

Serum or plasma samples were obtained from 8 patients with CD and 8 with UC attending the Alastair Frazer and John Squire Metabolic and Clinical investigation Unit, East Birmingham Hospital. The diagnosis was made using accepted criteria (2). Control sera were from 10 members of staff of the Departments involved in this study. The passive haemagglutination assays which allowed performance of the RCLAAR assays for detection of antibody classes, were performed as previously described (1). The indirect immunofluorescent assay used intact E.coli organisms at a concentration of 1×10^9 per millilitre of buffer. Fluorescein labelled sheep anti-human IgM, IgG, IgA and IgE antisera were obtained from Wellcome Reagents Ltd., England.

RESULTS

Using the RCLAAR assay, anti E.coli antibodies of IgM, IgG and IGA classes were detected in all sera [Table 1].

Table 1. Class of antibodies [anti E.coli 0127 B8 antibodies] detected by RCLAAR and indirect immunofluorescence [IgE anti E. coli 0127 B8 antibodies]

control sera	Antiglobulin [RCLAAR]					Fluorescence
	IgM	IgG	IgA	IgD	IgE	IgE
1	+	+	+	-(+)	-	-
2	+	+	+	-(+)	-	-
3	+	+	+	-	-	-
4	+	+	+	-	-	-
5	+	+	+	-	-	ND
6	+	+	+	-	-	ND
7	+	+	+	ND	-	-
8	+	+	+	ND	-	-
9	+	+	+	ND	-	-
10	+	+	+	ND	-	-

IBD sera		Antiglobulin [RCLAAR]					Fluorescence
	Diagnosis	IgM	IgG	IgA	IgD	IgE	IgE
1	CD	+	+	+	+	+	w+
2	CD	+	+	+	+	+	+
3	CD	+	+	+	-	+	w+
4	CD	+	+	+	-	+	w+
5	CD	+	+	+.	-	ND	w+
6	CD	+	+	+	-	-	-
7	CD	+	+	+	+	+	w+
8	CD	+	+	+	-	-	w+
9	UC	+	+	+	-	+	ND
10	UC	+	+	+	-	+	ND
11	UC	+	+	+	ND	+	w+
12	UC	+	+	+	ND	+	+
13	UC	+	+	+	ND	+	+
14	UC	+	+	+	ND	+	w+
15	UC	+	+	+	ND	-	-
16	UC	+	+	+	ND	+	w+

+ = positive agglutination/fluorescence. - = no agglutination/negative fluorescence. w+ = weak positive fluorescence. (+) = detection of IgD antibodies after absorption of sera with IgM, IgG and IgA (1). CD = Crohn's disease. UC = Ulcerative colitis.

however, only 3 [all CD] of 10 [8CD and 2UC] IBD sera, and 2 of 6 of control sera tested for IgD antibodies were positive - the latter only after absorption of the sera with polyvalent anti IgM, IgG and IgA. IgE antibodies could be demonstrated in 5 of 7 CD sera and 7 of 8 UC sera but in none of the 10 control sera. With respect to the indirect immunofluorescent test, again no IgE antibodies could be demonstrated in control sera, with one exception [Table 1] there was a good correlation using both assay systems.

DISCUSSION

Specific IgE antibodies to the E.coli 0127 B8 antigen have been found in the sera of patients with IBD but not in the control sera. It is highly likely that the serum IgE antibody detected was induced in immunocompetent tissue associated with the intestine. In terms of disease pathology, it is conceivable that the IgE antibody directed against an intraluminal microbial antigen, say E.coli, could induce relapse or perpetuate damage. Furthermore, it could also play a permissive role in the development or intensification of other hypersensitivity mechanisms.

REFERENCES
1. Sewell HF, Chambers L, Maxwell V, Matthews JB, Jefferis R. (1978) The natural antibody response to E.Coli includes antibodies of IgD class. Clin.Exp.Immunol.31:104-109
2. Schachter H, Kirsner JB. (1975) Definition of inflammatory bowel disease of unknown aetiology. Gastroenterology 68:591-602

FLUORESCENCE IMMUNO-ASSAY FOR MONITORING OF "ACTIVITY" OF GUT ASSOCIATED LYMPHOID TISSUE

H.K.F. VAN SAENE and D. VAN DER WAAIJ

INTRODUCTION

The Gut Associated Lymphoid Tissue [GALT] is considered to play an important role in infection prevention and in excluding the absorption of antigens [immune exclusion]. Secretory immunoglobulin A [S-IgA] on the mucous membranes may be involved in this protective GALT activity by interfering with bacterial adherence. Attachment to mucosal surfaces via fimbriae may be a prerequisite for many bacteria to colonize and to penetrate the digestive tract. Adherence of fimbriaeted bacteria is apparently inhibited by S-IgA, because the latter blocks interaction fimbriae and mucosal surface. The anti-adhesive or coating phenomenon of S-IgA may therefore be a more important measure of the functional characteristics of S-IgA than the simple quantitation of S-IgA in serum and secretions. In the present study we discuss an in vitro test system, the fluorescence immuno-assay [FIA] to determine the coating's incidence as a functional parameter of GALT activity [GALT-FIA].

MATERIALS AND METHODS

The procedures of GALT-FIA were described in detail elsewhere (1). The test consists of two stages: a first phase in which S-IgA coated faecal bacteria - after visualisation with conjugate - were detected by immunofluorescence and a second stage in which those IgA positive intestinal bacteria - after incubation at 37° C - were subcultured and subsequently identified and typed. For technical reasons, the faecal bacteria chosen for screening were the Enterobacteriacae.

To study "normal" values for the coating's incidence, ten healthy volunteers have screened by means of the technique.

They were sampled for approximately 8 subsequent weeks: 116 samples could be evaluated.

The group of patients in relapse of inflammatory bowel disease [IBD], 7 patients with Crohn's disease and 6 with ulcerative colitis included 141 faecal samples. All IBD patients were hospitalized for more than 4 weeks and all recieved sulfasalazine; no steroids, immunosuppressive or anti-diarrhoea drugs were given. In 7 Crohn patients the disease was active and in all there was colonic involvement.

RESULTS

From the 116 stool samples [an average of 11.6 per volunteer] a total of 2003 Enterobacteriaceae colonies were isolated and identified. 76% of these colonies were found to be resident: all resident types were Escherichia coli subtypes. Statistical analysis revealed that a coatings incidence of about 40% could be considered as the mean and that a percentage of 12.5 could represent the 95% confidence underlimit.

In 141 stool samples of the 13 IBD patients [an average of 10 samples per patient] 1193 Enterobacteriaceae colonies were isolated. Again more than 70% of the colonies were found to be resident. The isolated resident strains were typed as Escherichia coli, Enterobacter cloacae, Klebsiella pneumoniae and Citrobacter freundii. Only 6% of these Gram-negative bacilli were coated with IgA. In all 13 IBD patients the coatings incidence for all strains was found to be underneath the underlimit.

DISCUSSION

These observations that statistically reduced numbers of S-IgA coated Gram-negative bacilli are found in IBD patients possibly reflect a dysfunction of the Gut Associated Lymphoid Tissue, the apparatus controlling the colonization pattern of Enterobacteriaceae.

CONCLUSIONS

In IBD patients the coating's incidence of aerobic Gram-negative bacteria is apparently significantly reduced. This could play a role in the pathogenesis concerning a "leaky" digestive tube permitting antigen absorption leading to stimulation of the central immune sytem [T-and B-cells].

ACKNOWLEDGEMENTS

We wish to thank Mr. J. Krikken and Mrs. E.van Santen for technical assistance. We are also grateful to Dr. V. Fidler for statistical advice.

REFERENCE

1. Saene van HKF, Waaij van der D.(1979) A novel technique for detecting IgA coated potentially pathogenic microorganisms in the human intestine. J.Immunol.Methods 30:87-96

F18 Summary of Discussions relating to topics F16 to F17

Lloyd-Still: Why did Asquith decide to study E.coli 0127 and does he have data on other E.coli? We have also noted very high total IgE levels, but not specific to E.coli 0127.

Asquith: We looked at several antigens but the specific antibodies to the other antigens were fairly similar in control subjects, UC, CD, Coeliac disease and liver disease. CD patients seemed to have higher levels to E.coli 0127 and B8 and so we studied this antigen.

Gebbers: We find an increase of IgE cells near ulcers in CD and we find many granulocytes staining for a common coli antigen. It will be interesting to look for the specific E.coli 0127.

Douwes: What about patients with a damaged mucosa for reasons other than IBD?

Asquith: The diverticular disease group had a similar haemagglutination titre to the IBD patients; we were able to split them only by the more refined techniques.

Jewell: When I was using this test some years ago I got different results according to the method of coupling. How specific was your anti-IgE serum?

Asquith: Most commercial antisera have some non-specific reactivity. Our antiserum was evaluated by Stanworth in the Immune Standards Laboratory of the University of Birmingham and R.A. Thompson who also works in a standard reference laboratory for the preparation of specific immunoglobulin antisera.

F19 General Discussion and Conclusions
Reported by J.E. Lennard-Jones and J. Versteeg

The following points emerged from a detailed discussion:
Cytopathic effect

All workers agreed that a cytopathic effect can be demonstrated when Crohn's disease tissue homogenates or filtrates are inoculated into certain cell cultures. There was disagreement as to whether this effect is due to a virus or a toxic chemical. An exchange of materials, as is being done in the United States, was recommended to resolve some of the outstanding differences. It was emphasized that initial attempts to grow a virus, even when its presence is known, are often difficult until the optimal cell line is found. The difficulty in Crohn's disease [CD] is great because we do not know whether a virus is present or not.

Transmission experiments

Work on the mouse footpad and the rabbit ileum, despite much effort, have given disappointing results. The marked granulomatous reaction, alluded to in the discussion, when mouse peritoneal macrophages were exposed to CD tissue homogenates and then injected into the mouse cheek pad, deserves further study.

The induction of a lymphoma in thymus-deficient nude mice on injection of Crohn's tissue homogenates needs repeating on a large scale. In the experiments so far the incidence of lymphoma was at least four times that expected to occur spontaneously in this type of mouse at the age used. The increased frequency with which the tumours occur might be due to a number of factors. The observed cross-reaction between Crohn's tissue and mouse tumour and kidney tissue was promising, but more observations are needed on its specificity.

Faecal flora

It is not known whether the increased proportion of anaerobic gram-negative rods and coccoid rods in the faeces of patients with terminal ileal CD precedes or follows the onset of the disease. Epidemiological studies have shown that patients with CD tend to eat more refined carbohydrate than control subjects; the question was asked whether dietary factors might affect the faecal bacterial flora. The use of chemical methods to measure the metabolic activity of the intestinal flora was recommended.

Studies have shown a marked fall in the Bacteroides count and rise in the faecal Streptococci count during treatment with metronidazole, whether or not combined with co-trimoxazole, the significance of these changes is at present not clear.

Cell-wall-deficient bacteria

It was agreed that organisms in this form have rarely, if ever, been shown to cause disease, though it has been suggested that they can excite a granulomatous response. The finding of acid-fast organisms, possible derived from cell-wall deficient forms, in the draining mesenteric lymph nodes of intestine involved by CD or UC was noted with interest. The question was asked as to why, if the organisms play a role in pathogenesis, they excite a granulomatous response in patients with the manifestations of CD but not in those with UC.

Inter-action between enteric organisms and Host antibodies

Although IgA-coated bacteria were observed with decreased frequency in the faeces of patients with CD as compared with controls, it is not possible to interpret this finding because the mode of action of S-IgA in the protection of the mucosa is not clear. The specificity of IgD and IgE antibodies to E.coli 0127 B8 in CD was questioned. Further controls among patients with IBD other than CD of UC should be studied. The functional role of IgG is stimulating phagocytosis and the absence of opsonizing activity against certain bacteria in patients with CD could indicate a defective defence mechanism in some patients.

SECTION G

Immunological Aspects

Section Editor: W. Strober

320

Gut mucosal lymphocytes

METHODS FOR THE DETECTION OF CIRCULATING IMMUNE COMPLEXES

M.R. DAHA and L.A. VAN ES

INTRODUCTION

Immune complexes can cause glomerulonephritis and vasculitis in both man and animals (1). This conclusion is based on the detection of immune complexes in the circulation of patients with these abnormalities and also on the fact that antibodies, antigens and complement components have been found within the sites of inflammation. In addition, disease can be reproduced in experimental animals by inducing the formation of large quantities of immune complexes or by the intravenous infusion of pre-formed immune complexes.

In recent studies, wherein new assays have been employed for the detection of immune complexes, complexes have been found in the serum of patients not only with vasculitis and glomerulonephritis but also with many other diseases, such as serum hepatitis, infectious endocarditis, rheumatoid arthritis, ulcerative colitis, Crohn's disease and malignancies. It should be noted that the presence of circulating immune complexes not always leads to vasculitis and glomerulonephritis.

There are many methods to determine immune complexes in sera of patients with a wide variety of diseases. However, it is not always clear which type of immune complex, as regards size, antigen to antibody ratio etc. are detected by the various methods. By using standards in the assay procedure, it is possible to get some homogeneity in the expression of results. One of the accepted ways of expressing the amount of immune complexes present in a certain sample is, by comparison with aggregated human IgG. Good results have been obtained with soluble IgG aggregates of restricted size which are stabilized with bovine serum albumin (2). By constructing a standard curve for aggregated IgG, the level of immune complexes may be compared from day to day within one assay procedure. It is however not possible to relate results in one assay method with another method on a quantitative basis.

PROCEDURE

The determination of immune complexes [IC's] in the circulation may be based on:
a] their size; b] the presence of immunoglobulins in the immune complexes; c] the presence of complement components in the immune complexes.

a] Methods based on separation by size

Density gradient ultracentrifugation analysis may be applied for the separation of large complexes from the smaller plasma constituents. IC's may also be precipitated with polyethylene glycol [PEG]. The amount of precipitated protein may also serve as a measure of the amount of IC's present in the original sera.

Because the precipitation of some complexes is temperature dependent [cryoproteins], it is possible to isolate IC's found in such cryoprecipitates.

b] Methods based on the presence of immunoglobulins in
    IC's

Interaction with cells.

Platelets aggregate after their surface Fc receptors interact with IC or aggregated immunoglobulin. Based on this property, a platelet aggregation assay for detection of IC's has been developed. The method is sensitive, but is hindered by non-reproducable platelet preparations, and by aggregation with materials other than IC's such as rheumatoid factor.

The use of Raji cells, a Burkitt lymphoma-derived cell line with some B-cell properties, may also be used to detect IC's. Raji cells possess low affinity receptors for the Fc part of complexed IgG and high affinity receptors for C3b, C3d, C1q and possibly other complement components. IC's present in patient's serum may be bound to the cells and subsequently detected either with fluorescent or radiolabeled anti-immunoglobulin. The test is sensitive, but some sera containing antibodies against Raji cells may give rise to false positive results.

In a fashion similar to the Raji cells, guinea pig peritoneal macrophages has been used to detect IC's. These cells have Fc and C3 receptors and are capable of phagocytizing IC's present in sera. The internalized IC's can be detected with anti-IgG or anti-C3.

The inhibition of antibody dependent cellular cytotoxicity [ADCC] a cytotoxicity reaction based on interaction of immunoglobulin with Fc receptors on effector cells [K-cells] has been used to detect IC's. In this case, the IC's interfere with the arming of K-cells for the cytotoxicity reaction.

The direct polymorphonuclear phagocytosis test is based on the detection of immunoglobulin [IgG, IgA, IgM] and complement factors [Clq, C3] in the leucocytes in peripheral blood of patients with IC's. On the indirect test, normal PMN's, are incubated with patients serum, and subsequently assessed for internalized IC's by measuring fluorescence with FITC-labeled anti-IgG or anti-complement.

Several methods for the detection of IC utilizing monoclonal or polyclonal rheumatoid factor [RF] have been described. Monoclonal RF's, mostly readily obtained from patients with lymphoproliferative diseases precipitate IC in gel more efficiently than polyclonal RF. The disadvantage is, that monoclonal RF's vary greatly in the amount of monomeric IgG that inhibits RF interaction with complexed immunoglobulin.

The monoclonal RF inhibition radioimmunoassay described by Gabriel and Agnello (5) is based on the ability of IC to inhibit the binding of ^{125}I-labeled monoclonal RF to an insoluble substrate, IgG-Sepharose. The use of monoclonal RF with a high avidity for complexed IgG minimizes any interference by polyclonal RF or monomeric IgG. In a similar way Ig specific IC assays were developed by preparing low affinity IgM antibodies with specificity for IgG or IgA (2).

c] Methods based on interaction of IC's with complement.

It is known that certain IC's are capable of activating the complement system. By incubation of patient's sera with an exogenous source of complement, IC's present in the patient's sera may induce complement consumption. The amount of complement consumed serves as a measure of the amount of IC's present. This assay is used very often; it is extremely sensitive to day-to-day variation.

One of the most sensitive, reliable and rapid method of detection IC's is the fluid phase Clq-binding assay. This method is based on the observation that ^{125}I-labeled-Clq reacts with the Fc portions of IgG and IgM in complexed form. The complex of ^{125}I-Clq-IC may be precipitated with PEG, and the amount of ^{125}I-Clq precipitated serves as a measure for the concentration of IC (3). A disadvantage of the method is that polyanions, DNA, endotoxin, C-reactive protein, and heparin bind Clq and may interfere with the assay.

Clq bound to plastic tubes may be used to detect IC's (4). In this assay bound Clq is interacted with serum containing IC and subsequently washed. The IC bound to the Clq are detected by using ^{125}I-labeled anti-IgG or by Elisa techniques. This technique has proven to be reliable and accurate; however, for reasons that are not clear, there is no correlation between this method and the fluid phase Clq binding method.

Since it is known that IC may activate complement in the circulation, the levels of complement may provide information on the presence of IC. On the other hand, the amount of complement consumption may be too low to be detected as a decrease in overall complement levels. In these cases, the determination of C3 breakdown products, namely C3d, may be helpful. It should be noted however, that complement activation may not only be caused by IC, but also by other products, such as bacteria and other complement activating reagents.

IC may activate complement and acquire C3 breakdown products. These types of IC may be detected by the conglutinin binding assay. Conglutinin is a bovine plasma protein, capable of reacting with C3 breakdown products. In this assay purified bovine conglutinin is absorbed to plastic tubes; sera containing IC bearing C3 breakdown products will bind to the conglutinin and may subsequently be detected with anti-IgG, anti-IgA or anti-IgM. This assay is very reproducible and seems to detect IC which are released from vessel walls by the action of complement.

CONCLUSIONS

From the description of techniques for the detection and measurement of IC's in biologic fluids, it is clear that no universal reagent is available for demonstrating IC's. The application of various methods simultaneously in longitudinal studies in disease, should allow evaluation of the various IC-assays. When used together the existing IC-assays may yield complementary information because of their different properties and reagents. The use of stabilized aggregated IgG as a reference standard may allow comparisons between laboratories as long as the same methods are used.

REFERENCES
1. Cochrane CG, Koffler D. (1973) Immune complex disease in experimental animals and man. In: Advances in Immunology Eds. Dixon FJ, Humphrey JH. Acad.Press, New York Vol 16 pp 185-264
2. Kauffmann RH, Es van LA, Daha MR. (1979) Aggregated human immunoglobulin G stabilized by albumin: a standard for immune complex detection J.Immunol.Meth. 31:11-22
3. Zubler RH, Cange C, Lambert PH, Miescher PA. (1976) Detection of immune complexes in unheated sera by a modified 125I-Clq binding test. J.Immunol. 116:232-235
4. Hay FC, Nineham LJ, Roitt JM. (1976) Routine assay for the detection of immune complexes of known immunoglobulin class using solid phase Clq. Clin.Exp.Immunol. 24:396-400
5. Gabriel A Jr, Agnello V. (1977) Detection of immune complexes. The use of radioimmuno assays with Clq and monoclonal rheumatoid factor. J.Clin.Invest. 59:990-1001

CIRCULATING IMMUNE COMPLEXES IN CROHN'S DISEASE

R.D. SOLTIS

INTRODUCTION

Despite recent studies to the contrary we have been un-succesful in detecting immune complexes [IC] in Crohn's disease [CD]. Our negative result (1) is supported by a recent WHO collaborative study, in which no differences between CD and normal sera were demonstrated in 18 different IC assays (2). In most previous positive studies the IC reactivity in CD sera could be explained by a variety of factors other than IC. First, Clq precipitins in CD sera are small [μ 4S] and may not therefore represent IC (1). Second, activated Cl is present after fractionation of both normal and CD sera and produces anticomplementary activity (3). Third, recent studies suggest that Cl, rather than IC, affects the agglutination of IgG-latex by Clq or rheumatoid factor and therefore that these agglutination inhibition assays are probably incapable of detecting IC (4). Finally, heat inactivation of serum at 56°C produces immunoglobulin aggregates [AGG], the quantity being directly proportional to IgG and inversely proportional to albumin [ALB] concentrations; sera with abnormalities in the concentrations of these proteins, a common finding in CD, may give false-positive results in IC assays following heat-inactivation, due to formation of AGG (5).

In addition to these factors, we have suggested that AGG may form in vivo in conditions associated with hypergammaglobulinemia and hypoalbuminemia. Our previous studies demonstrated that monomeric IgG, when added to buffer or normal serum and incubated at 37°C under sterile conditions, underwent aggregation, but the addition of ALB inhibited such aggregation (6). In active CD, hypoalbuminemia is common, but serum IgG concentrations may be normal or slightly decreased, presumably due to enteric loss.

The present study sought to determine: 1] whether native IgG in normal serum, present in low-normal concentrations, would aggregate at 37°C in the presence of hypoalbuminemia; 2] whether structural IgG alterations in IgG, such as desialation, would facilitate IgG aggregation and 3] whether high molecular weight IgG could be detected in CD sera and, if so, whether it had characteristics of AGG rather than antigen-antibody complexes [AG-AB CX].

PROCEDURE AND RESULTS

Aggregation of endogenous IgG in hypoalbuminemic serum. Normal serum, depleted of ALB by absorption with Affi-gel Blue [4°C x 4 hrs] was reconstituted with ALB or saline, sterile filtered, and incubated at 37°C. 200 µl aliquots were fractionated on 10-40% sucrose density gradients and high molecular weight IgG [>11S] was quantitated by RIA [Table 1].

Table 1. Amount of high molecular weight IgG found in > 11S Fraction

	ALB= 15 g/l IgG= 3.6 g/l	ALB= 32 g/l IgG= 3.0 g/l
No incubation	71 µg/ml	76 µg/ml
37°C x 6 days	164 µg/ml	55 µg/ml
37°C x 12 days	454 µg/ml	78 µg/ml

The results shown in table 1 demonstrate that endogenous IgG, even at low-normal concentration, aggregates in the presence of hypoalbuminemia, when incubated at 37°C.

Aggregation of desialated IgG. CD sera were treated with neuraminidase to desialate IgG and other glycoproteins [0.01 unit neuraminidase/mg protein, or buffer, in 0.1 M acetate, pH=5.1, 37°C x 4 hrs, followed by dialysis against 0.1 M TRIS-NaCl-EDTA, pH=6.8] and tested for ^{125}I-Clq binding [Fig.1]. The increase in ^{125}I-Clq binding was associated with an increase in high molecular weight IgG [>11S] as demonstrated by ultracentrifugation.

330

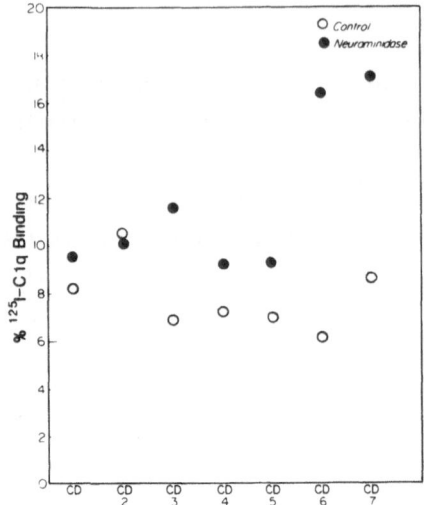

Figure 1. ^{125}I-Clq binding by neuraminidase-treated or control-treated sera.

High molecular weight IgG in CD sera: Preliminary studies sought features which might distinguish AG-AB complexes from AGG. We found that IgG AGG are almost totally dissociated at pH=3.0, reaggregation at 4°C is slow [days], and is inhibited by the presence of ALB. By contrast, although soluble AG-AB CX formed in antigen excess are dissociated at pH=3.0, soluble complexes formed near equivalence or in antibody excess are not dissociated. Soluble AG-AB complexes reassociate rapidly [hours], and this is not inhibited by ALB (manuscript submitted for publication).

To determine if either AG-AB complexes or AGG, might be present in CD, sera were dialysed against pH=7.4 or pH=3.0 buffers. After 16 hours at 4°C each was diluted 1:2 with 1% ALB and then dialysed against pH=7.4 buffer for 24 hours at 4°C. 200 µl aliquots were fractionated on 10-40% sucrose density gradients, pH=7.4, containing 1% ALB. ^{125}I-thyroglobulin and catalase were used as internal reference markers in each gradient. IgG was quantitated by RIA in fractions >19S and in fractions 11-19S from each gradient. Figure 2 summarizes the methods used and the expected results for AG-AB complexes and AGG. As shown in Figure 3, increased amounts of 11-19S IgG were present in three CD sera which, after dissociation at pH=3.0, did not reassociate at pH=7.4 in ALB. Thus, the high molecular weight IgG present in these sera behaved like AGG rather than AG-AB complexes.

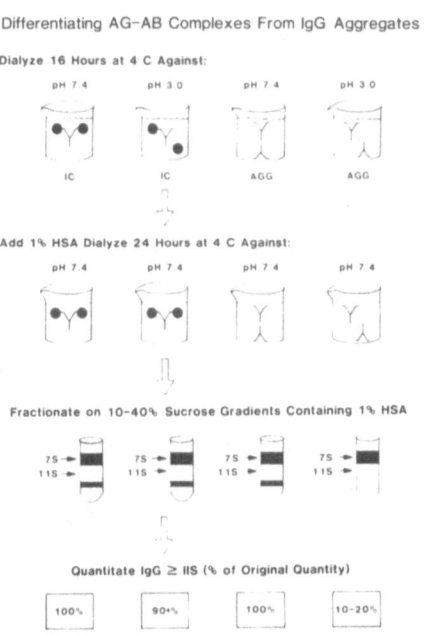

Figure 2. Differentiation of AG-AB CX from AGG by dissociation at pH=3 and reassociation at pH=7.4 in the
presence of ALB.

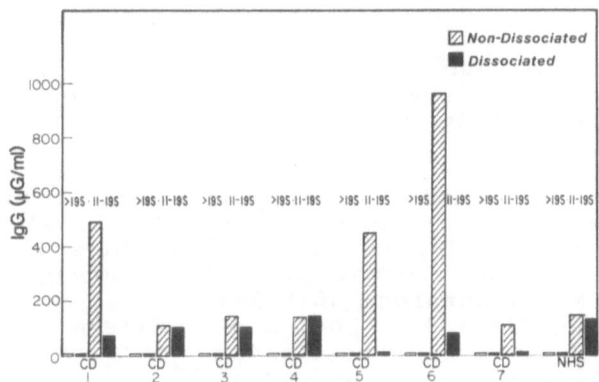

Figure 3. High molecular weight IgG in CD sera at pH=7.4 or
following preliminary dissociation at pH=3.0

DISCUSSION AND CONCLUSIONS

Although IC reactivity in CD sera has been previously reported, this reactivity may have been due to other serum components such as small Clq precipitins, activated Cl or IgG aggregated *in vitro* by heat-inactivating serum. In addition, we have suggested that IgG may aggregate *in vivo*. Factors which would facilitate IgG aggregation include: 1] hypergammaglobulinemia; 2] hypoalbuminemia, even with low-normal serum IgG concentrations; and 3] desialation of IgG, which may occur in various infectious and inflammatory conditions. All three factors may be present in active CD and could lead to IgG AGG formation in vivo.

Preliminary studies have shown the presence of increased amounts of high molecular weight IgG in three of seven CD sera tested. Following dissociation at low pH, this IgG did not reassociate at neutral pH in the presence of ALB. These results suggest that this IgG has characteristics of IgG AGG rather than AG-AB complexes.

ACKNOWLEDGEMENT

Supported by USPHS grant number AM-26086.

REFERENCES
1. Soltis RD, Hasz DE, Morris MJ, Wilson ID. (1979) Evidence against the presence of circulating immune complexes in chronic inflammatory bowel disease. Gastroenterology 76:1380-1385
2. Lambert PG, Dixon FJ, Zubler RH, et al. (1978) A WHO collaborative study for the evaluation of eighteen methods for detecting immune complexes in serum. J.Clin.Lab. Immunol. 1:1-15
3. Soltis RD, Hasz D, Morris MJ, Wilson ID. (1979) Studies on the nature of heat-labile anti-complementary activity in normal human serum. Clin.Exp.Immunol. 33:310-322
4. Hallgren R. (1979) Human serum inhibits the interaction between Clq or rheumatoid factor and IgG-coated latex particles. Immunology 38:529-537
5. Soltis RD, Hasz DE, Morris MJ, Wilson ID. (1979) The effect of heat inactivation of serum on aggregation of immunoglobulins. Immunology 36:37-45
6. Soltis RD, Wilson ID. (1979) Are immune complexes immunoglobulin aggregates? In: Protides of the Biological Fluids, Ed. H. Peeters, Pergamon Press, Oxford 26:127-130

COMPLEMENT ACTIVITY IN CROHN'S DISEASE

D.P. JEWELL, B.J. POTTER, D.J.C. BROWN, H.J.F. HODGSON and A.S. MEE

INTRODUCTION

The mechanisms inducing the inflammation of Crohn's disease [CD] are unknown. Antigen-antibody reactions may be one such mechanism as there is an increase in the immunoglobulin-producing cells and an increase in immunoglobulin synthesis within the inflamed mucosa. Since complement activation plays a major role in immune complex-mediated tissue injury, we investigated the complement system in these patients.

PROCEDURE

A] Serum concentrations of complement components

Concentrations of Clq, C4, C3 and Factor B were measured by single radial immunodiffusion. The inhibitors of the complement cascade, ClINH, C3bINA and β_{1H} were determined by rocket immunoelectrophoresis.

B] Metabolic studies

Clq and C3 were purified from fresh human serum (1,2). Both substances were labelled with ^{125}I and tested for immunological and biological activity. Following injection into patients, serial serum samples were taken and all urine and faeces collected. Plasma disappearance curves of radioactivity were analysed by multi-exponential analysis.

C] Immunoconglutinin concentration

Sera were decomplemented by heat inactivation and absorbed with sheep erythrocytes. Serial dilutions were made and immunoconglutinins detected by the addition of EAC43 antrypol (human) reagent. A titre of greater than 1 in 4 was regarded as positive.

RESULTS

A] Serum concentration of complement components

The mean concentrations of C3 [1460 ± 43 mg/l] and Factor B [232 ± 9.0 mg/l] were significantly higher in CD patients than in control subjects[1040 ± 50 mg/l, 165 ± 10 mg/l respectively, p<0.05]. Patients with active CD had significantly higher concentrations than those in remission. Concentrations of Clq were not significantly altered. ClINH was elevated [390 ± 29 mg/l n=35] in CD patients compared with controls [261 ± 18 mg/l n=28] and also behaved as an acute phase reactant. Patients with either active or quiescent CD had significantly higher concentrations of C3bINA [p<0.01] than controls but there was no differences among the patients [Active 182 ± 16% normal pool[NP] n=21; quiescent 173 ± 17% NP n=14; controls 108 ± 6% normal pool n=28]. β_{1H} values in CD patients did not differ from controls [CD 460 ± 28 mg/l, n=32; Controls 417 ± 23 mg/l, n=26].

Table 1 shows that in six CD patients coming to surgery, the concentrations of C3, ClINH and C4 in portal venous blood were similar to those in peripheral blood.

Table 1. Mean and range [mg/l] of complement levels

	C3	ClINH	C4
Portal blood	942	303	374
	[590 - 1200]	[205 - 435]	[240 - 570]
Peripheral blood	932	323	382
	[590 - 1080]	[255 - 450]	[180 - 620]

B] Metabolic studies

In metabolic studies utilizing iodinated Clq and C_3 the mean fractional catabolic rates of Clq and C3 in CD were 5.99 ± 1.14 and 3.23 ± 0.14% IV pool/hr respectively compared with values of 2.34 ± 0.23 and 2.05 ± 0.19% IV pool/hr in healthy control subjects. This increased catabolism in CD was not accounted for by faecal losses. The turnover data showed increased extra vascular sequestration of complement in the patients as compared to controls.

C] Immunoconglutinin concentration

Immunoconglutinin titres greater than 1 in 4 were present

in 29% of 41 patients with CD compared with 25% of 32 healthy controls. Nevertheless, the presence of immunoconglutinins correlated with disease activity [Table 2].

Table 2. Immunoconglutinins and disease activity
    Active disease   [n=27]   37% positive
    Remission   [n=14]   14% positive

DISCUSSION

The rise in serum C3 and Factor B in patients with active CD has been previously noted but there is little change in the concentration of Clq. The metabolic studies, clearly indicate increased catabolism of Clq and C3 in patients with active disease as well as extra-vascular sequestration of the complement components. The latter is presumed to occur in the inflamed intestine. Complement activation in patients with active disease is supported by the increased incidence of antibodies to activated complement components with these immunoconglutinins directed towards activated C3 and C4 for the most part. One explanation for increased complement activation would be a failure to modulate the complement system. However, this study shows that there is no deficiency of the major complement regulators in CD. Lake et al. (3) have suggested a functional disorder of the alternate complement pathway during relapses of the disease. The relationship between this finding and the raised concentrations of C3bINA but normal β_{1H} levels, requires further study.

CONCLUSIONS

There are no deficiencies of the major complement components or their regulators in CD. Complement activation is suggested by increased metabolism of Clq and C3, and by the association of immunoconglutinins with active disease.

REFERENCES
1. Hodgson HJF, Potter BJ, Jewell DP. (1977) C3 Metabolism in UC and CD. Clin.Exp.Immunol. 28:490-495
2. Potter BJ, Hodgson HJF, Mee AS, Jewell DP. (1979) Clq Metabolism in UC and CD. Gut 20:1012-1019
3. Lake AM, Stitzel AE, Urmson JR, Walker WA, Spitzer RE. (1979) Complement alterations in inflammatory bowel disease. Gastroenterology 76:1374-1379

G4 Summary of Discussions relating to topics G1 to G3

Hermon -   Soltis, why didn't you use two-dimensional
Taylor: electrophoresis isoelectric focusing to analyse your
             separated aggregates? This would have given you the
             ability to identify dissociated poly-peptides and
             the altered pI associated with the loss of the nega-
             tive charge in the desialation of the oligosaccha-
             ride moiety chains. If you apply peptide mapping to
             your aggregates, you would also be able to finger-
             print any antigens that were present in immune com-
             plexes.

Soltis: I think that is a very good suggestion.

Strober: I wonder if you have examined the more classi-
             cal diseases that have been associated with immune
             complexes to determine if in those cases also the
             complexes are, in reality, IgG aggregates.

Soltis: I have been intrigued for the past two years
             with the fact that so many diseases (132 at last
             count) are associated with immune complexes in the
             circulation. These conditions are always character-
             ized by hypergammaglobulinemia or hypoalbuminemia,
             particularly if the diseases are active; I suspect
             that perhaps even in classical immune complex dis-
             eases such as lupus, in part what is being detected
             are aggregates. A few years ago we naively asked why
             antigen-antibody complex assays were developed which
             utilize aggregates rather than antigen-antibody com-
             plexes, as the assay standard. We found that it is
             relatively difficult to form antigen-antibody com-
             plexes in the test tube and to react in these assays
             whereas aggregates are highly reactive. I suspect
             that is one reason why they have been used. Since

these assays were designed to detect aggregates, it is not unfair to suggest that that is what they primarily detect. I have been told by my colleagues that perhaps we have re-invented the sedimendation rate.

Strober: Have you examined the sera of CD that have extra-intestinal manifestations for the presence of immune complexes?

Soltis: In our study reported last year we did measure IC in CD patients with the extra-intestinal manifestations and did not find serum IC.

Tijtgat: In support of Soltis' presentation I would like to add that we too, in collaboration with the Central laboratory in Amsterdam for Blood transfusion were unsuccesful in finding circulating immune complexes in a large group of patients with active CD.

Thayer: I would also like to answer Strober's question. In our negative study we used the Clq inhibition assay and we used as controls lupus and rheumatoid patients. They were often positive whereas the Crohn's patients were negative. Primary biliary cirrhosis is positive in about 50% of cases in our assay.

Booth: What light does this throw on mechanisms of tissue damage, I have never really believed immune complex cause tissue damage.

Soltis: There is evidence from in vitro studies of what aggregates could do but there have been relatively few studies of what aggregates can do in vivo. Some of them have been inadvertent: patients with agammaglobulinemia were given gammaglobulin, but unfortunately it was found that anaphylaxis and <u>in vivo</u> complement activation are quite frequent following such therapy and we know now that the Cohn fraction preparations contain a large quantity of aggregates of IgG and that presumably is what is activating the complement system. Chenais showed that IgG aggregates actually formed cryoglobulins when injected into rabbits and that human IgG, rabbit IgG and rabbit complement can be found by the next day deposited in the rabbit kidney. It is conceivable then that aggregates could play a biologically important role in disease and may not be simply an epiphenomenon.

Jewell: Firstly, I think one does have to remember that the so-called complexes that we find in UC and CD are in fact of small molecular weight. Therefore, it does become very pertinent to question which techniques have been used when negative studies are being reported. As has been shown by many groups now, tests that rely on Clq binding are in fact only activated by high molecular weight complexes. We have always made the point that you can not really say you are dealing with an immune complex in any assay until you have actually defined the antigen. Aggregated IgG, aggregating <u>in vivo</u> is obviously a possiblity. What does surprise me however, is that we and others have been unable to correlate the findings that we get with our various tests with the serum IgG level or total immunoglobulin concentration or indeed even with the serum albumin level. The other question I have is that when Soltis was showing us how IgG could aggregate in the presence of hypoalbuminemia his test system was set at an albumin level of only 15 g/l; patients with CD have to be very sick to get down to that level and most of the patients where we find assays of immune complexes positive have albumin levels of 30-35 g/l.

Soltis: In the past a few people have tried to correlate results of immune complex assays with serum IgG concentrations, but often that has not been successful. I am not aware of anyone devising an IgG: albumin ratio and trying to correlate that with results of assays. We did that with the seven patients reported here. There were 4 patients that had an abnormal IgG: albumin ratio; three of them had high molecular weight IgG and the fourth had relatively low high molecular weight IgG at pH 7.4, but it entirely disappeared after pH 3 treatment and I am not sure what to make of that. I think the point is that there are probably several other factors that could influence the formation of aggregates in vivo. Immunoglobulin and albumin concentration are two such factors, the functional capacity of the reticulo-endothelial system and other changes in IgG such as in vivo desialation that might occur in vivo are yet others. In addition, there is some evidence that not just albumin inhibits aggregation of IgG but globulins also inhibit; in vivo IgG aggregation may therefore be a multi-factorial event that two variables would not define terrible well. To answer your question about the very low albumin level in my test system, I picked out this particular set of data because I thought it was the most impressive. However, we have done many other studies in which both albumin and IgG concentration were varied and it appears that even very subtle differences in either IgG or albumin concentration will be associated with a greater or lesser degree of aggregation.

Kraft: It has been reported that in idiopathic pneumonitis immune complexes are found in the subgroup who have cellular infiltrates in the lung biopsy whereas immune complexes were absent in the subgroups who had a fibrotic lung biopsy. The first subgroup tended to respond to steroids but the second did not. I am wondering if the people who have been measuring immune complexes in CD have made a similar correlation. Was there a correlation with the response to steroids or with the histologic type of CD?

Jewell: All I can say is that most of the tests of immune complex levels that we have used, such as, inhibition of K-cell cytotoxicity and the Clq binding have all tended to correlate with disease activity; in other words, we get positive results in patients with active disease and near normal results when the patients go into remission. Hodgson showed in one or two patients and we subsequently showed in a few more, that patients who have uveitis and erythema nodosum in CD nearly always have strongly positive anticomplementary activity as well as a large amount of high molecular weight IgG on gel filtration. They are not always the patients that have high IgG and low albumin levels. So we have postulated that there did seem to be a relationship between certain of these extra-intestinal manifestations and the tests for immune complexes.

LYMPHOCYTOTOXIC ANTIBODIES IN PATIENTS WITH CROHN'S DISEASE AND FAMILY MEMBERS

INEKE KUIPER, IRENE T. WETERMAN, I. BIEMOND, RIA C. CASTELLI, J.J. VAN ROOD and A.S. PEÑA

INTRODUCTION

The aetiology of Crohn's disease remains unknown. It has been suggested that genetic predisposition, environmental factors and immunological abnormalities play a role in the pathogenesis of the disease.

Lymphocytotoxic antibodies [LCA] have been found in the sera of patients with Crohn's disease [CD] and their relatives (1-3). Similar antibodies were first described by Mottironi and Terasaki in a variety of diseases (4). More recently, LCA have also been found in patients with lupus erythematosus (5), rheumatoid arthritis (8) and many other diseases (9). Finally, healthy subjects after vaccination or viral illnesses may have LCA transiently (10).

For several years it has been assumed that these antibodies resulted from modified surface proteins present on virus-infected cells and it was suggested that they may represent markers of infectious agents. In support of this concept, some evidence has come forward that a viral agent is involved in the aetiology of CD (11-13); however, recently this evidence has been brought into question (14). Yet, another hypothesis that has been advanced concerning LCA is that they are antibodies directed against immunoglobulins on the surface of the B-lymphocytes; as such they play a role in regulation of the immune response (15).

We would like to report the results of a study of LCA conducted in unrelated patients with Crohn's disease and their first-degree relatives.

342

MATERIALS AND METHODS

Sera were obtained from 136 patients with CD, 53 healthy relatives including 23 mothers, 5 fathers, 12 children, 13 sibs, 10 spouses and 119 controls [bloodtransfusion donors]. The sera were screened against a panel of 29 to 31 lymphocytes of normal donors with different HLA phenotypes and against a panel of 20 lymphocytes of HLA typed patients with Crohn's disease. The microcytotoxicity test described by Mittal et al. (5) was used. The percentage of dead lymphocytes was, after staining with Eosin, read under an inverted light microscope. We also used the two colour fluorescence technique [TCF] described by Van Rood et al. (16). In both tests a reaction was considered positive if 20% or more cells of one donor were killed. If 10% of the donor panel's members were positive, the serum was considered to have lymphocytotoxic antibodies. To identify the immunoglobulin class of LCA, sera of three patients were subjected to fractionation on a Sephacryl S300 superfine column [90cm x 2.5cm] equilibrated with 0.15M phosphate buffered saline. The protein peaks corresponding to the IgM and IgG fractions were concentrated to the original serum volume [2 ml] and were tested for cytotoxicity with the TCF technique.

RESULTS

Sera from 119 patients were screened with both microcytotoxicity tests. In the test described by Mittal et al.(5) only 14 of 119 patients had antibodies in their sera, when they were tested against lymphocytes of 37 controls. However, when the same sera were tested with the TCF technique it was found that 68 of the 119 were positive for T cells; this included the four positive sera found in the microcytotoxicity test. By contrast, only four sera from 119 healthy blood transfusion donors were positive with both techniques [Table 1].

Table 1. Cytotoxicity of sera of patients with CD and of
controls against a panel of control lymmphocytes.
Comparison of two methods

Crohn's disease sera   Control sera
Microcytotoxicity test   Microcytotoxicity test

          +   -   +   -

     + 14   54   + 3   1

TCF   TCF
     - 0   51   - 1   114
     P= 0.208 X 10^{-3} P= 0.693

Later 17 patients with CD were added to the series so
that in total 136 sera of unrelated patients were screened
with the TCF technique against the control panel and the
results are shown in table 2. As can be seen the cytotoxic
activity against T cells is much lower than against B cells.

Table 2. Lymphocytotoxic antibodies against B and T cells

sera of	Number tested sera	Cell panel	Number tested cells	% positive B cells	% positive T cells
CD patients	136	C	29	64	36
	64	CD	20	64	22
Family members	61	C	28	64	22
	61	CD	21	50	28
Controls [C]	119	C	31	4	4

Also shown in table 2 is the fact that 64 of 136 CD sera
were screened against a panel of 20 lymphocytes of patients
with CD. No difference in cytotoxicity was seen between the
two different panels. However, four sera reacted significantly more against the the control B cells than Crohn's B cells
and five sera reacted significantly more against the T lymphocytes of the Crohn's panel [see table 3].

In addition, LCA were also detected in the sera of family
members, 61 sera of family members were tested against the
lymphocytes of 28 controls - 64% was positive for B cells and
22% for T cells - and against the lymphocytes of 21 CD patients - 50% was positive for B cells and 28% for T cells.

Table 3. Cytotoxicity for B- and T-lymphocytes of sera of CD
         patients

Serum	B-cell panel		T-cell panel	
	Control	Crohn's	Control	Crohn's
no.	% pos	% pos	% pos	% pos
1	79	0*	66	0*
12	66	35*	31	6*
26	62	24*	48	6*
44	48	6*	17	0*
3	38	18	31	0*
10	34	24	24	0*
13	34	12	28	0

* Significant χ^2-test

We also determined the reactions of sera of 23 mothers of
Crohn's patients against a control and Crohn's panel of lymphocytes. Two mother's sera reacted significantly more a-
gainst the panel of Crohn's patients than the controls, 24%
[B] and 4% [T], 38% [B] and 7% [T] respectively. However, the
serum reactions were mostly weak and the positive reactions
could not be correlated with defined HLA specificities. As
previously observed with the patient's sera, the activity of
maternal sera against B lymphocytes was stronger than against
T lymphocytes. Finally, three sera which were known to be
cytotoxic with the TCF technique were fractionated on Seph-
acryl-S300 and it was found that the IgM fraction and not the
IgG fraction contained the cytotoxic antibodies[see table 4].

Table 4. Cytotoxicity as percentage of three positive react-
         ing individuals of the control panel fractioned sera
         from patients with CD against control lymphocytes

Serum before fractionation		IgM fraction		IgG fraction	
B cells	T cells	B cells	T cells	B cells	T cells
77%	54%	62%	23%	0	0
60%	15%	54%	18%	0	0
54%	23%	8%	0%	0	0

DISCUSSION

The present study has confirmed previous observations
that the sera of patients with Crohn's disease and their

relatives are very often cytotoxic for lymphocytes of controls and patients with Crohn's disease (1,2,3). As in prior studies, these antibodies are not directed against well defined HLA specificities and they are more active against B lymphocytes than against T cells (3). Our limited studies with fractionation of the sera indicate that these antibodies are predominantly of the IgM class as previously reported (17).

One cannot explain the presence of LCA as a secondary manifestation of the inflamed and abnormal gastrointestinal tract as relatives of the patients, without intestinal disease, have the antibodies in the same frequency. These LCA are likely to be heterogenous with multiple specificities, since they react with normal T and B lymphocytes. In addition, since they do not react with lymphocytes from HLA-typed donors and patients, in a way that correlates with any known HLA specificities, probably do not interact with conventional HLA antigens. However, in SLE the lymphocytotoxic activity was significantly inhibited by preincubating target lymphocytes with Fab_2 fragments of xeno antisera against microglobulin or the heavy chain of the HLA-A,B,C antigenic molecular complex (18). This indicates that although we have not performed the cytotoxicity reactions at 5^oC, the LCA in CD share many features with IgM cold cytotoxins found in a variety of diseases. In this regard Cicciarelli et al. (15) has postulated recently that such antibodies can function as autoregulatory feedback antibodies.

Finally, a role for lymphocytotoxic antibodies in the causation of the low number circulating T lymphocytes subsets recently shown in CD (18,20) should be further investigated.

CONCLUSIONS
1. We have confirmed previous observations that the sera of patients with Crohn's disease and relatives are cytotoxic for normal lymphocytes and lymphocytes of patients with CD.
2. Whereas the cytotoxicity is directed against both B and T cells, cytotoxicity against B cells is more prominent; the

346

cytotoxicity is not directed against well defined HLA specificities.

3. It is suggested that in common with other diseases where
LCA are found, these antibodies are a manifestation of a
subtle immunological abnormality rather than markers of viral
agents or disease associated antigens.

ACKNOWLEDGEMENT

This present work was supported in part by a grant from
the National Foundation for Ileitis and Colitis, Inc. New
York, U.S.A.

REFERENCES
1. Korsmeyer S, Strickland RG, Wilson ID, Williams RC Jr.
   (1974) Serum lymphocytotoxic and lymphocytophilic antibody activity in inflammatory bowel disease. Gastroenterology 67:578-583
2. Korsmeyer SJ, Williams RC Jr, Wilson ID, Strickland RG.
   (1975) Lymphocytotoxic antibody in inflammatory bowel
   disease - A family study. New Engl.J.Med. 293: 1117-1120
3. Strickland RG, Friedler EM, Henderson CA, Wilson ID,
   Williams PC Jr. (1975) Serum lymphocytotoxins in inflammatory bowel disease. Studies of frequency and specificity for lymphocyte subpopulations. Clin.Exp.Immunol.
   21:384-393
4. Mottironi VD, Terasaki PI. (1970) Lymphocytotoxins in
   disease. In: Infectious Mononucleosis, Rubella and
   Measles. Histocompatibility Testing Ed. Terasaki PI,
   Munksgaard Copenhagen pp 301-308.
5. Mittal KK. Rossen RD, Sharp JT, Lidsky MD, Butler WT.
   (1970) Lymphocyte cytotoxic antibodies in systemic lupus
   erythematosus. Nature 225:1255-1256
6. Persellin JE, Messner RP, DeHoratius RJ, Troup GM. (1977)
   Antilymphocyte Antibodies in Systemic Lupus Erythematosus: Familial Clustering of Lymphocyte antigens. J.Reuma-
   tol. 4:11-14
7. Malave I, Papa R, Layrisse Z. (1976) Lymphocytotoxic
   antibodies in SLE patients and their relatives. Arthritis
   Rheum. 9:700-704
8. Winchester RJ, Winfield JB, Siegal F, Wernet P, Bentwich
   Z, Kunkel HG. (1974) Analysis of lymphocytes from patients with Rheumatoid Arthritis and Systemic Lupus Erythematosus. J.Clin.Invest. 54:1082-1092
9. Ozturk G, Terasaki PI. (1979) Non-HLA Lymphocyte Cytotoxins in various diseases. Tissue Antigens 14:52-58
10. Kreisler MJ, Hirata AA, Terasaki PI. (1970) Cytotoxins in
    Disease. III Antibodies against lymphocytes produced by
    vaccination. Transplantation 10:411-415
11. Gitnick GL, Arthur MH, Shibata I. (1976) Cultivation of
    viral agents from Crohn's disease. Lancet 2: 215-217

12. Whorwell PJ, Beeken WL, Philips CA, Little PK, Roessaner KD. (1977) Isolation of reovirus-like agents from patients with Crohn's disease. Lancet 1: 1169-1171
13. Das KM, Valenzuela I, Morecki R. (1980) Crohn's disease lymphnode homogenates produce Murine lymphoma in athymic mice. PNAS 77:588-592
14. Phillpotts RJ, Hermon-Taylor J, Teich NM, Brooke BN. (1980) A search for persistant virus infection in Crohn's disease. Gut 21:202-207
15. Cicciarelli JC, Chia D, Terasaki PI, Barnett EV, Shirahama S. (1980) Human IgM anti-IgM cytotoxin for B lymphocytes. Tissue Antigens 15:275-282
16. Rood van JJ, Leeuwen van A, Ploem JS. (1976) Simultaneous detection of two cell populations by two colour fluorescence and application to the recognition of B-cell determinants. Nature 262:795-797
17. Henderson CA, Greenlee L, Williams Jr RC, Strickland RG. (1976) Characterization of anti-lymphocyte antibodies in inflammatory bowel disease. Scand.J.Immunol. 5:837-844
18. Messner RP, DeHoratius RT, Ferrone S. (1980) Lymphocytotoxic antibodies in systemic lupus erythematosus patients and their relatives. Reactivity with the HLA antigenic molecular complex. Arthritis Rheum. 23:265-272.
19. Hodgson HJF, Victorino RR. (1980) T lymphocyte subpopulations and immunoregulation in inflammatory bowel disease. These proceedings
20. Peña AS, Cnossen J, Damsteeg WGM, Weterman IT, Meijer CJLM. (1980). T-cell subpopulations in Crohn's disease. These proceedings

G6 Summary of Discussions relating to topic G5

Jewell: We have obtained rather similar results just
               recently using the standard microcytotoxicity-test.
               We tested four of our most cytotoxic sera against
               autologous and allogeneic (normal) lymphocytes and
               found that the sera killed a greater percentage of
               allogeneic cells than autologous cells. However,
               you could increase the autologous cytotoxicity by
               pre-treating the autologous lymphocytes with tryp-
               sin or pronase. The same patients were then studied
               during remission and to our surprise their sera
               became highly reactive against the autologous
               cells. These studies suggest that in active disease
               there is something on the surface of the T- or the
               B-cells, possibly immunoglobulin or immune com-
               plexes, which prevents the antibody from killing
               the cell. We found that a panel of IBD lymphocytes
               [either whole peripheral blood cells or isolated
               T-cells] were relatively resistant to sera which
               were highly reactive against a panel of non-IBD,
               normal lymphocytes. However, we did not determine
               the effect of pronase or other protease digestion
               on the IBD cells to see whether they could be made
               more susceptible to killing. Further, we did not
               note any specific relationship between susceptibi-
               lity to killing and disease activity.

MacDermott: We have also done studies looking at LCA in
               IBD. Of the 120 patients we looked at, half had
               anti-lymphocytotoxic antibodies. Of those patients
               all had anti-lymphocytotoxic antibodies, directed
               against B-cell and the majority (80%) against both
               B- and T-cells. We did't find any patient who had

antibodies only against T-cells. In most instances, if the antibody was directed against B-cells, it was also directed against macrophages. In collaboration with Dean Mann (NIH) we found that anti-B-cell antibodies could kill cells bearing any of several D locus antigens. In CD this was usually DRw3, DRw5 and DRw6 and in UC this was usually DRw4, DRw6 and DRw7.

Phillpotts: Cold reactive lymphocytotoxic antibodies are also found in something like 19 percent of post-partum women. Could these antibodies be modulators of the immune response?

Peña: It has indeed been suggested that one of the possible roles of these antibodies is that they are either directed against various idiotypes or that they act simply against immunoglobulin. When their are directed against T-cells they may in fact be directed against certain populations of T-cells that play regulatory roles of the immune response. We have no data on that yet in CD. In Rheumatoid Arthritis' sera Meijer and co-workers have found antibodies against T-cells with Fc receptors for IgM.

Gebbers: We found an abundant number of necrotic plasma cells in the inflammatory infiltrate in UC and CD. Might this be due to the cytotoxic lymphocyte antibodies?

Strickland: Most of the antibody activity _in vitro_ is in the cold; very few of the activity occurs at 37°. This makes it unlikely that the antibodies cause tissue destruction _in vivo_.

Strober: Strickland reported that there was less reactivity against cells obtained from patients with common variable hypogammaglobulinemia. I was wondering whether Strickland or anyone else investigated that further. Is it not more reasonable to suppose that these lymphocytotoxic antibodies are directed against public HLA specificities rather than at private HLA specificity? The only evidence that the specificity is not for an HLA coded-antigen is that the antibodies react with cells from a number of individuals with differing HLA types. However, those individuals could share public HLA specificities.

Strickland: We did indeed test some of our most positive sera against a panel of cells obtained from patients with common variable hypogammaglobulinemia patients. We found that these cells exhibit the same degree of resistance to lysis as the IBD lymphocytes. However, this resistance was not present across the board; cells from only 3 of 6 patients showed this resistance. We had hoped to be able to show a relationship between suppressor-cell activity and the reduced reactivity of the anti-lymphocyte antibody. Unfortunately at that time, we were not able to show such a correlation; that is as far as we have taken it.

Das: Are these LCA unique to IBD or are they found in other chronic GI-disorders?

Strickland: We have studied sera from 20 disease controls. These were patients with amoebiasis, Shigellosis, coeliac disease and radiation enteritis. The incidence of the LCA in those sera, was not different from the healthy controls.

MacDermott: Certainly these antibodies are not unique to IBD. We have found that patients with malaria, dengue fever, rubella, hepatitis, multiple sclerosis, SLE also have lymphocytotoxic antibodies of the kind described in IBD. LCA seemed to be associated with an immune response to a wide variety of agents and insults. In terms of GI -disease, there is one report of LCA in primary biliary cirrhosis.

Jewell: We have found LCA in a wide range of liver diseases and also in one or two coeliac sera.

Asquith: Do sera of unaffected relatives of people with these other diseases also contain antibodies?

Strickland: The only situation I am aware of is SLE. Here the pattern of familial occurrence is very similar to that seen in inflammatory bowel disease.

NEUTROPHIL ABNORMALITIES IN CROHN'S DISEASE

C. O'MORAIN, D. WALKER and A.J. LEVI

INTRODUCTION

A striking abnormality of neutrophil function has been described in Crohn's disease [CD] in that there is diminished neutrophil accumulation at the site of an abrasion (7). It was proposed that this phenomenon predisposes the patient to acquiring the disease. A similar defect has been described in sarcoidosis. The failure of neutrophils to accumulate may be explained by the presence of increased amounts of chemotactic factor inactivators in the serum (6). Chronic granulomatous disease is an inherited illness which when it affects the gastrointestinal tract is indistinguishable from CD (2). In this condition there is a documented neutrophil defect in that they are incapable of phagocytosing certain organisms which cause repeated infection. In this paper we have attempted to elucidate the abnormality of neutrophil function in CD.

MATERIAL AND METHODS

a] Skin Window Tests

In order to perform skin window tests two areas 0.8 mm in diameter were abraded on the forearm with the aid of a battery-powered dental drill. The area size was kept uniform by using a template. A skin window chamber was glued in place over each abraded area and the number of neutrophils migrating into the chambers was counted after 5 h. Initial skin window tests were performed on 34 healthy controls and 38 patients with Crohn's disease. The diagnosis of CD was made by finding characteristic histological lesions or on typical clinical and radiological features. Further skin window tests were carried out in 18 patients with CD and 18 healthy controls. In these studies four abrasions were made and covered by skin window chambers. In two of the chambers autologous serum and in the other two Zymosan-activated serum were used as the chemotactic agents. Zymosan-activated serum [ZAS] was prepared by incubating AB serum [Au antigen negative] with Zymosan 1 mg/ml at 37°C for 60 min and then at 56°C for 30 min. The zymosan was removed by centrifugation and the ZAS was stored at -20°C. AB serum [Au antigen negative] was used as the chemotactic agent in another 10 patients with Crohn's disease.

b] Neutrophils Migration In vitro

Neutrophils were isolated from patients with Crohn's disease. Neutrophil migration was measured by a modification of the Boyden chamber technique (1). The leucocyte suspension [0.25 ml] was added to the upper chamber and inverted onto a 3 μm pore size Millipore filter which had been placed on an antibiotic disc saturated with 0.2 ml of a chemotactic agent. After incubation for 1 to 2 h at 37°C [depending on the chemotactic agent used], in a humidified chamber, the filters were removed and stained with Harris haematoxylin. Migration was measured by the leading front method (10) taking the average of five reading per filter. All assays were performed in duplicate. Chemotactic agents were prepared as follows: Casein [BDH Ltd] was dissolved in alkaline balanced salt solution at a concentration of 1.0 mg/ml following in which the pH was brought to 7.4; Zymosan activated serum was prepared as outlined above; E.coli derived chemotactic factor was prepared by culturing E.coli overnight in Medium 199 [Flow Lab] and centrifuging at 2000 g for 30 min and filtering the culture medium through a Millipore filter. Checkerboard assays were carried out using the method of Zigmond and Hirsh (10) in which different concentrations of the chemoattractant were placed above and below the filter to give a concentration gradient. E.coli supernatant (6) and ZAS (3) were preincubated for 30 min at 37°C with 5% serum from patients with CD and 5% serum from healthy controls before testing their ability to attract neutrophils through the filter. To test for the presence of a cell-directed inhibition of movement, control cells were pre-incubated at $37^{\circ}C$ for 30 min in the presence of 10% serum from patients with CD.

c] Oxygen Consumption by Neutrophils during Phagocytosis

The neutrophils from 10 patients with Crohn's disease and 10 healthy controls were exposed to latex particles [Difco 0.8μ diameter] at a concentration of 2 x 10^7 cells/ml and opsonized with human IgG [Lister Institute] (8); Similarly, neutrophhils were exposed to heat killed E.coli and opsonized with pooled AB serum. Oxygen comsumption during phagocytosis of latex on E.coli was measured in a closed, plastic chamber attached to a Clarke type oxygen electrode [Rank]. Skin window fluid aspirated after 5 h of being in contact with the abraded area was assayed for bradykinin, histamine and prostaglandin E_2 [Dr Kabza-Blac].

RESULTS

The number of cells migrating into skin windows after 5 h was significantly lower in patients with Crohn's disease [0.77 ± 1.07 x 10^6/ml, mean $\pm$ SD, n = 58] than normal controls [1.95 ± 1.45 x 10^6/ml, mean $\pm$ SD, n = 34], p < 0.001 [Wilcoxon Rank test]. There was no relationship of cell migration to disease activity, site of involvement or treatment.

The checkerboard assay suggested that ZAS and casein were chemotactic, that cells moved along a positive concentration gradient and that serum at a concentration greater than 10% was chemokinetic with cells migrating even in the absence of a positive concentration gradient. We found no significant difference in distance migrated by cells isolated from controls and Crohn's disease. To rule out the possibility of an intrinsic cellular defect in patients with Crohn's disease, all possible combinations of neutrophils and serum were used. However, no significant difference in migration was seen in any combination. There was no evidence of cell-directed inhibition in that there was no significant difference in the migration of neutrophils suspended and pre-incubated in 10%

control serum or 10% serum obtained from patients with CD. Similarly, there was no evidence of an inactivator of chemotactic factor in that there was no significant difference in the distance migrated when ZAS and E.coli supernatant was pre-incubated in 5% serum from controls and 5% serum from patients with Crohn's disease.

Further studies with skin windows showed that AB serum did not enhance migration in patients with CD. An increase in migration did occur with Zymosan-activated serum but was significantly lower [P < 0.001, Wilcoxon Rank test] when compared to healthy controls. A plot of the square root transformation of the mean showed that enhanced response to ZAS in CD was identical to that in healthy controls.

Neutrophils isolated from Crohn's disease showed the same response as neutrophils from healthy controls in oxygen consumption when exposed to immunoglobulin-coated latex particles or E.coli.

There was no significant difference in histamine content of skin window fluid from controls and normals. However, prostaglandin E_2 and bradykinin-like substance levels were too low to be recorded in both groups by a bioassay method.

DISCUSSION

In our investigation we have confirmed that in patients with CD neutrophils do not migrate normally. This behaviour is not affected by site, severity or treatment of the disease and appeared to be exclusive to CD. Our in vitro investigations failed to show any intrinsic defect in the neutrophils. Neutrophils from patients with CD showed a normal oxygen consumption response when exposed to opsonized latex particles and bacteria and therefore the abnormality in neutrophil function is different from that occurring in chronic granulomatous disease. We chose different chemotactic agents in our in vitro studies since each agent may have act through different receptor sites on the neutrophils. We used serum as a chemokinetic agent as it has been suggested that chemotaxis and chemokinesis of neutrophils can be controlled by distinct cellular mechanisms. Serum from patients with CD did not inhibit neutrophil migration. This suggests that there is no inhibiting factor or chemotactic inactivator in the serum of CD. Increased amounts of inactivators have been found using a similar technique in patients with sarcoidosis (6), Hodgkin's disease (9) and cirrhosis of the liver (5). Further evidence to support the finding that serum in CD is not the factor responsible for the skin window abnormalities comes from additional skin window studies: AB serum in the skin window chambers failed to enhance neutrophil accumulation.

We failed to show any difference in histamine levels at the site of abrasion in CD and controls but it is possible that in CD patients there is a relative decrease in the amount of chemotactic agents which we were unable to measure. The enhanced response to Zymosan activated serum, a powerful chemotactic agent, in patients with Crohn's disease would be evidence in favour of this hypothesis.

This neutrophil migration abnormality could be a primary event in CD. In this regard, the patient's neutrophils may be unable to deal with either dietary antigens or infective agents that cross the mucosal barrier. This defect would explain the granuloma formation and the high recurrence rate following surgery, even when all macroscopic lesions are removed.

ACKNOWLEDGEMENTS
    The author thanks Dr. A Kabja-Black of the Institute of Dermatology, London for the bioassay results.
C. O'Morain is an Eaton Research Fellow.

REFERENCES
  1. Agget HPJ, Harries JT, Harvey BAN, Soothill JF. (1979) An inherited defect of neutrophil mobility in Schwachmann's syndrome. J. Paediatr. 94:391.
  2. Ament ME, Ochs HD. (1973) Gastrointestinal manifestations of chronic granulomatous disease. New Engl.J.Med. 288: 382-387.
  3. Blumenfeld W, Territo M. (1979) A chemotactic inhibitor produced by blast cells and present in serum of a patient with acute lymphoblastic leukemia. Blood. 54:412.

4. Keller HU, Wissler JH, Hess MW, Cottier H. (1978) Distinct chemokinetic and chemotactic responses in neutrophil granulocytes. Eur. J. Immunol. 1:1-7.
5. Maderazo EC, Ward PA, Quintiliani R. (1976) Defective regulation of chemotaxis in cirrhosis. J. Lab. Clin. Med. 85:621-630.
6. Maderazo EC, Ward PA, Woronick CL, Kubik MA, De Graff AC. (1976) Leucotactic dysfuntion in sarcoidosis. Ann. Int. Med. 84:414-419.
7. Segal AW, Loewi G. (1976) Neutrophil dysfunction in Crohn's disease. Lancet, 2:219-221.
8. Segal AW, Coade SB. (1978) Kinetics of oxygen consumption by phagocytosing human neutrophils. Biochem. Biophys. Res. Comm.84:611-617.
9. Ward PA, Berenberg JL. (1974) Defective regulation of inflammatory mediators in Hodgkin's disease. New Engl.J. Med. 290:76-80.
10. Zigmond SH, Hirsch JC (1973) Leucocyte locomotion and chemotaxis: New methods for evaluation and demonstration of cell-derived chemotactic factor. J. Exp. Med. 137:387-410.

LOCAL LEUCOCYTE MOBILIZATION IN CROHN'S DISEASE

J.H. WANDALL and VIBEKE BINDER

INTRODUCTION

Non-caseating epithelioid cell granulomas and Langhans' type giant cells are a predominant and distinguishing factor of the local inflammatory reaction of CD.

A similar histologic picture in the reticuloendothelial system is found in chronic granulomatous disease [CGD]. The fundamental cause of CGD has been shown to be an inherited defect in bactericidal capacity of the neutrophil granulocyte macrophage – allowing some bacteria to remain alive inside first the neutrophils later the macrophages.

There are examples of a granulomatous reaction in sites where foreign material gains access to the tissue, such as foreign body granuloma, tuberculosis and leprosy.

With this as background a hypothesis of a defect primary defence system in Crohn's disease was formed and studies on the neutrophil granulocyte function in vivo and in vitro were carried out. Simultaneously a decreased leucocyte mobilization to skin windows of 5 hours' duration was found in Crohn's disease by Segal and Loewi (1).

METHODS

As an in vivo model of the inflammatory primary reaction we used a skin window, i.e., abrasion of the epidermal layer in a small area [approx. 3 cm^2] of the forearm. The mechanical trauma of the abrasion elicits the inflammatory reaction. A chamber filled with autologous serum was placed over the abrasion and the serum was changed every second hour in 48 hours according to a method previously described (2). The number of cells that migrated to the chamber fluid was counted and expressed as migration per hour per cm^2 abrasion [leucocyte migration rate: LMR] and as cumulated leucocyte migration per cm^2 [CLM].

In vitro tests were carried out to measure the chemotactic, phagocytic and nitroblue tetrazolium [NBT] reduction activity as described in detail previously (3). The chemotactic response of the circulating neutrophil granulocytes was measured using a Boyden technique where the chemotactic gradient is formed inside a Millipore [R] filter with a pore size of 3μm. The chemotactic response was quantitated by the leading front method, viz., the maximal length the cells had migrated into the filter. Casein was used [5 mg/ml] as a strong complement independent chemotactic agent.

The phagocytic activity was measured as the initial rate of phagocytosis of Oil-Red-O coloured paraffin emulsion. Engulfed oil was extracted from the granulocytes, quantitated colourimetrically and expressed as mg oil taken up per min. per 10^7 granulocytes. Spontaneous phagocytosis and phagocytosis after stimulation by opsonins in autologous serum was measured.

As a measure of the metabolic activity which accompanies the bactericidal and particle sequestration reaction, reduction of nitroblue tetrazolium to formazan was determined colorimetrically.

MATERIAL

Twenty patients with CD, 9 men and 11 women aged 13 to 74 years with a median of 32 years. The localization of disease was ileocolonic in 10 patients, only ileum in 5 and only colon in 5. Sixteen patients had a typical histologic pattern with epithelial granulomas, 3 had typical X-ray findings and fistulae, and 1 had typical X-ray findings alone. The disease was inactive in 9, slightly active in 6, and moderately active in 5 patients. Further the activity index given by Harvey and Bradshaw (4) was used. The patients had activity scores from 1 to 11.

All patients were without medical treatment at the time of the investigation and no steroids had been given for at least 6 months, no sulphasalazine for at least 2 weeks, and no other anti-inflammatory drugs for at least 8 days.

The control group comprised 21 volunteers without any symptoms or signs of disease, aged from 20 to 68 years with a median of 30 years.

A further 20 patients with ulcerative colitis [UC]and 15 patients in the second day after a small operation [herniotomy] served as not normal controls.

RESULTS

The _in vivo_ migration in Crohn's disease and normal controls is shown in fig. 1 expressed as LMR and in fig. 2 as CLM after 24 and 48 hours respectively.

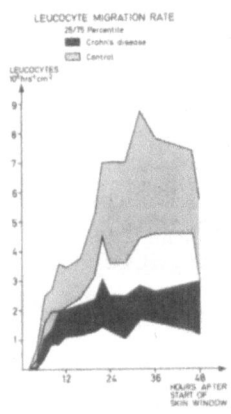

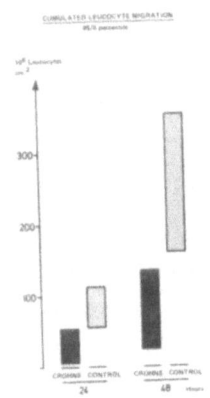

Figure 1. Leucocyte migration rate in CD and controls

Figure 2. Cumulated migration rate in CD and controls

The number of cells that migrate into the skin window chamber is diminished in patients with CD almost without overlap to the normal controls. LMR as well as CLM was found to be independent of activity, duration, and localization of the disease.

The _in vitro_ tests on circulating leucocytes are given given in table 1.

Table 1. Median and range of migration, phagocytosis and NBT
          reduction on circulating leucocytes

	Crohn's disease	Normal controls
Migration [µm]		
-random	85	75
	[40 - 121]	[57 - 112]
-stimulated	131	132
	[105 - 152]	[107 - 158]
Phagocytosis [mg.oil/min/10^7]		
-spontaneous	0.087	0.056
	[0.027-0.273]	[0.011-0.139]
-serum-dependent	0.255	0.180
	[0.159-0.336]	[0.124-0.284]
NBT-test [OD/8 min/10^7]	0.2941	0.1539
	[0.0963-0.6387]	[0.0200-0.4437]

It is seen that, the chemotactic response and random migration value following exposure to casein was normal. The chemotactic response was independent of whether the leucocytes were washed several times in a balanced solution or they were in a plasma solution, thus indicating that no inhibiting or stimulating factor occurred in the plasma. The phagocytic capacity was slightly elevated in the patients with CD compared to normal controls and there was a slight but significant correlation between disease activity and phagocytic response [r = 0.4654, p < 0.05]. NBT reduction in resting granulocytes was slightly elevated in patients with CD but no correlation to activity could be demonstrated.

The control groups of UC and postoperative patients both showed reduced leucocyte mobilization to skin windows compared to normal controls. Patients with CD, however, showed significantly reduced mobilization also compared to these 2 groups after 24 hours but without significant difference after 48 hours to postoperative patients.

DISCUSSION
The initial hypothesis of a defect primary defense system in CD seems to be confirmed. The present findings are in agreement with that of Segal and Loewi. Similar findings in patients with sarcoidosis have been reported, but in that case a leucocyte defect was associated with a plasma inhibi-

ting factor (5). *In vitro* migration by leucocytes in our study was normal without presence of inhibitors in plasma. The question remains whether the defect is primary or secondary to the disease. The lack of correlation between leucocyte mobilization and activity, duration or localization of disease points to a primary role. On the other hand the tendency towards the same phenomenon in newly operated patients points to the opposite. The possible reasons for defective leucocyte mobilization are 1] a defective granulocyte response to normal humoral tissue factors released by different invasive procedures [infective, traumatic]; 2] a defective humoral mediator system not releasing sufficient mediators for the normal cells migration; 3] presence of an inhibitor either in the circulating blood plasma or in the interstitial fluid. These findings point to a defect primary defense which may allow foreign material from the gut to gain access to the intestinal tissue, thereby causing a chronic inflammatory reaction.

CONCLUSIONS

CD is associated with a defect granulocyte mobilization. Defective humoral mediators or local inhibitors are postulated since *in vitro* cellular function was preserved.

ACKNOWLEDGEMENTS

The skillful technical assistance of Mrs. H.Kargaard, Mrs. H.Furhauge and Miss A.L. Poulsen is gratefully acknowledged. This study was supported by the Danish Medical Research Council.

REFERENCES
1. Segal AW, Loewi G. (1976) Neutrophil dysfunction in Crohn's disease. Lancet 2:219-221
2. Wandall JH. (1980) Leucocyte mobilization to skin lesion. Acta Path.Microbiol.Scand. C, in press
3. Wandall JH, Binder V, Friis B, Bech B. (1979) Functional characteristics of neutrophil granulocytes from children with recurrent respiratory infections. In: "Inborn Errors of Immunity and Phagocytosis" MTP Press, Lancaster pp 341-348
4. Harvey RF, Bradshaw JM. (1980) A simple index of Crohn's diseae activity. Lancet 1:514
5. Gange RW, Black MM, Carrington P, McKerron R. (1977) Defective neutrophil migration in sarcoidosis. Lancet 2:379-381.

WHITE CELL MOTILITY AND ITS INHIBITION BY SERUM FACTORS AND DRUGS

J.M. RHODES and D.P. JEWELL

INTRODUCTION

Segal and Loewi found a marked diminution of neutrophil chemotaxis into skin-window chambers containing the patient's own serum (1). Their results could be explained by an intrinsic defect in neutrophil chemotaxis or motility as well as by the presence of serum inhibitors or abnormalities in vascular permeability or coagulation. We have therefore studied the random motility and chemotaxis of isolated neutrophils from patients with Crohn's disease [CD] and have also looked for chemotaxis inhibitory activity in CD sera. Patients with ulcerative colitis [UC] have been used as a disease control group.

We have also investigated the effects of a number of drugs on leucocyte motility in vitro. The drugs tested were prednisolone, sulphasalazine, its metabolites 5 amino-salicylic acid and sulphapyridine and indomethacin.

PROCEDURE

Patients

Neutrophil random motility and chemotaxis have been studied in 20 patients with CD, 20 with UC, and 20 healthy controls. Serum inhibitory activity was studied in 42 CD patients, 20 with UC and 20 healthy controls. Disease activity was evenly distributed between inactive, mild, moderate and severe. Approximately half the patients were receiving sulphasalazine or prednisolone at the time of study. Patients receiving other forms of drug therapy were not studied.

Cell isolation and chemotaxis assay

Neutrophils were isolated from venous blood by dextran sedimentation followed by Ficoll-Hypaque density gradient centrifugation. They were suspended at 2×10^6 cells/ml in Gey's medium containing 1 mg/ml pure human serum albumin [Behringwerke]. Modified Boyden chambers (2) containing 3 pore diameter filters [Millipore] were used for the chemotaxis assay. Casein [Sigma] 4 mg/ml was the chemotactant except in the study of the serum fractions when complement C5a and the lymphokine LDCF were used as chemotactants. Random motility was assayed in the presence of human serum albumin [Behringwerke] 1 mg/ml. The distance moved by the leading cell front was measured after 40 minutes [chemotaxis] or 75 minutes [random motility]. For each assay the mean of 15 observations were taken.

Serum studies

Whole sera were examined for the presence of cell-directed and chemotactic factor directed inhibitors. Cell directed inhibition was detected by comparing the chemotaxis of neutrophils incubated in 10% test serum with the chemotaxis of neutrophils from the same cell population incubated in Gey's medium. Anti-chemotactic factor activity was assayed by determining the inhibitory effect of test serum on the chemotactic activity of dilute normal serum.

Sera from patients with severe CD [3] and severe UC [2] were fractionated by Sephadex G 200 gel filtration and 40% ammonium sulphate precipitation. The fractions were tested for cell directed inhibition and chemotactic factor inactivation.

Drug studies

Pure preparations of prednisolone sodium phosphate, sulphasalazine, 5 amino-salicylic acid, sulphapyridine and indomethacin were studied. Drug stock solutions in Gey's medium were made on the morning of test and corrected as necessary to pH 7.2 using 0.05 M Tris/HCl buffer. The drug under test was added to both cell suspension and chemotactant so as to give the same final drug concentration above and below the filter. Seven serial dilutions of each drug were studied.

RESULTS

Leucocyte motility

There was no significant difference in neutrophil chemotaxis between normals [76μ ± 10.8], CD patients with [74μ ± 16.4] and UC patients [69μ ± 18.4]. There was also no significant difference in neutrophil random motility between the groups: normals 34.6μ ± 8.3, CD 35.2μ ± 7.2 and UC 38.4μ ± 10.7.

Serum inhibitors

The chemotactic activity of 10% normal serum was significantly lower [p<0.05] after the addition of sera from CD patients than after the addition of sera from different normal controls or sera from UC patients. The degree of inhibitory activity of the Crohn's disease sera correlated with increasing disease severity [r=0.40, for b=0:t= 2.79]. There was no correlation between inhibitory activity and drug therapy.

When complement C5a was used as the chemotactant, inhibitory activity was found in the gel filtration fraction corresponding to the second optical density peak in the sera from 2 healthy controls [mean inhibition 23%], 2 patients with severe UC [mean inhibition 40%], and 2 patients with severe CD [mean inhibition 60%]. No significant inhibition of lymphokine [LDCF] directed chemotaxis was found in any serum fraction.

Sera from three patients with severe CD and two with severe ulcerative colitis were subjected to 40% ammonium sulphate precipitation. While only one of these sera [from a CD patient] proved inhibitory [32%] when tested whole, two of the CD sera and both the UC sera yielded precipitates with ammonium sulphate that were strongly inhibitory [41 to 43%]. None of the supernatants were significantly inhibitory [+1 to −16%].

Neutrophil chemotaxis towards casein was similar after incubation in CD sera [88.65μ ± 13.4] and control sera [88.2μ ± 11.3], but was reduced after incubation in sera from UC patients [79.25μ ± 14.3], p<0.05. There was no correlation with disease activity or drug therapy.

Effect of drugs

Dose response curves were plotted for the percentage
inhibition of leucocyte motility caused by serial dilutions
of each test drug. By interpolation the drug concentrations
required for 50% inhibition were sulphasalazine 2.51 μmol/ml,
5 amino-salicylic acid 32.7 μmol/ml, and prednisolone
1,45 μmol/ml. Sulphapyridine caused no significant inhibition
at 40 μmol/ml, a concentration considerably greater than
that occurring in the colon of patients receiving sulphasalazine (3). Indomethacin caused no significant inhibition at
a concentration [0.028 μmol/ml] greater than that required to
cause 100% inhibition of prostaglandin synthesis (4). Similar drug concentrations caused inhibition of neutrophil random motility and again sulphapyridine [40 μmol/ml] and indomethacin [0.028 μmol/ml] had no effect.

DISCUSSION

These results show that isolated neutrophils from CD patients move normally. However, serum in CD contains one or
more inhibitors of chemotaxis. The fact that the C5a directed
chemotactic factor inactivator is also present to a lesser
extent in the same fraction of normal sera suggests that this
inhibitor may represent increased activity of a normal serum
globulin. The presence of serum inhibitors in CD may explain
the skin window results. These inhibitors may also be important in the regulation of the inflammatory reaction that
occurs in CD.

The results with the drugs show that sulphasalazine and 5
amino-salicylic acid inhibit leucocyte motility at concentrations which are similar to those found in the colon of treated patients. Indomethacin is not effective suggesting that
this inhibition is independent of any action on prostaglandin
synthesis. Sulphapyridine has no effect on leucocyte motility even at very high concentrations and this accords with its
lack of therapeutic effect when given as an enema (5).

CONCLUSIONS

In CD isolated neutrophils move normally in vitro. Serum inhibitors of chemotaxis occur particularly in active disease. They probably represent increased activity of one or more normal plasma globulins.

Sulphasalazine and 5 amino-salicylic acid inhibit leucocyte motility. This action is independent of inhibition of prostaglandin synthesis.

ACKNOWLEDGEMENTS

J.M.R. is a Stanley Johnson research fellow. This work was generously funded by the British Digestive Foundation.

REFERENCES

1. Segal AW, Loewi E. (1976) Neutrophil dysfunction in Crohn's disease. Lancet 2: 219-221
2. Wilkinson PC. (1974) In: Chemotaxis and inflammation. Churchill Livingstone. p44
3. Peppercorn MA, Goldman P. (1973) Distribution studies of salicylazosulfapyridine and its metabolites. Gastroenterology 64:240-245
4. Vane JR. (1971) Inhibition of prostaglandin synthesis as a mechanism of action for aspirin-like drugs. Nature 231:232-235
5. Azad Khan AK, Piris J, Truelove SC. (1977) An experiment to determine the active therapeutic moiety of sulphasalazine. Lancet 2:892-895

G10 Summary of Discussions relating to topics G7 to G9

Gilat:　　　　What happens after resection of CD? Also, what happens with this test in other granulomatous diseases?

Binder:　　　Six of our 20 Crohn's patients had had resection and all six had a depressed leucocyte migration independent of the disease activity so I do not think anything happens after resection in respect to leucocyte function.

O'Morain:　　Twelve of our patients had had resection. As I stressed that was not related to disease activity. As far as other granulomatous diseases are concerned the same phenomenon has been observed in sarcoidosis for example. However, in these cases they did find chemotactic factor activators in the serum and could correlate the presence of such factors with the condition of the patient.

v.d. Meer:　　The discrepancy between these in vivo and in vitro data, suggest to me that we should look more at the kinetics of the granulocytes. I think in this respect recent data produced by John Gallin and co-workers at the NIH are of great interest. They have shown that the circulating neutrophils are composed of different populations, those cells forming rosettes with sheep red cells and those not forming rosettes. In abscess fluid almost all cells are rosette forming. As for functional activity the rosette-forming neutrophils are the cells most capable of phagocytosis and reponses to C5a-mediated chemotaxis. Whereas both kinds of neutrophils

participate equally in random migration latex phagocytosis, the latter function is not Fc-mediated
and is the kind of phagocytosis that you are looking at in the skin window test. Interestingly in
hemodialysis patients there is selective sequestration of rosette forming granulocytes in the lung.
Similar kinds of selective sequestration could
occur in the GI tract in CD.

Elson: Guinea pigs which are infected with BCG became
anergic to skin testing with the relevant antigen;
nevertheless the lymph nodes contain large numbers
of antigen-reactive cells; in other words, the guinea pigs demonstrate a compartmentalization of the
immune response. I wonder if that is what you are
seeing in patients with CD rather than a granulocyte defect.

O'Morain: We also think that there are two populations of
neutrophils. We have observed in studies of chemotaxis that some cells migrate and some do not. We
are looking into the question of functionally distinct granulocytes by studying the capacity of
cells to adhere to glass, a property which is essential to migration of cells out into the skin
window chamber.

Bienenstock: Rhodes mentioned that in gel filtration studies the antichemotactic factor came out in the
same place as IgA. Ralph Williams has suggested
that IgA aggregates may be antichemotactic. Do you
have any evidence that this was the case in your
patients?

Rhodes: We have looked at IgA, IgE and alpha-1-anti-
trypsin levels. We found no correlation of antichemotactic activity with levels of IgA or IgE which

in fact were within the normal range. We did find a correlation in both UC and CD between monocyte directed inhibitory activity and alpha-1-antitrypsin levels. However, this may have been the same thing as saying that there is a correlation with disease activity and does not necessarily establish alpha-1-antitrypsin as a chemotactic inhibitor.

Bienenstock: Has anybody done a skin window on mucosa? If not, why not? That might answer the question as to what is going on in the local situation.

Kraft: Along the same lines I would like to ask Binder what the in vitro assays of neutrophils obtained from the skin window show?

Binder: We performed the same in vitro tests on exudate cells and found normal function in all assays, normal phagocytosis and normal NBT reduction or even a slightly elevated NBT reduction.

Strickland: Several years ago Van Epps and I described an IgA chemotactic inhibitor in a group of patients with liver disease. I wonder if there is any correlation with the presence or absence of liver disease in these patients.

Rhodes: All of the patients studied had normal liver function; we did not test any with overt liver disease.

Asquith: Did those patients showing granuloma formation show the most inhibition of chemotaxis?

Binder: Sixteen out of 20 patients with CD had granulomas at a time before the test was carried out. The remaining four patients had no histologic diagnosis and we therefore did not know whether they had granulomas or not.

Dourmashkin: The preparation of serum by the usual means can produce activation of complement. Thus the varying results of the speakers might be due to the varying amounts of chemotactic agent in serum obtained by ordinary means. Use of EDTA plasma or purified C5a as an attractant may overcome this problem.

Rhodes: We tried to get around this problem by subtracting from the chemotaxis value obtained with normal serum, the value obtained with normal serum and CD serum. In this way we hope that we have corrected for any differences in intrinsic chemotactic activity produced while the serum is being obtained. We tried using EDTA plasma but that led to a lot of problems such as fibrin formation and plugging of the filter.

Jeejeebhoy: Have the speakers excluded the presence of something like essential fatty acid or zinc deficiency as being the cause of the abnormality?

O'Morain: We measured serum zinc levels in CD patients as part of study of infertility due to salazopyrine. The patients we tested had normal levels of zinc yet still had abnormal skin window tests.

Jeejeebhoy: Unfortunately the plasma levels of zinc have no relevance to deficiency.

Jewell: Most of the studies in CD have shown serum zinc levels to be within the normal range except in the very poorly nourished patients. However, we need to know about intracellular zinc levels, and as far as I know there is no data on that in CD.

Gebbers: Have you looked for ingested immunoglobulins in the neutrophils which could indicate ingestion of immune complexes?

Binder: We have not, but I think that is a very interesting idea and should be followed up.

Hermon-   Binder's studies suggest that the defect in
Taylor: granulocyte migration may be on the side of reception of signal rather than with the effector component. That being so, I would like to know if the polyamines have any effect on C5a-induced chemotaxis?

Rhodes: Polyamines have not been tested in our assay.

Das: I would like to ask Rhodes if, in his in vitro studies with sulphasalazine and its metabolites, he checked the pH of the solution.

Rhodes: We corrected the pH to 7.2 with TRIS/HCL buffer before adding to the cell suspension, but we did not check the pH throughout the incubation period. Moreover, after incubation with sulphasalazine and with the other drugs (except 5-aminosalicylic acid) there is no alteration in chloride membrane gradient and no alteration in trypan blue. So we do not think that the effects observed were due to damage to the cells except possible in the case of 5-aminosalicylic acid.

MONOCYTE FUNCTION IN CROHN'S DISEASE

D.P. JEWELL, A.S. MEE and J.M. RHODES

INTRODUCTION

Macrophages are a predominant feature in the inflammation of Crohn's disease [CD] and it is probable, by analogy with animal studies, that many of them derive from peripheral blood monocytes. These cells have received little study in CD patients although an absolute monocytosis has been reported (1). It is also known that their turnover is increased (2) and that they have an increased receptor activity for IgG and C3 (3). We have therefore examined absolute monocyte counts, lysosomal enzyme activity, phagocytosis and cell locomotion in CD patients.

PROCEDURES

Absolute Counts

Monocytes were detected in peripheral blood smears using the specific cyto-chemical staining technique for non-specific esterase. Total white counts were obtained from a Coulter counter.

Lysosomal Enzyme Activity

The activity of the specific lysosomal enzyme, N-acetyl-D-glucosaminidase, was measured using a fluorogenically labelled substrate following lysis of a cell suspension containing 85% monocytes. Enzyme activity was also measured in cells which had been incubated with endotoxin [lipopolysaccharide extract of E. coli 0127.B8] and with immune complexes [HSA-anti HSA complexes made at equivalence and in antigen excess].

Phagocytosis and Intracellular Killing

A monocyte-enriched population of cells was incubated with Staph. aureus opsonized with AB negative serum. Phagocytosis was determined by colony counts before and after this period of incubation. Intracellular killing was derived from the number of organisms phagocytosed and the number of surviving intracellular organisms determined by colony counts of the lysed cells after killing extracellular organisms with lysostaphin.

Cell locomotion

Chemotaxis of monocytes towards casein was performed in modified Boyden Chambers using an 8 μmillipore filter. Random motility was assayed in the presence of purified human serum albumin. Cell movement was assessed by measuring the distance moved through the filter by the leading cell front.

RESULTS

The absolute monocyte count in 40 CD patients was 634 ± 49/μl compared with 525 ± 38 cells/μl in 37 healthy control subjects. This difference was not significant. Patients with active disease had higher counts than those in remission but this also did not reach significance. There was no correlation between the monocyte count and the total white cell count. In contrast, patients with ulcerative colitis [UC] had significantly higher counts which correlated with disease activity and with the total white cell count.

The mean activity of β-D-glucosaminidase was 4.54 n mol/hr/10^4 cells [± 0.28, n = 21] in CD patients which was significantly [p<0.01] higher than that found in the control group [3.09 ± 0.09 n mol/hr/10^4 cells, n = 21]. Patients with active disease showed greater lysosomal enzyme activity than those in remission.

Incubation of monocytes from CD patients with immune complexes, at equivalence or in antigen excess, caused a rapid fall in intracellular enzyme activity so that after three hours incubation only about 50% of the original enzyme activity remained. This was significantly less than when cells were incubated in medium alone. Similar changes occurred using monocytes from healthy subjects. This accelerated fall in intracellular enzyme activity did not occur with endotoxin although endotoxin did cause a significant rise in supernatant activity.

The mean percentage [± SEM] of **Staph.aureus** phagocytosed in 2 hours by monocytes from CD patients [n = 15] was 53.8 ± 5.2% compared with 39.9 ± 2.6% by monocytes from healthy controls [n = 28] [p<0.02]. There was no correlation with disease activity but numbers are small. Over 95% of ingested organisms were killed by monocytes from CD patients and from the controls.

Random motility of monocytes from CD patients was similar to that of control monocytes but chemotaxis towards casein was enhanced although this did not reach significance [CD n = 20, 121 ± 14µ ; Controls 115 ± 14µ ; p = n.s.]. Monocytes from UC patients, however, showed a significant increase in chemotaxis [126 ± 12µ , n = 20, p<0.05] which correlated with disease activity.

DISCUSSION

These studies suggest that peripheral blood monocytes in CD patients are circulating in an activated state since there is enhancement of lysosomal enzyme activity, phagocytosis and directional motility. In animal studies, similar activity can be induced in monocytes by incubating them with endotoxin, immune complexes and lymphocyte derived factors.

Since these stimuli probably occur in the blood of CD patients, it seems likely that the monocytes are activated secondarily to mucosal inflammation. The trigger which causes them to leave the circulation and localize in the intestine, if that is indeed what happens, is unknown. However, once in the tissues, the release of their tissue damaging lysosomal enzymes by antigen-antibody complexes may be an important factor in the development of a chronic inflammation.

CONCLUSIONS

CD Patients tend to have an absolute monocytosis in the peripheral blood. These cells possess increased lysosomal enzyme activity and show enhanced phagocytosis. They also show enhanced directional motility but this was not statistically significant. Immune complexes are a potent stimulus releasing lysosomal enzymes and it is suggested that this may be one effector mechanism in the pathogenesis of the intestinal inflammation. There is no evidence that defective monocyte function is a factor in the development of granulomata.

REFERENCES
1. Thayer WR, Charland C, Field CE. (1976) The subpopulations of circulating white cells in inflammatory bowel disease. Gastroenterology 71:379-384
2. Meuret G, Bitzi A, Hammer B. (1978) Macrophage turnover in Crohn's disease and ulcerative colitis. Gastroenterology 74:501-503
3. Schmidt ME, Douglas SD. (1977) Monocyte IgG receptor activity. Dynamics and modulation - normal individuals and patients with granulomatous diseases. J.Lab.Clin.Med. 89:332-339

G12 Summary of Discussions relating to topic G11

Booth: First I would be interested to know if the en-
              zyme activity was expressed in terms of protein or
              DNA rather than simply by a cell count. Second we
              all make the assumption that lysosomal enzyme re-
              lease necessarily cause tissue damage. I would like
              to know whether there is evidence for that.

Jewell: I don't actually have the data for the enzyme
              expressed per milligram of protein or DNA. There
              are a number of problems with doing that in this
              particular system.

v.d. Meer: I think that the concept that lysosomal enzyme
              release is necessarily followed by damage to the
              tissues is based on very limited evidence.

Hodgson: Jewell, can your changes be due to the fact
              that they are simply a young population of cells?

Jewell: This is always possible. Other people have
              shown in animal studies that as monocytes mature
              their lysosomal enzyme activity increases. Our
              findings could be due to the fact that an older
              population of cells is present. However, that is
              very unlikely when you remember the kinetic studies
              which show that in CD, monocytes are turning over
              more rapidly so that you would expect a younger
              population of cells with lower enzyme levels than
              normal.

v.d. Meer: Has anybody determined enzyme activity of skin
              window macrophages in CD patients?

O'Morain: We did differential counts of cells migrating into skin windows and found that 95% were neutrophils. Therefore, in CD there are very few macrophages to do any work on.

v.d. Meer: If you change your technique and apply just a glass cover slip on the abrasion, you might see an increased number of monocytes.

Binder: We also find a surprisingly small number of macrophages in the skin window when the chamber technique is used. We have also done skin window with only a cover slip and found a much larger number of monocytes.

v.d. Meer: Could it be that the monocytes are adhering to the chamber and that is the reason you don't see them?

Binder: We have looked at that possibility, but that doesn't explain the great difference using cover slips and chambers.

Dourmashkin: Alison and Feluga did some experiments a few years ago in which they showed that released enzymes from macrophages did not cause cell killing. Also I would like to ask Jewell if he has tested the macrophages in CD for cell-mediated cytotoxicity?

Jewell: No.

Verspaget: Did you look at the tissue macrophages in the gut?

Jewell: We have not as yet managed to isolate gut macrophages sufficiently well to be confident that we can do anything with them.

MacDermott: I would agree that investigation of the macrophages in the lamina propria would be of great interest, particularly with regard to cellular cytotoxicity. In the limited studies that we have performed, gut macrophages certainly do have cytotoxic capabilities against red cell targets but not against cell line targets.

van Saene: Are there data available about monocyte activity in CD after surgery?

v.d. Meer: I do not think anybody has data on that point.

CON A INDUCED SUPPRESSOR CELL ACTIVITY IN IBD AND OTHER INFLAMMATORY DISEASES[*]

W. KNAPP, J.S. SMOLEN, G. LANZER, R. BERGER, E.J. MENZEL, G. GRABNER and A. GANGL

INTRODUCTION

During the past several years the regulation of the immune response, particularly regarding suppressor cell activity, has met with considerable interest, and a number of different suppressor cell systems, some specific, others nonspecific, have been described (Reviewed in 1,2). For the study of suppressor cell function in man, two test systems were mainly used: the measure of T cell controlled in vitro proliferation, differentiation, and immunoglobulin production of human B lymphocytes following polyclonal activation with pokeweed mitogen [PWM] and the investigation of the ability of in vitro concanavalin A [Con A] - activated lymphocytes to suppress proliferation responses of autologous or allogeneic responder cells (3,4).

We have studied the Con A induced suppressor cell activity for proliferative responses in several inflammatory diseases including inflammatory bowel disease [IBD]. The results of these studies are herein presented.

MATERIALS AND METHODS

Patients.

Inflammatory bowel disease [IBD] group. Thirteen patients with IBD [10 with Crohn's disease and 3 with ulcerative colitis] were investigated in this test series and compared with 8 healthy adult controls. The diagnosis was based on past and present history, physical examination, intestinal X-ray stu-

[*]Supported by Fonds zur Forderung der wissenschaftlichen Forschung in Österreich

dies, endoscopy and histological examination of tissue obtained at colonoscopy or at surgery. Disease activity in CD patients was assessed by the Crohn's disease activity index. For UC patients the same index was used, however, an examination for occult or overt blood in stool was carried out instead of or in addition to the examination for a possible or definite palpable mass in the ileocoecal region. An AI = 100 was set as borderline between active and inactive disease. Treatment with steroids, azathioprine and sulfasalazine was discontinued at least 2 weeks prior to the immunological investigation.

Inflammatory uveal disease [IUD] group. Twenty patients with IUD as well as twenty-two healthy adults were tested for Con A induced suppressor cell activity in this test series. Seventeen patients suffered from acute anterior uveitis, two from additional peripheral uveitis and one presented with severe panuveitis. Nine patients were studied during the acute stage of the disease, eleven patients were examined during a period of remission.

Rheumatoid arthritis [RA] group. Thirty-five patients with classical or definite RA according to the diagnostic criteria of the American Rheumatism Association (5) were tested together with twenty-five healthy individuals who acted as controls. Disease activity was assessed according to clinical criteria [number of swollen joints, duration of morning stiffness, grip strength] and erythrocyte sedimentation rate. All patients were treated with nonsteroid antiinflammatory drugs [indomethacine, diclofenac or tolmetine]. In addition, fifteen patients had received longterm treatment [at least during the last six months] with gold-thiomalate, D-penicillamine or chloroquine.

Suppressor cell assay

The Con A induced suppressor cell activity was estimated essentially as described before (6). Patients from each series were in all instances studied under identical conditions and compared with healthy adult controls.

The Con A preparations and final Con A concentrations were different in the three test series. These variations will be described together with the results.

RESULTS

Con A induced suppressor cell activity in patients with IBD. Con A induced suppressor cell activity in IBD patients was studied in an allogeneic test system. MNC from the peripheral blood of IBD patients and healthy adult controls were incubated for 3-4 days with either Con A [Sigma, St. Louis, Mo., USA] [25 µg/ml] or medium alone and then tested simultaneously for SC activity with Con A [Sigma] [5 µg/ml] stimulated allogeneic MNC from healthy adult controls. Results are shown in Fig.1. Simultaneously tested control persons in this test series showed a mean suppression of 23.4 ± 4.4%. This is not different from the mean suppression of IBD patients [12.2 ± 6.7%]. If, however, Con A induced suppressor cell activity is evaluated according to the activity of the respective patient's disease, the mean suppression of 2.1 ± 3.3% in the group of patients with active disease is significantly [p<0.02] lower than that of patients with inactive disease [28.8 ± 10.8%] and of simultaneously investigated healthy controls [23.4 ± 4.4%;p<0.001].

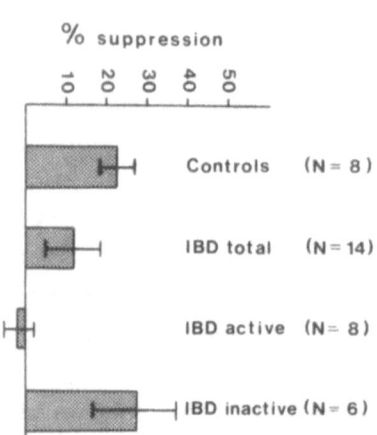

Figure 1. Con A induced suppression in IBD patients and controls [mean ± SEM]

Con A induced suppressor cell activity in patients with inflammatory uveal disease.

Suppressor cell activity in this test series was studied in an autologous test system and with a different source [Pharmacia, Uppsala, Sweden] and concentration [12.5 µg for activation of SC and 1 µg for stimulation of responder cells by Con A. Results are shown in Fig. 2.

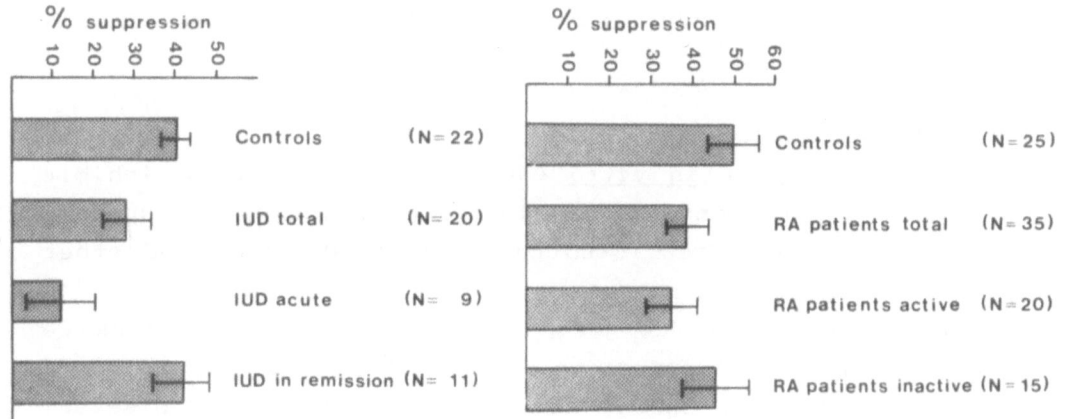

Figure 2. Con A induced suppression in IUD patients and controls [mean ± SEM]

Figure 3. Con A induced suppression in RA patients and controls [mean ± SEM].

Under these conditions the Con A induced suppressor cell activity of simultaneously studied control persons was found to be 40.8 ± 3.7%. Also in this test series the mean suppressor cell activity of all patients [28.4 ± 6.1%] was not significantly different, while patients tested during the acute stage of an inflammatory uveal disease showed a significant reduction of Con A induced suppressor cell activity [12.4 ± 8.5%] when compared to controls [p<0.01] or to patients during an inactive stage of disease [42.7 ± 5.9%; p<0.05].

Con A induced suppressor cell activity in patients with rheumatoid arthritis [RA]

Suppressor cell activity in this series was studied in an allogeneic test system using Pharmacia Con A for both activation [12.5 µg/ml] of SC and stimulation of responder cells. Results are shown in Fig. 3. Con A activated MNC from 25 healthy individuals tested together with RA patients gave a 50 $\pm$ 6% suppression of the proliferative response of allogeneic responder cells. The suppression observed in 35 RA patients [39 $\pm$ 5%] was not significantly different. In contrast to the other two groups of patients studied, no significant difference was observed between clinically active [35 $\pm$ 6% suppression, N=20] and inactive [46 $\pm$ 8% suppression, N = 15] disease stages.

DISCUSSION

The ability of _in vitro_ Con A activated MNC to inhibit proliferative response of autologous or allogeneic responder cells has already been found to be impaired in SLE and other potential autoimmune diseases (7,8).

In two of the three groups of patients studied by us we found an impaired suppressive or inhibitory capacity of Con A activated MNC only during the active stage of the disease. As far as the IBD group is concerned this is in agreement with the results of Hodgson (8), however, the other two groups of patients have not been investigated comparably, as far as we were able to ascertain.

Suppressor cells deficiencies are considered to be of potential pathogenic importance in certain autoimmune diseases. The demonstration of deficient suppressor cell activities with the Con A test system in diseases such as SLE supports the hypothesis that dysregulations of the immune system play a major role in the pathogenesis of autoimmune diseases. At the same time these results seem to indicate that the Con A suppressor cell assay is a practical and reliable system for screening for suppressor cell deficiencies in patients. However, it is now clear that lower proliferation responses in cocultures of Con A activated mitomycin treated MNC with fresh autologous responder MNC as compared to cocultures of medium cultured MNC with fresh responder MNC could be due to several mechanisms and the active suppression of responder cell proliferation is only one possibility. For instance, Con A activated cells might be inhibitory because they absorb out helper factors [e.g., IL-2] more efficiently than non activated cells. In addition, they might provide less help or be less stimulative than non-activated cells. The observation of lower "suppressor" activity of Con A activated MNC in certain disease groups, therefore, does not necessarily prove that these patients have a suppressor cell defect. It indicates, however, that in these patients differences from the normal situation exist. These differences should be studied further and analyzed carefully.

REFERENCES
1. Gershon RK. (1974) T cell control of antibody production. Contemp.Top.Immunobiol. 3:1
2. Waldmann TA, Broder S. (1977) Suppressor cells in the regulation of the immune response. Prog.Clin.Immunol. 3:155-199
3. Waldmann TA, Broder S, Blaese RM, Durm M, Blackman M, Strober W. (1974) Role of suppressor T cells in pathogenesis of common variable hypogammaglobulinaemia. Lancet 2:609-613
4. Shou L, Schwartz SA, Good RA. (1976) Suppressor cell activity after concanavalin A treatment of lymphocytes from normal donors. J.Exp.Med. 143:1100-1110
5. Steinbrocker O, Traeger CH, Battermann RC. (1949) Therapeutic criteria in rheumatoid arthritis (1. Classification of progression of rheumatoid arthritis.) JAMA 140: 659-662
6. Knapp W, Posch B. (1980) Concanavalin A-induced suppressor cell activity: opposing effects of hydrocortisone. J.Immunol. 124:168-172
7. Sakane T, Steinberg AD, Green I. (1978) Studies of immune functions of patients with systemic lupus erythematosus. I. Dysfunction of suppressor T-cell activity related to impaired generation of, rather than response to, suppressor cells. Arthritis Rheum. 21:657-664
8. Hodgson HJF, Wands JR, Isselbacher KJ. (1978) Decreased suppressor cell activity in inflammatory bowel disease. Clin.Exp.Imm. 32:451-458

G14 Summary of Discussions relating to topic G13

Hodgson: Wands and I first applied the Con A suppressor test because it was practical and applicable; but clearly it is a highly artificial test and we do not know about the possible effects of macrophages which are also in the cell population being studied. We now need a new generation of tests of suppressor cell function in which we can put a lot more confidence. What we are measuring in this test is non-specific suppression of lymphocyte proliferation and it is not clear that this has any relevance to the immune responses which we assume are taking place in the mucosa against either mucosal antigens or gut antigens. The latter are likely to be of more importance in IBD.

Strober: Would you agree that it is still possible, that the non-specific abnormalities determined with the tests presently available could be important as background factors in disease pathogenesis?

Hodgson: With the tests available at the moment we can not prove it.

Fiocchi: I was most impressed by Knapp's work regarding the variability he obtains with the different doses of Con A. We really should try to standardize the Con A dose or use different doses of Con A and come up with the optimal suppressor dose.

Strober: I think the point that Knapp made concerning base line suppression is very important and it is worth repeating, namely that when one calculates percent suppression one is using as a base line the value obtained with cells that have not been activated by Con A; if those non-activated cells have pre-existent abnormal levels of inhibition then the final suppressor cell value obtained will be less than normal. This will give the artificial impression that you are dealing with decreased suppression. Have any of the various investigators actually determined whether non Con A-treated cells of CD patients are more inhibitory than cells of normals?

Hodgson: I have not done that experiment. However, spontaneously active suppressor cells may be short-lived in culture and therefore 48 hours incubation might remove background suppressor activity initially present.

Knapp: There is one problem I see with the short-lived suppressor cells: when you incubate for 24 hours you get a high response in the Con A proliferative assay but in the pokeweed mitogen assay you get the reverse: inhibition of pokeweed mitogen-induced B-cell differentiation and immunoglobulin secretion. Thus, at the same time you lose suppressor cells, or whatever it is that leads to a higher proliferation in the presence of Con A, you create something which suppresses pokeweed mitogen-induced immunoglobulin secretion.

MacDermott: We have looked at peripheral blood antibody synthesis and secretion and in a twelve day in vivo pokeweed mitogen-induced system. We found that peripheral blood mononuclear cells from CD patients as well as SLE and UC patients make large amounts of immunoglobulins even without addition of mitogen. This is particularly true for immunoglobulin A.

This suggests that there is a lack of suppressor cells, or that there is a primary B-cell defect. Ginsburg, Master and Falchuck recently reported that the autologous mixed leucocyte reaction was depressed in both CD and UC. We have done similar studies and in five active, untreated Crohn's patients was found that the autologous mixed leucocyte reaction is markedly depressed. Therefore I think that in other systems, in addition to the Con A-induced system there are abnormalities of a potentially immunoregulatory nature.

Fiocchi: It is important to remember that we have a different subset of cells in the circulation and that in the lamina propria the subsets may have different spontaneous suppressor cell activity. We have done a very limited number of experiments where we suppressed the proliferative response of blood lymphocytes using gut mucosal lymphocytes without adding Con A. In addition, the gut mucosal lymphocytes can suppress the response of the autologous peripheral blood lymphocytes to phytohemagglutinin.

Elson: I just want to add one further problem with the Con A system, and that is that this Con A is known to activate multiple subsets of cells including both helper and suppressor cells. Thus the addition of Con A pre-treated cells which do not result in suppression of these various subsets, may result in the proliferation of a cell that is ultimately going to suppress Ig synthesis. In other words, there is no functional equivalent of the suppressor of proliferation that you can directly apply to one of the arms of the immune response. You might end up by not suppressing a cell that will be a suppressor, so that even though you are looking at a lack of suppression in terms of proliferation the ultimate results might be enhanced suppression in a functionally meaningful system.

Auer: I briefly want to comment on the suggestion which was made to correlate spontaneous T suppressor cell activity with suppressor T-cell activity generated by Con A. I can only say that preliminary data do not show there is an inverse relation between spontaneous suppressor T-cell activity and the suppressor T-cell activity which can be activated *in vitro*.

Strober: Are you implying that you do not find a spontaneous suppressor T-cell?

Auer: Yes, but there is no inverse relation as it was suggested.

Knapp: I must say we have no clear data yet because the situation changes with the cell concentration used in the test system: with low cell concentrations one has a completely different situation than with high cell concentrations.

REGULATION OF IMMUNOGLOBULIN SYNTHESIS IN VITRO IN CROHN'S DISEASE: "COVERT" SUPPRESSOR T-CELLS

C.O. ⌐LSON, A.S. GRAEFF, S.P. JAMES and W. STROBER

INTRODUCTION

Crohn's disease [CD] is generally assumed to have an immunologic pathogenesis, but the mechanisms involved in the disease remain obscure. One hypothesis is that CD may be due to a defect in immune regulation which leads to an altered reactivity to enteric antigens. For this reason we asked whether CD patients have an abnormality of suppressor T cells regulating immunoglobulin synthesis.

PROCEDURE

Because nutritional depletion, infection and steroid therapy can have their own effects on tests of immune function, we chose to study only patients whose disease was well compensated. Peripheral blood was obtained from sixteen patients with mild or inactive CD. As a group, the patients had had the disease of average of 13 years, and five had an intestinal resection. Fourteen were known to have intestinal lesions on X-ray: in the small intestine in five, in the colon in one, and in both the small intestine and colon in eight. Despite this history, at the time of study disease activity was mild or inactive as assessed by the Crohn's activity index (1). Thirteen had a score of <150 and three had a score of approximately 200. Eleven were taking sulfasalazine; none were taking corticosteroids. Our control group consisted of randomly chosen normals in the same age range as the patients; peripheral blood cells from controls were studied concurrently with those from the patients.

Peripheral blood lymphocytes [PBL] were obtained by centrifugation over Ficoll-Hypaque. In some experiments the PBL were put directly into culture after thorough washing to remove any immunoglobulins. In other experiments, the PBL were separated into T cells and B cells by passage through an anti-immunoglobulin [anti-Fab] affinity column. After washing, the T cells and B cells were added back together and cultured. All cultures contained pokeweed mitogen to stimulate immunoglobulin synthesis. With this mitogen T cells play a critical role by helping or suppressing the transition of B cells into immunoglobulin secreting plasma cells. After seven days incubation the culture supernatants were collected and the amount of IgM present in them was measured using a specific double-antibody radioimmunoassay as previously described (2).

RESULTS

The synthesis of IgM in the pokeweed mitogen stimulated cultures of PBL from the patients, geometric mean 956 ng/culture x÷1.43 SEM, was not statistically different from that synthesized in the concurrent cultures of peripheral blood lymphocytes from normal controles, geometric mean 1667 ng/culture x÷1.34 SEM.

To determine whether PBL from patients contained altered regulatory cell activity, PBL from patients were mixed 1:1 with PBL from normal controls and cultured as before. There was no significant difference between the observed synthesis of IgM in such mixtures as compared to that which was expected from the synthesis of IgM obtained when each was cultured separately. Thus there was no evidence of altered suppressor cell activity in these cultures of whole, unseparated cell populations.

Because in previous studies we had found that cultures of purified B cells and T cells are a more sensitive method of assessing regulatory T cell influences, these cell populations were purified and then cultured together at multiple T cell to B cell ratios. In contrast to the previous studies using unseparated PBL, the synthesis of IgM in cultures of B cells and T cells from the patients [at an optimal T cell to B cell ratio of 5:1], was greatly decreased, geometric mean 290 ng/culture x÷1.31 SEM, compared to that seen in cultures of B cells and T cells from normal controls, geometric mean 1366 ng/culture x÷1.28 SEM. This difference was highly significant [p<0.005] by the Mann-Whitney two sample rank test. Because the cultures of B cells plus T cells from six of the patients had no detectable synthesis of IgM, further studies focused particularly on these six patients.

In the next set of experiments, B cells from normal controls were cultured with T cells from patients and vice versa. The synthesis of IgM in these mixtures was then compared to that in cultures of autologous B cells and T cells. There was no synthesis of IgM in cultures of normal B cells plus patient T cells, whereas there was good synthesis of IgM in cultures of patient B cells plus normal T cells in half of the patients studied; the other half did not show IgM synthesis even with normal T cells in the mixtures.

These data are consistent with either of two possibilities that the purified T cells from the patients have reduced helper activity or that they have increased suppressor activity. To resolve this question purified T cells or B cells were added to an indicator culture consisting of normal B cells plus normal irradiated [helper] T-cells. In these experiments the added B cells were irradiated prior to culture to prevent them from synthesizing immunoglobulin and the T cells were futher purified by sheep RBC rosetting prior to addition. The addition of either normal B cells or patient B cells had little or no effect on the synthesis of IgM by the indicator cells. The addition of normal T cells also had little effect. In contrast, addition of patient T cells markedly suppressed in the synthesis of IgM by the indicator cell culture [Table I]. Since this suppressor T cell was not evident in co-cultures of patient and normal PBL, we infer that it was generated during the cell separation procedure. For this reason, we have used the term "covert" to describe this suppressor T-cell because its activity is seen only after purification. We cannot discern whether it became evident during cell separation because of in vitro stimulation, or because a counter-acting cell population was removed in the cell purification procedure.

Table 1. The effect of purified B cells and T cells to an indicator culture of normal B cells plus irradiated normal T cells.

Indicator culture	Purified cells added	IgM ng/culture Expt.1	Expt.2
Normal B and T*	None	1713	2492
"	Normal B cells*	1581	2704
"	Crohn's B cells*	922	5251
"	Normal T cells	1598	9048
"	Crohn's T cells	<80	<80

*given 1500 R prior to culture

DISCUSSION AND CONCLUSION

We concluded that CD patients do not have a deficiency of suppressor T-cells regulating immunoglobulin synthesis. On the contrary, many CD patients have "covert" suppressor T-cells which only become evident after cell purification step in vitro. This cell has not been previously described in any study of human regulatory function. The significance of these findings is yet to be determined. It seems likely that covert suppressor T cell activity in vitro is probable the reflection of similar reactivity in vivo, perhaps as circulating PBL are separated as they filter through tissues. Regarding the role of these cells in the pathogenesis of this disease, two hypothesis are worthy of mention. First, the "covert" suppressor T-cell may represent a mechanism to control the disease by limiting the immune reaction in the intestine. Second, it may play a primary role in the disease by inhibiting an antibody response to some antigen or antigens, resulting in an ineffective immune response and chronic inflammation.

REFERENCES
1. Best WB, Becktel JM, Singleton JW, Kern F.Jr. (1976) Development of a Crohn's disease activety index. National cooperative Crohn's disease study. Gastroenterology 70:439-444
2. James SP, Elson CO, Jones EA, Strober W. (1980) Abnormal regulation of immunoglobulin synthesis in vitro in primary biliary cirrhosis, Gastroenterology 79:242-254

G16 Summary of Discussions relating to topic G15

Bienenstock: Could you tell us about the other immunoglobulin isotypes, IgG and IgA?

Elson: We are currently assaying the samples for IgG.
However, we feel it would be very unlikely that
there is going to be a difference among the Ig
classes.

Bienenstock: This might be one of the reasons that one finds
excessive numbers of IgG-containing cells in the
intestine of CD.

Hermon-   Were there any morphological changes in the
Taylor: target B-cells whose release of IgM had been inhibited by CD derived T-cells? This would help to
decide whether it was suppression of transcription
or whether it was modification of posttranslational
processing and transport.

Elson: No, we have no data on the morphology of the
B-cells.

Hodgson: The patients studied by Elson had either mild
or inactive disease and in fact were similar to the
group of patients in whom we, and Knapp found no
suppressor cell alteration. Did Elson looked at a
few patients who had active disease.

Elson: I can not say whether the more severely ill patients show less suppression or whether it gets
more enhanced.

MacDermott: We have looked at active, untreated patients and controls with regard to 12 day in vitro immunoglobulin synthesis. Control peripheral blood mononuclear cells have low spontaneous IgG and IgM immunoglobulin synthesis and PWM induces a marked increase. On the other hand, cells from patients with active CD or SLE all have increased spontaneous IgG and IgM synthesis and no major increase induced by PWM. With regard to IgA these findings are even more pronounced: the spontaneous synthesis and secretion of IgA by patients cells is as great or greater than seen after PWM activation of controls. Addition of PWM does not increase and in some instances suppresses this spontaneous activity.

Peña: Elson had some patients that were abnormal and others were normal. Do you think that this might suggest that there may be heterogeneity in this disease?

Elson: It is not clear right now whether all patients with CD have this suppressor T-cell to a varying extent or whether only a subset has it. However, IgM synthesis by culture of T and B cells from patients were generally lower than culture of normal cells, so that the patient population was much more uniform than it might appear.

Strober: In one or two cases one could find this suppressor cell without the necessity of separating the cells into T- and B-cell fraction so there is definitely a spectrum here ranging from patients in whom the cell is not demonstrable at all, to patients in whom they are demonstrable after cell separation, to patients in whom they are demonstrable without cell separation.

Knapp: Could you speculate on the mechanism of suppression of these cells?

Elson: What we think is going on is that during our cell purification procedure we are taking out another cell, an "anti-suppressor cell", which prevents the expression of the suppressor cell.

Hodgson: It seems to me that perhaps the simplest interpretation is that Elson's suppressor cell has disappeared during activity and that is why all those immunoglobulins are being made.

Elson: My guess is that it is going to be more complicated than that. If you have tremendous drive you get a lot of helper cells. It is quite possible that pokeweed is triggering the suppressor cell in this instance.

Jewell: If you take normal T-cells, and you incubate them with the IgM lymphocytotoxic antibody you depress the T-cell rosetting. It is therefore possible that in a group of patients with lymphocytotoxic antibodies in their serum for example, then in your initial cell extraction, you may get a different result when you look at cell function than when you go through a number of manipulative procedures. Immunoglobulin may be washed off the lymphocyte surface and reveals new functions and new activity. I just wondered what you thought about that?

Elson: By the nature of our assay we must remove the immunoglobulins from the cells before culture and to accomplish this we extensively wash these cells. Also we do not know what is occurring _in vivo,_ I don't think we have any idea. There is a great deal of evidence that much of the communication between subsets of T cells is going on through soluble mediators; thus expansion of suppressor T-cell subset could result from soluble mediators. However, whatever the mechanism, the patients clearly seem to be very distinct from the normals.

Jeejeebhoy: Firstly, I wonder whether some of your patients with clinically inactive CD who have shown the suppressor activity in fact had a segment of bowel left which was still inflamed, although clinically inactive. Secondly, one should consider the possibility of nutritional factors affecting the membrane, for instance, essential fatty acid deficiency which may be sub-clinical in these patients.

Elson: The patients were all actively working and carrying on their occupations. They were all eating well, they all looked well; it is hard to believe and even harder to prove that they had subclinical nutritional deficiency. Is is a very difficult problem to control these studies. Which group do you look at? Do you look at the ones who are hospitalized and are with a huge inflammatory mass? We chose to try to eliminate the nutritional, infectious and drug-related side-effects, by selecting a patient population with non-active disease. I think it is probably as good as a population as you are going to get if you are interested in primary factors unless you were able to study pre-symptomatic Crohn's patients.

T-CELL SUBSETS, IMMUNOREGULATORY CELLS AND LYMPHOCYTE RESPONSIVENESS IN CROHN'S DISEASE

H.J.F. HODGSON and R.M.M. VICTORINO

INTRODUCTION

Studies of cellular immune function in Crohn's disease have pursued two lines: 1) there is evidence of a generalised depression of cellular immune function, as evidenced by skin testing, in vitro lymphocyte responses and skin sensitization techniques (1); whether this is merely a non-specific concomitant of illness, or persists in remission, is still uncertain; 2) in contrast to this depression in the general level of cell-mediated immunity, there is evidence of enhanced specific cellular immune responses against gut bacteria, intestinal contents and, most strikingly, colonic epithelium (2). Expression of these specific immune responses may contribute to the tissue damage of inflammatory bowel disease.

The concept that Crohn's disease may involve cellular auto-immune reactions to the gut has lead to the investigation of immunoregulation as much recent evidence suggests that the development of auto-immunity follows a loss of suppressor cell activity. Studies of peripheral blood concanavalin A-induced suppressor cell activity, which reflects the function of a specific subpopulation of T-cells which develop suppressor activity in vitro, indicated that during active disease Con A-induced suppression is decreased (3).

Recently, subsets of T cells in man have been delineated which can be differentiated by the possession of Fc receptors for IgM [Tμ cells] or IgG [Tγ cells]. These cells have immunoregulatory functions _in vitro_, Tμ cells helping and Tγ cells suppressing immunoglobulin synthesis (4).

The purpose of the present study was to enumerate circulating Tμ and Tγ cells in patients with Crohn's disease [and ulcerative colitis] and correlate the findings with a simul-

taneous measurement of suppressor activity of the cell population. We used a test designed to reflect the spontaneous
suppressor function present (5) rather than Con A-induced
activity. We also explored the relation between cellular
immune responsiveness, as measured by lymphocyte transformation in response to mitogens, T cell subsets and suppressor
activity.

PROCEDURE

T_μ and T_γ cells: these were measured in patients and
controls by counting the proportion of T cells rosetting with
ox erythrocytes coated with sub-agglutinating doses of IgM or
IgG antibody (4).

Short-lived suppressor cell activity: This test is based
on the demonstration that spontaneously active suppressor
cells are short lived in culture, and the response of cells
to mitogen stimulation immediately after isolation is less
than the response of cells which have been incubated for 24
hours. Results are expressed as a suppressor index [S.I.] and

$$S.I. = \frac{\text{cpm in cells stimulated after 24 hours}}{\text{cpm in cells stimulated immediately}}$$

higher indices reflect greater spontaneous short-lived suppressor activity initially present (5).

Lymphocyte responsiveness to mitogens [Con A, Phytohaemagglutinin and pokeweed]: this was measured using a micro-
culture technique.

RESULTS

Total T cell numbers did not differ between patients with
Crohn's disease [2,097 [+198 SEM] per μl] and control individuals [2,030 + 118 per μl] Similarly T_γ cells did not differ
between these groups, but there was a striking reduction in
T_μ cells [Table 1]. This reduction was seen in patients whose
disease was active and in patients in remission, and whether
or not patients were on treatment with systemic corticosteroids.

Table 1. T_μ and T_γ cells in peripheral blood of inflammatory bowel disease, in absolute no/μl. Figures in parenthesis equal as % of total T cells $\pm$ SEM

	T_μ	T_γ
Controls [n=25]	980$\pm$ 53 [44.4$\pm$1.5%]	291$\pm$33 [13.8$\pm$0.9%]
Crohn's disease [n=23]	615$\pm$ 73 [29.5$\pm$1.7%]	269$\pm$35 [13.1$\pm$1.1%]
Ulcerative colitis [n=8]	420$\pm$114 [29.5$\pm$4.4%]	220$\pm$33 [17.2$\pm$1.5%]

Patients with inflammatory bowel disease [19 with Crohn's disease, 7 with ulcerative colitis] had a mean suppressor index of 1.78 $\pm$ 0.18 indicating a significant [p<0.01] reduction in spontaneous suppressor cell activity compared to controls whose mean suppressor index was 2.94 [$\pm$ 0.18]. The loss of suppressor cell activity was much more marked amongst patients with active disease [mean 1.6 $\pm$ 0.12] than patients with inactive disease [2.55 $\pm$ 0.48]; it was seen both in patients on treatment with systemic corticosteroids and in those without. There was however no correlation between suppressor activity and the number of circulating T_μ or T_γ cells.

Lymphocyte hyporesponsiveness to phytohaemagglutinin [PHA], Con A and pokeweed mitogen [PWM] [using eight different doses in all] was confirmed in both Crohn's disease and ulcerative colitis, when compared with healthy controls. Furthermore, there was a striking correlation between lymphocyte responsiveness [in cpm of ^{3}H-thymidine incorporated] and the absolute numbers of T_μ cells present [Table 2]. No correlation between T_γ cells and lymphocyte responsiveness was found.

Table 2. Correlation between no. of Tμ cells and lymphocyte
responses to mitogens in vitro.

		r	p
Con A	[15 μg/ml]	0.67	<0.05
Con A	[50 μg/ml]	0.84	<0.001
Con A	[250 μg/ml]		n.s.
PHA	[2.5μg/ml]	0.78	<0.01
PHA	[25 μg/ml]	0.69	<0.01
PHA	[250 μg/ml]		n.s.
PWM	[4 μg/ml]	0.54	<0.02
	[40 μg/ml]	0.60	<0.01

DISCUSSION

These results extend the previous observations on induced
suppressor cell function and indicate that spontaneous suppressor cell activity is reduced during active inflammatory
bowel disease. These measurements are made on peripheral
blood cells, and use in vitro assessments of suppressor activity, but they suggest that abnormal immunoregulation exists
in inflammatory bowel disease, and may permit the expression
of damaging immune responses directed against the gut. These
abnormalities in suppressor function merit further attention,
as potentially alteration of the activity of immunoregulatory
cells could provide an alternative means of therapy in inflammatory bowel disease.

We also describe a significant imbalance amongst T cells
in patients with Crohn's disease, independent of disease
activity or therapy. This did not provide the basis for the
suppressor cell abnormalities described, but correlated well
with the lymphocyte responsiveness found in this condition.
The correlation between diminished Tμ cells and low mitogen
responsiveness might reflect the loss of the helper activity
present in this population, but it seems more likely that
many of the lymphocytes responding to the mitogens reside
within the Tμ cell population. We do not know whether
Tμ cells are diminished as a primary abnormality, or by sequestration or loss into the gut, but we suggest that the
reduction in circulating Tμ cells is the cellular basis for
depressed cell-mediated immunity in Crohn's disease.

CONCLUSION

Patients with Crohn's disease have abnormal T cell subpopulations, with reduced numbers of Tμ cells, but normal numbers of total Tγ cells. A different test of suppressor cell activity from that used previously (3) confirmed deficient activity during active disease; the activity of the short-lived suppressor cell however did not correlate with numbers of either Tμ or Tγ cells in peripheral blood. Lymphocyte hyporesponsiveness correlated well with diminished numbers of circulating Tμ cells. Whilst this could reflect a loss of helper activity of Tμ cells, it seems more likely that the Tμ cells themselves are those largely responsible for mitogen responses _in vitro_. We suggest that a reduction in circulating Tγ cells is the cellular basis for depressed cell-mediated immunity in Crohn's disease.

ACKNOWLEDGEMENT

This work was supported by a grant from the Medical Research Council of the U.K.

REFERENCES
1. Sachar DB, Taub RN, Ramachander K, Meyers S, Forman SP, Douglas SD, Janowitz HD. (1976) T and B lymphocytes and cutaneous anergy in inflammatory bowel disease. Am.N.Y. Acad.Sci. 278:565-570
2. Shorter RG, Cardoza M, Huizenga KA, ReMine SG, Spencer RJ. (1969) Further studies of in vitro cytotoxicity of lymphocytes for colonic epithelial cells. Gastroenterology. 57:30-35
3. Hodgson HJF, Wands JR, Isselbacher KJ. (1978) Decreased suppressor cell activity in inflammatory bowel disease. Clin.Exp.Immunol. 32:451-488
4. Moretta L, Webb S, Grossi C, Lydyard P, Cooper M. (1977) Functional analysis of the two human T cell subpopulations help and suppression of B cell responses by T cells bearing receptors for IgM or IgG. J.Exp.Med. 146:184-200
5. Bresnihan B, Jasin HE. (1977) Suppressor function of peripheral blood mononuclear cells in normal individuals and patients with systemic lupus erythematosus. J.Clin. Invest. 59:106-116.

T-CELL SUBPOPULATIONS IN CROHN'S DISEASE

A.S.PEÑA, JETSKE CNOSSEN, MIEKE G. DAMSTEEG, IRENE T.WETERMAN and C.J.L.M. MEIJER

INTRODUCTION

Human T lymphocytes bearing receptors for the Fc portion of rabbit IgG[T_γ] and rabbit IgM[T_μ] have been identified (1,2). The T_μ subclass appears to help B-cell differentiation induced by pokeweed mitogen. T_γ cells after interaction with IgG immune complexes suppress B-cell differentiation (3).

T_μ cells are typical small- or medium-sized lymphocytes with distinctive cytoplasmic accumulations with one or two spots of nonspecific acid esterase activity (4). Although Fc-IgM receptors do not appear to be markers for distinct T cell subsets under some conditions as transition of T_γ to T_μ cells has been observed, e.g., after immune complex interaction (5), T cells are theophylline-resistant and have a helper function in the induction of plaque forming cells, specific for sheep red blood cells or ovalbumin (6). It is possible that within the T_μ subpopulation different subsets with different functions exist. In this regard, it has been shown that a] when purified T_μ cells were treated with neuraminidase, a small population expressed later both T_μ and T_γ (7); b] using monoclonal antibodies against T cells that the T_μ subpopulation contained both inducer and cytotoxic/suppressor populations (8).

The study of T cell subsets in Crohn's disease [CD] might be important not only in understanding the immunological abnormalities observed in this disease but also in the study of genetic markers as the presence of T cell antigen polymorphisms has recently been shown in man (4,5).

MATERIAL AND METHODS

Sixteen patients with CD and 22 controls have been studied using a mixed rosette assay for the detection of Tμ and Tγ in unfractionated carbonyl-iron monocyte depleted lymphocyte suspensions (6). In this test T lymphocytes are detected with neuraminidase treated sheep erythrocytes [SRBC]; Ox erythrocytes [ORBC], labelled with fluorescein isothiocyanate and sensitized with either rabbit IgM or anti-ox antibodies, are used as indicator erythrocytes for rabbit Fc bearing lymphocytes. For counting the rosette forming cells the mononuclear cells are stained with acridine orange. At least 200 lymphocytes were counted. A mixed rosette was scored when two or more erythrocytes of each kind adhered to a lymphocyte. Four types of lymphocytes are recognized:

a] Lymphocytes with SRBC and ORBC which are T cells with receptor for the Fc fragment of IgG or IgM;

b] Lymphocytes with SRBC but without ORBC which are T cells without receptors for IgG or IgM;

c] Lymphocytes without SRBC but with ORBC which are B cells which have receptors for the Fc fragment of IgG; and also N or K cells

d] Lymphocytes without SRBC or ORBC which represent a subpopulation of B cells.

RESULTS

T cells were determined one hour and 24 hours after incubation at $4^{\circ}C$. No significant differences were observed between patients and controls. However, within the T cells subpopulations the T_μ and the T_γ cells were significantly depressed in the patients [see table 1 and table 2]. The total Fc receptor cell population was also decreased in the patients but this was due exclusively to the T_μ fraction.

No significant differences were observed between the patients in an active phase of the disease and those in remission. No correlation was found between the T-cell counts and the E.S.R., Haemoglobin, serum Iron and serum total iron binding capacity. Some patients not receiving corticosteroids or salazopyrin had low T_μ percentages as well.

Table 1. Percentage of T cells, T cell subsets and other Fc receptor-bearing cells in lymphocytes of patients with Crohn's disease and controls

cells	patients [n=16]		controls [n=10]		T*	p
	x[%]	s[%]	x[%]	s[%]		
T	71.81	6.52	70.95	5.21	0.4519	n.s
Fcμ	29.95	8.00	43.86	3.75	7.1745	<0.0001
Tμ	36.50	8.73	56.86	5.56	8.7820	<0.0001
Fcγ	23.0	8.95	23.05	3.44	0.0240	n.s.
Tγ	10.75	2.27	12.52	1.69**	2.7218	<0.001

*student's t-test, **N=21

Table 2. Absolute number per mm^3 of T cells and cell subsets in the peripheral circulation of Crohn's patients and controls

cells	patients [n = 14]		controls [n = 7]		T*	p
	x	s	x	s		
T	1066	239	1404	178	3.2956	<0.001
Tμ	386	132	1056	203	9.1659	<0.0005
Tγ	113	30	229	46	6.9932	<0.0005

* Student's t-test

DISCUSSION AND CONCLUSIONS

The present work has shown that in spite of normal total number of T cells in the peripheral blood of CD patients, significant imbalances in T-cell subsets do exist, namely, Tμ and Tγ cells are significantly decreased.

Low percentages of Tμ cells have been found in progressive systemic sclerosis (12), in aging humans (13) and more recently, Meijer et al.(14) have found very low percentages of Tμ in active rheumatoid arthritis. As shown in table 1 the Fcγ cells were normal. As the Tγ were decreased this suggest that NK cells or non-fagocytic cells of the monocytic series bearing Fcγ receptors are increased. As no functional tests were carried out sofar and we don't have data about the distribution of these T-cell subsets in the lamina propria of the affected bowel, no prediction can be made at present about the significance of these findings in the pathogenesis of CD.

REFERENCES

1. Ferrarini M, Moretta L, Abrile L, Durante M.(1975) Receptors for IgG molecules on human lymphocytes forming spontaneous rosettes with sheep erythrocytes. Eur.J.Immunol. 5:70-72
2. Gmelig-Myeling F, Ham van der M, Ballieux RE.(1976) Binding of IgM by human T lymphocytes. Scand.J.Immunol. 5:487-495
3. Moretta L, Webb SR, Grossi CE. Lydyard PM, Cooper MD (1977) Functional analysis of two human T-cell subpopulations: help and suppression of B-cell responses by T cells bearing receptors for IgM or IgG. J.Exp.Med. 146:184-200
4. Grossi CE, Webb SR, Zicca A, Lydyard PM, Moretta L, Mingari MC, Cooper MD.(1978) Morphological and histochemical analysis of two human T-cell subpopulations bearing receptors for IgM or IgG. J.Exp.Med. 147:1405-1417
5. Pichler WJ, Lum L, Broder S. (1978) Fc-receptors on hum T lymphocytes. 1.Transition of T to T cells. J.Immunol. 121:1540-1548
6. Shore A, Dosch HM, Gelfand EW. (1970) Induction and separation of antigen-dependant T helper and T suppressor cells in man. Nature [London] 274:586-587
7. Schulof RS, Fernandes R, Good RA, Gupta S. (1979) Neuraminidase treatment of human T lymphocyte subpopulations. Effect on expression of Fc receptors for IgM and IgG. Fed Proc. 38:1273
8. Reinherz EL, Moretta L, Roper M, Breard JM, Mingari MC, Cooper MD, Schlossman SF.(1980) Human T lymphocyte subpopulations defined by Fc receptors and monoclonal antibodies. A comparison. J.Exp.Med. 151:969-974
9. Ferrara GB.(1979) Identification of new cell surface markers in man: the problem of immunogenicity.Transplant. Proc. XI:715-721
10. Leeuwen van A. (1979) Alloantibodies that react with subsets of human T cells. Tissue Antigens 14:437-443
11. Cnossen J, Lafeber CJM, Damsteeg WGM, Meijer CJLM.(1980) Mixed rosette assay for the detection of T and T lymphocytes. J.Immunol.Meth. 36:197-210
12. Gupta S, Good RA.(1979) Subpopulation in human T lymphocytes.IX Imbalance of T cell subpopulations in patients with progressive systemic sclerosis. Clin.Exp.Immunol. 38:342-347
13. Gupta S, Good RA. (1979) Subpopulation of human T lymphocytes. X Alterations in T, B, Third population cells and T cell with receptors for IgM or IgG in ageing humans. J.Immunol. 122:1214-1219
14. Meijer CJLM, Lafeber CJM, Cnossen J, Damsteeg M, Cats A.(1980) T lymphocyte subpopulations in rheumatoid arthritis. Submitted for publication

G19 Summary of Discussions relating to topics G17 to G18

Elson: In view of MacDermott's findings about the high IgA synthesis in isolated gut mucosal lymphocytes it would be interesting to study the T cell bearing Fc-receptors for IgA. In relation to the significance of the changes in the T population, I think that unless we can get a better assessment of functional activity, we do not know whether the T cells are immunoregulating or causing tissue damage, or whether the T cells simply shunt off into the mucosa.

Meijer: We found a good correlation between the activity of Rheumatoid Arthritis as expressed in the Ricchi index, the erythrocytes sedimentation rate and the levels of the T_μ cells: when disease activity was high, T_μ cell levels were low.

Strober: There is now a set of antisera available, which appears to be able to differentiate among the various classes of immunoregulatory cells. In particular, the OK 4 antiserum appears to recognize distinct markers on helper cells whereas OK 5 and 8 recognize distinct markers on suppressor-cytotoxic cells. So perhaps the means of identifying immunoregulatory cells on a more definite basis is now at hand.

IS THERE PHA HYPORESPONSIVENESS IN THE INFLAMMATORY BOWEL DISEASES?

W.R. THAYER and C. CHARLAND

INTRODUCTION

Lymphocyte stimulation by phytohemagglutinin in [PHA] has been extensively studied in both Crohn's disease [CD] and ulcerative colitis [UC]. However, there are considerable discrepancies in the published results. Many investigators report diminished reactivity of lymphocytes, primarily in CD (1-5), but also in UC (2,6,7). On the other hand, an equal number of investigators have reported normal reactivity to this same mitogen (6, 8-16). Since most of the investigators used a conventional single optimal PHA stimulating dose with lymphoid cells from patients with varying disease duration, activity, extent and treatment, the resulting heterogeneity makes it even more difficult to reconcile the results. Furthermore, in the PHA stimulation studies, the amount of "optimal" mitogen used and the length of the incubation period have varied.

It has been shown that lymphocyte transformation by widely different, especially lower, PHA concentrations can elicit a better spectrum of lymphocyte capabilities than the conventional optimal single dose PHA stimulation (17). This approach, especially when used with Hodgkin's disease, can detect the early presence of an intrinsic functional lymphocyte defect (18,19). In an effort to quantitate the supposed immune defect in the inflammatory bowel diseases, this study examines the response of the lymphocytes from these patients and an age- and sex-matched control population, to suboptimal doses of PHA.

PROCEDURE

Eleven CD and nine UC patients who were either untreated,

or had been off all medication for the previous month were studied. To rule out malnutrition-induced PHA suppression, only patients with a normal serum albumin were tested. Run concurrently with the 20 IBD patients were 23 healthy controls matched to the age and sex of the patients.

Lymphocytes were separated on Isolymph^{TM} as described previously (29) and were adjusted to 2×10^6 cells/ml in media containing 40% pooled or autologous human serum. Highly purified PHA, diluted from a stock concentration, was used as the mitogen. The optimal dose of PHA, 2.5 μg/ml, was determined by establishing a dose response curve in pooled human serum using lymphocytes from 26 additional healthy controls. PHA stimulation was carried out using standard techniques and all measurements were done in duplicate (21).

RESULTS

The results of the 26 standardizing controls showed that the optimal stimulating dose of PHA was 2.5 μg/ml. At this concentration the mean count per minute of these normal lymphocytes was 24,380±1,286 with a range between 8,630 to 37,731. The 23 concurrently run controls when tested in pooled human serum had a mean of 28,520±1,714 with a range of 12,528 to 45,201, while in autologous serum, the mean was 21,654±2,200 with a range of 8,797 to 41,924. There was no significant difference between the control groups and the standardizing controls.

At the optimal concentrations of PHA in either pooled human or autologous serum, the IBD patients showed no significant difference compared to concurrently run controls. In pooled human serum, the 11 CD patients had a mean of 28,838 ±2,537 with a range of 18,199 to 50,293; while the 9 UC patients had a mean of 30,973±5,332 with a range of 8,508 to 55,032. In autologous serum, the CD group showed a mean of 19,014±2,600 with a range of 11,188 to 31,134, while the UC group showed a mean of 25,497±2,188 with a range of 16,989 to 38,206. Neither subgroup was significantly different from each other or its concurrently run controls when tested in either pooled human or autologous serum.

When suboptimal doses of PHA were employed in an effort to detect mild degrees of hyporesponsiveness, the dose response curves constructed for the CD and UC patients did not differ significantly from that of concurrently run controls.

When each point on the curve was analyzed separately, no significant differences appeared for either UC or CD when compared to controls or to each other.

DISCUSSION

These results are similar to the well controlled studies of Ropke, where different concentrations of PHA and different culture times in both autologous and pooled human serum were used (12). Others have also dose response curves, but it is difficult to interpret their data in regards to suboptimal PHA concentrations. The reason for the discrepancies in PHA responsiveness reported by various investigators is not readily explained. Some of he variability could be caused by extraneous factors. For instance, in at least one study post-surgical patients were used (22) and surgery has been implicated in depressed immune responsiveness (23). In other studies, it is unclear whether the patients were on steroids, a medication that can suppress PHA responsiveness (24). Finally, the nutritional state of the patient may be important. Since malnutrition can effect PHA responsiveness (25), the malnutrition which many of these patients suffer because of anorexia, malabsorption, fever, protein-losing enteropathy, and fistulae, may be responsible for the diversity of results. Since none of our patients were studied post-operatively or while on steroids, and since all had normal nutrition as judged by a normal serum albumin, these factors did not affect our results. In view of these facts, our results indicate the unlikelihood that diminished responsiveness could be much of a factor in the pathogenesis of IBD.

CONCLUSIONS

The results of this investigation do not give any support to the contention that anergy plays an important role in the pathogenesis of either UC or CD.

ACKNOWLEDGEMENTS

From the Department of Medicine, Brown University, Providence, RI Supported by the National Foundation for Ileitis and Colitis.

REFERENCES
1. Parent K, Barrett J, Wilson ID. (1971) Investigation of the pathogenic mechanisms in regional enteritis with in vitro lymphocyte cultures. Gastroenterology 61:431-439
2. Sachar DB, Taub RN, Brown SM, Present DH, Korelitz BI, Janowitz HD. (1973) Impaired lymphocyte responsiveness in inflammatory bowel disease. Gastroenterol. 64:203-209
3. Guillou PJ, Brenman TG, Giles GR. (1973) Lymphocyte transformation in the mesenteric lymph nodes of patients with Crohn's disease. Gut 14:20-24
4. Walker JG, Greaves MF. (1969) Delayed hypersensitivity and lymphocyte transformation in Crohn's disease and proctocolitis. Gut 10:414
5. Cave D, Brooke BN. (1973) A study of lymphocyte function in Crohn's disease using the mitotic index. Brit.J.Surg. 60:319
6. Asquith P, Kraft SC, Rothberg RM. (1973) Lymphocyte responses to nonspecific mitogens in inflammatory bowel disease. Gastroenterology 65:1-7
7. Chiba M. (1977) Cellular immunological studies in chronic ulcerative colitis. Hirosaki Igaku 29:1-14
8. Bird AG, Britton S. (1974) No evidence for decreased lymphocyte reactivity in Crohn's disease. Gastroenterology 67:926-932
9. Meuwissen SGM, Schellekens PA, Huismans L, Tytgat G. (1975) Impaired anamnestic cellular immune response in patients with Crohn's disease. Gut 16:854-860
10. McHattie J, Magil A, Jeejeebhoy K, Falk RE. (1971) Immunoresponsiveness of lymphocytes from patients with regional ileocolitis [Crohn's disease] by in vitro testing. Clin.Res. 19:779
11. Aas J, Huizenga KA, Newcomer AD, Shorter RG. (1972) Inflammatory bowel disease:lymphocytic responses to nonspecific stimulation in vitro. Scand.J.Gastroenterol. 7:299-303
12. Ropke C. (1972) Lymphocyte transformation and delayed hypersensitivity in Crohn's disease. Scand.J.Gastroenterol. 7:671-677
13. Bolton PM, James SL, Newcombe RG, Whitehead RH, Hughes LE. (1973) The immune competence of patients with inflammatory bowel disease. Gut 15:213-219

14. Bolton PM, James SL, Hughes LE. (1973) Is there impaired immunity in patients with Crohn's disease? Brit.J.Surg. 60:319
15. Townsend C, Sakai H, Ritzmann SE, Fiske JC. (1972) Lymphocyte reactivity in patients with regional enteritis. Surg.Forum 23:394-396
16. Stefani S, Fink S. (1967) Effect of E.coli antigens, tuberculin and phytohaemagglutinin upon ulcerative colitis lymphocytes. Gut:249-252
17. Fitzgerald M. (1971) The establishment of a normal human population dose response curve for lymphocytes cultured with PHA [phytohaemagglutinin] Clin.Exp.Immunol. 8:421-425
18. Faguet GB. (1975) Quantitation of immunocompetence in Hodgkin's disease. J.Clin.Invest. 56:951-957
19. Levy R, Kaplan HS. (1974) Impaired lymphocyte function in untreated Hodgkin's disease. New Engl.J.Med. 290:181-186
20. Thayer WR, Charland C, Field CE. (1976) The subpopulations of circulating white blood cells in inflammatory bowel disease. Gastroenterology 71:379-384
21. Sibbitt W, Bankhurst A, Williams R. (1978) Studies of cell subpopulations mediating mitogen hyporesponsiveness in patients with Hodgkin's disease. J.Clin.Invest. 61:55-63
22. Brown SM, Taub RN, Present DH, Janowitz HD. (1970) Short-term lymphocyte cultures in regional enteritis. Lancet 1:1112
23. Riddle PR, Berenbaum MC. (1967) Postoperative depression of the lymphocyte response to phytohaemagglutinin. Lancet 1:746-748
24. Claman HN. (1972) Corticosteroids and lymphoid cells. New Engl.J.Med. 287:388-397
25. McFarlane H, Hamid J. (1973) Cell-mediated immune response in malnutrition. Clin.Exp.Immunol. 13:153-164

G21 Summary of Discussions relating to topic G20

Booth: Knight has shown that one of the major consi-
            derations that has to be given to this sort of
            study, is the initial concentration. Do you think
            that that might explain the enormous variation of
            results that people are obtaining?

Thayer: That is a possibility. We have looked at other
            concentrations of cells and do not find any differ-
            ences. We originally set out to do this study be-
            cause we thought that the way you could explain the
            results in the literature was that there were two
            populations of patients which might differ clini-
            cally. However, we did not find significant differ-
            ences in the Crohn's populations.

Elson: We can confirm this observation. For the pa-
            tient group that we studied in the immunoglobulin
            synthesis system, we did also performed prolifera-
            tion studies. Their values were normal.

Hodgson: Although total T-cell numbers are generally
            normal, Thayer did suggest that there is a sub-
            group of patients with CD who had very low numbers
            of T-cells. I wonder whether any of these patients
            were included in the proliferation studies?

Thayer: We did some studies in which we divided the
            PHA-stimulation by the total number of T-cells in
            our incubation media. We did not find any signifi-
            cant difference from the normals.

Asquith: Thayer makes an important point about the dif-
                ference in methodology used in the various popu-
                lation studies. If you look at the 200 publications
                on this issue, they differ in the number of cells
                cultured and the dose of PHA. So it is not a sur-
                prise that there is such a variation. Did you check
                the nutritional status of the patients?

Thayer: I have not used the sub-optimal PHA dose in
                studying patients with active disease. We have
                correlated PHA responsiveness to the CDAI and did
                not find any correlation, although the CDAI was not
                to high because we did not study anybody who is on
                steroids. So, that may be a point.

Strober: That could be a significant point, because per-
                haps only the very severely ill patients, will show
                the defect.

Thayer: It has been shown in Hodgkin's disease that the
                sicker the patients, the more the PHA response is
                depressed. But even with Hodgkin's disease of low
                clinical activity you can show a depressed response
                to PHA by using a sub-optimal dose. So, even if PHA
                responsiveness is decreased in patients with very
                active CD, does that have any real significance?

MacDermott: Mitogenic lectins are firstly very non-specific
                and secondly are themselves very variable. PHA is
                actually composed of substances including erythro-
                phytohemagglutinin, a leucoagglutinin and other
                non-specific materials; the same goes for PWM which
                can be split into five different active molecules.
                Lectins also differ on the bases of their source.
                Israeli wheat germ agglutinin is much different
                than wheat germ agglutinin which is made in the
                U.S. in its mitogenic properties and its cytotoxic

induction properties. So there are differences not only in some of the techniques used, but also in the mitogenic lectins themselves.

Thayer: We were well aware of this and we therefore used a constant batch of the purified PHA.

Strober: Some years ago we studied patients with intestinal lymphangiectesia who have loss of T-cells into the GI-tract. In severely ill CD patients you may also have such loss. In the intestinal lymphangiectesia patients there was a great reduction in capacity to respond to mitogens as well as antigenic substances. Do you think that T-cell loss into GI tract might play a role in some of the more severely ill CD patients?

Thayer: We checked that by counting the number of T-cells in our preparation and dividing the PHA stimulation by the total number of T-cells.

Strober: That procedure would not correct for GI loss of selected T-cell population.

Bos: Do you have specific data on the zinc status of your patients? It is known that the phytohemagglutinin stimulation test is influenced by zinc levels in the medium.

Thayer: I do not have any data on the zinc levels.

INABILITY TO DEMONSTRATE ANTIBODY-DEPENDENT CELL CYTOTOXICITY
AGAINST COLON LIPOPOLYSACCHARIDE ANTIGEN BY INFLAMMATORY
BOWEL DISEASE SERA

W.R. THAYER and P. PERLMANN

INTRODUCTION

Although circulating antibodies, reactive with colonic
mucosa, have been repeatedly demonstrated in patients with
both ulcerative colitis [UC] and Crohn's disease [CD]
(1,2,3), these antibodies do not appear to be cytotoxic even
with the addition of complement (4). However, antibodies,
complexing to target cells could induce cell cytotoxicity by
a mechanism called antibody-dependent cell cytotoxicity
[ADCC] (5). These antibodies, responsible for the ADCC reaction, are almost invariably in the IgG class (6), but recent
evidence suggests that the IgM antibodies can occasionally
participate (7). Since circulating anticolon antibodies can
be found in the IgG class (8), this study was undertaken to
see if these antibodies could be responsible for the colon
cytotoxicity by an ADCC mechanism.

The antigen to which these antibodies bind was first
demonstrated in lipopolysaccharide extracts of human fetal
colon (1). However, similar cross-reacting antigens have been
demonstrated in extracts of colon and feces from germ free
rats (9) and also appear to be related to the common enterobacterial antigen of Kunin (9).

PROCEDURES

Blood was collected from 20 UC and 12 CD patients with
varying degrees of disease activity as well as from 15 healthy controls and allowed to clot at room temperature before
removal of the sera. Sera was first inactivated at $56^{\circ}C$ and
then absorbed with a equal volume of washed chicken red blood
cells [CRBC] to remove any potential CRBC antibodies. Anti-

GFRC antibody titers of the patients and control sera were determined by use of a previously described hemagglutination technique (2,3).

Lipopolysaccharide antigen was extracted from germ free rat feces, human fetal colon, and E. coli 0:14 with the phenol water method using a modification of Westphall's method (1). Anti-GFRC, anti-E. coli 0:14 and anti-human fetal colon antisera was prepared in rabbits by repeated intravenous immunizations (10).

Freshly drawn CRBC were incubated with solubilized antigen. Coating of the CRBC could be demonstrated using a standard hemagglutination assay against the appropriate rabbit antisera. After coating, the cells were incubated with $Na_2{}^{51}CrO_4$. Normal human peripheral lymphocytes, the effector cells, were purified by gelatin sedimentation, passage through a nylon wool column and centrifugation on a Ficoll-Isopaque gradient (4). The ADCC assay was performed according to the method of Perlmann and Perlmann (6) by incubating 0.5 ml of the lymphocyte suspension containing 5×10^6 lymphocytes/ml, 0.5 ml of the test serum in various dilutions and 0.5 ml of the antigen ^{51}Cr-coated CRBC [2×10^5 CRBC/ml]. This gave an effector to target ratio of 25:1. Positive and negative controls were established with GFRC antisera and normal rabbit sera respectively at a dilution of 1×10^{-5}. Controls using ^{51}Cr-labeled CRBC without absorbed antigen and controls without lymphocytes were run concurrently. Upon completion of incubation for 18 hours, the cells were centrifuged and 1 ml of each tube was withdrawn and transferred to a fresh tube. Radioactivity in both the sediment and supernatant was then counted and isotope release calculated as:

$$\% \text{ Release} = \frac{c \times 100}{a + b} \qquad \begin{array}{l} a = \text{Activity in Supernatant} \\ b = \text{Activity in Sediment} \\ c = a \times 1.5 \end{array}$$

All 32 patients and 15 controls were tested against the GFRC antigen. Five of the patients [3 UC, 2 CD] and five controls were tested against the human fetal colon and E. coli 0:14 antigens.

Cytoxicity inhibition studies were also performed by

preincubating the GFRC antigen coated CRBC in either inflammatory bowel disease sera, control sera or buffer, and then performing the ADCC assay using the heterologous anti-GFRC antibody at a 10^{-6} dilution. Percent inhibition was then determined as :

$$\% \text{ Inhibition} = \frac{a - b}{a}$$ a = Cytotoxicity of CRBC in buffer
B = Cytotoxicity of CRBC in studied sera

RESULTS

Only one of the 13 tested controls had GRRC titers above 1:16, while 8 of the 16 UC and 5 of the 12 CD patients showed titers above this value. None of the controls or patients demonstrated ADCC to either GFRC, E. coli 0:14 or human fetal colon antigen coated CRBC, while the heterologous antisera always caused more than 70% cytotoxicity.

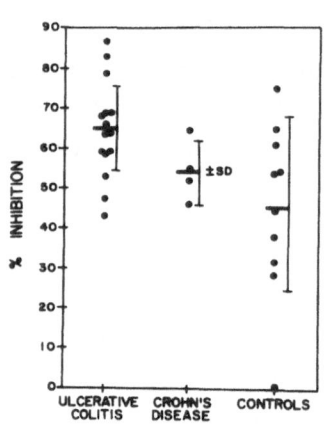

In the inhibition experiments, all three groups [UC, DC, and controls] showed inhibition. The UC sera averaged 65.1±11.1 SD [range 47.4-86.7], the CD sera showed a mean of 54.1±7.3 [46-63.5], and controls 45.2±21.6 [0-75]. The UC sera was statistically different from the controls [p<0.01] by Student's t-test. [fig.1]

Figure 1. Inhibition of ADCC by IBD and control sera

DISCUSSION

The results indicate that despite the presence of anti-colon antibodies in the sera, no in vitro cytotoxicity could be induced in normal lymphocytes against either GFRC, human fetal colon or E.coli 0:14 coated target cells. The earlier work of Broberger et al. (4) suggested that these antibodies, although binding to the target cells, were not cytotoxic. However, further work by Shorter et al.(11) suggests that a factor in the sera of IBD patients is capable of activating lymphocytes to become cytotoxic to colon epithelial cells. More recent investigations by this group suggest that the activated lymphocyte is a K-cell and the mechanism of target cell destruction is possible ADCC (12). These results, then, would suggest that the antigen and antibody involved in the in vitro cytotoxicity do not appear to be the lipopoly-saccharide antigen and antibody system first described by Broberger and Perlmann (1). However, these results do not rule out other antigen-antibody system which might be cyto-toxic.

The inhibition experiments, on the other hand, are diffi-cult to interpret since, although in UC there is a statisti-cally increased inhibition of rabbit antisera induced ADCC to the GFRC antigen, some inhibition is found in almost all sera tested. Antigen-antibody complexes present in the sera of patients with UC have been shown to competitively inhibit the ADCC test (13). In this case, the inhibition would be direc-ted at the effector cell, since the complexes inhibit by binding to an Fc receptor on the white blood cell. Similarly blocking seen with other substances such as anti-IgG (14), anti-Fc, staphylococcal protein, and rheumatoid factor (15) seem to be directed against the immunoglobulin bound to the target cell. This type of inhibition would also not be detec-ted in our assay.

CONCLUSION

These results show that IBD sera does not induce cyto-toxicity to the lipopolysaccharide colon antigen by uncom-mitted lymphoid cells. Whether there is any biological sig-nificance to the blocking of this reaction noted with UC sera is unclear at the present time.

420

ACKNOWLEDGEMENTS

Department of Medicine, Brown University, Providence, RI USA and Department of Immunology, Wenner-Gren Institute, University of Stockholm, Stockholm, Sweden.
Supported by the National Science Foundation, Washington, DC USA.

REFERENCES
1. Broberger O, Perlmann P. (1959) Autoantibodies in human ulcerative colitis. J.Exp.Med. 110:657-674
2. Lagercrantz R, Hammarström S, Perlmann P, Gustafsson BE. (1966) Immunological studies in ulcerative colitis. III. Incidence of antibodies to colon-antigen in ulcerative colitis and other gastro-intestinal diseases. Clin.Exp. Immunol. 1:263-276
3. Thayer WR, Brown M, Sangree MH, Katz J, Hersh T. (1969) Escherichia coli 0:14 and colon hemagglutinating antibodies in inflammatory bowel disease. Gastroenterology 57:311-318
4. Broberger O, Perlmann P. (1963) In vitro studies of ulcerative colitis. I. Reactions of patient's serum with human fetal colon cells in tissue cultures. J.Exp.Med. 117:705-716
5. Perlmann P, Holm G. (1969) Cytotoxic effect of lymphoid cells in vitro. Adv.Immunol. 11:117-193
6. Perlmann P, Perlmann H. (1970) Contactual lysis of antibody coated chicken erythrocytes by purified lymphocytes. Cell.Immunol. 1:300-315
7. Lamon EW, Skurzak HM, Andersson B, Whitten HD, Klein E. (1975) Antibody-dependent lymphocyte cytotoxicity in the murine sarcoma virus system: activity of IgM and IgG with specificity for MLV determined antigen(s). J.Immunol. 114:1171-1176
8. Harrison WJ. (1965) Autoantibodies against intestinal and gastric mucous cells in ulcerative colitis. Lancet 1:1346-1350
9. Perlmann P, Hammarstrom S, Lagercrantz R, Gustafsson BE. (1965) Antigen from colon of germ free rats and antibodies in human ulcerative colitis. Ann.N.Y.Acad.Sci. 124:377-394
10. Carlsson H, Hammarstrom S, Santeli M. et al. (1971) Antibody induces destruction of colon antigen-coated chicken erythrocytes by normal human lymphocytes. Eur.J.Immunol. 1:281-285
11. Shorter RG, Huizenga KA, ReMine SG, Spencer RJ. (1970) Effects of preliminary incubation of lymphocytes with serum on their cytotoxicity for colon epithelial cells. Gastroenterology 58:843-850

12. Stobo JD, Tomasi TB, Huizenga KA, Spencer RJ, Shorter RG. (1976) *In vitro* studies of inflammatory bowel disease. Surface receptors of the mononuclear cell required to lyse allogeneic colonic epithelial cells. Gastroenterology 70:171-176

13. MacLennan ICM. (1972) Competition for receptors for immunoglobulin on cytotoxic lymphocytes. Clin.Exp.Immunol. 10:275-283

14. Trinchieri G, Bauman P, deMarchi M, Tokes Z. (1975) Antibody-dependent cell-mediated cytotoxicity in humans. I. Characterization of the effector cell J.Immunol. 115:249-255

15. Austin RM, Daniels CA. (1976) Inhibition by rheumatoid factor, anti-Fc, and staphylococcal protein A of antibody-dependent cell-mediated cytolysis against Herpes simplex virus-infected cells. J.Immunol. 117:602-607

G23 Summary of Discussions relating to topic G22

Strober: Is it possible that you were simply looking at the wrong antigens?

Thayer: I think that is what I said. It does not appear to be the antigen-antibody system first described by Broberger and Perlmann, but I am sure that there are other Ag-Ab systems that should be investigated. For instance, workers at Duke University have been able to show antibody-dependent cell cytotoxicity against a mucopolysaccaride antigen in IBD.

Das: We have data supporting the existence of an antibody dependent cell mediated mechanism in IBD cytotoxicity using three different human cell lines as the target cells. Normal volunteers were the source of the effector cells and the sera were obtained from 25 patients with UC, 18 with CD, 16 normal subjects, 7 rheumatoid arthritis patients. The three cell lines used were RPMI 4788, an established human colon cancer cell line, HeLa, a human cervical cancer cell line and A7, which is a human smooth muscle cell line. We found that the UC sera had a significant higher cytotoxicity against RPMI 4788 compared with the sera obtained from patients with CD and controls. Indeed, the cytotoxicity with the sera from patients with CD were similar to the spontaneous cytotoxicity obtained when no serum was added to this system. Using the other two cell lines, namely the HeLa and A7 no cytotoxicity was obtained with any of the sera. We absorbed three UC sera with colonic mucosal homogenates from UC patients, CD colonic mucosal extracts, normal colon and cancer colon tissue extracts. The cytotoxicity obtained with these three sera ranged between 30 to 40 when no absorption was done. However, following absorption of these sera with the colitis colonic mucosal homogenates the cytotoxicity decreased significantly, whereas absorption with other homogenates resulted in no appreciable change in the cytotoxicity. To conclude, I think these studies show that ADCC could be a mechanism of cytotoxicity, at least in UC.

Jewell: There are a number of possibilities which can explain Thayer's results. Antibody dependent cellular cytotoxicity is mediated by different populations of lymphocytes according to what target cell you are using; the role of monocytes in the system is therefore pertinent. Have you repeated some of these studies using a mononuclear cell population containing monocytes?

Thayer: We have studied cell populations that have not been through the nylon column and we have looked at the monocytes directly and again have not found ADCC. As you know certain classes of immunoglobulin G antibodies do not mediate antibody-dependent cell cytotoxicity and some of them inhibit ADCC. Our antibodies were both IgG and IgM but we did not determine the subclass.

DECREASED IN VITRO NATURAL KILLER [NK] CELL ACTIVITY IN
CROHN'S DISEASE [CD] IN PERIPHERAL BLOOD

I.O. AUER, E. ZIEMER and H. SOMMER

INTRODUCTION

In the course of studying the immune status of CD patients we were particularly interested in the functional
state of the NK cells for the following reasons. Firstly, on
the one hand in CD viral agents, defined by cytopathic effect, have been found (1), and on the other hand NK cells may
play a role in defence against viral infections (2). Secondly, in CD a slightly, but statistically significant increased
propensity to malignancy has been shown (3). In this regard
it has been suggested that NK cells might be linked to in
vivo resistance against tumor growth (4,5,6). Therefore we
investigated NK cell activity in peripheral blood [PB] of
patients with CD and of normals. In order to be able to differentiate possible alterations of the NK cell activity as
primary and thus possibly even predisposing for the disease,
or as secondary to the disease, a group of patients with inflammatory bowel disease other than CD or ulcerative colitis
[group D] was studied.

MATERIAL AND METHODS

Patients and Controls

Patients with CD [group CD]. The 34 patients with CD consisted of two subgroups, group CD1 and CD2. Group CD1 was a
selected consecutive series of 16 "virgin Crohn's", who thus
had never been treated by SASP, steroids or azathioprine and
most of whom had shortstanding disease [$\bar{x}+SE$: 24.8$\pm$6.7
months]. In group CD2 18 CD patients were collected who had
longstanding disease [$\bar{x}+SE$: 59.7 $\pm$ 8.0 months] and who had
previously been drug treated. At the time of testing all
patients had been off these drugs for at least 3 weeks.

Disease activity and the site of disease were comparable in group CD1 and CD2. About one half of the patients were active [CDAI>150] and inactive [CDAI≤150], respectively, in either group.

Diseased controls [group D]. These subjects suffered from salmonella gastroenteritis [n=5], non specific gastroenteritis [n=3], diverticulitis [n=3] and bacterial overgrowth [n=1].

Normal controls [N groups]. For each patient one normal control subject was matched for both sex and age and was tested simultaneously with the corresponding CD or D patient. These 45 healthy subjects composed the normal control groups NCD [NCD1, NCD2] and ND.

Effector cells were isolated form heparinized PB by means of a Ficoll density gradient. After these cells have been depleted of phagocytic and plastic adherent cells, they were termed "purified cell suspensions".

NK cell activity was demonstrated in microtiter plates in triplicate cultures by a 4 hour ^{51}Cr-release assay with a human lymphoblastoid cell line [LIK-line] as target as described in (7) and (8) and modified according to (9). NK cell activity was evaluated both by means of "% specific ^{51}Cr-release" [R] and by "absolute number of cells needed for a specific release of 10 % in the given time of incubation". R was calculated by:

$$R = \frac{SCMC\ [cpm] - S\ [cpm]}{T\ [cpm] - S\ [cpm]} \times 100$$

The antibody dependent cell mediated cytotoxic [ADCC] activity was determined in a ^{51}Cr-release assay as described in (10) using a human lymphoblastoid cell line [LIK-line] as target, which was coated with an allogenic IgG-antibody against an HLA-determinant on the target.

Statistics

Results are given as mean [x̄] ± 1 standard deviation, unless otherwise stated. It was necessary to use non-para-

426

metric statistical tests. Thus, Wilcoxon's matched pairs
signed rank test was used to evaluate the significance of
difference between the various patients [CD and D patients,
respectively] and the corresponding, simultaneously tested
normals, while Wilcoxon's two sample rank test [U-test] was
applied for the other comparisons.

RESULTS

In unseparated leucocyte suspensions NK cell activity was
significantly lower in group CD than in the corresponding
controls [Fig. 1]. Very similar data were obtained in group
CD1 and CD2. Also group D showed a significantly lower NK
cell activity than ND [Fig. 1].

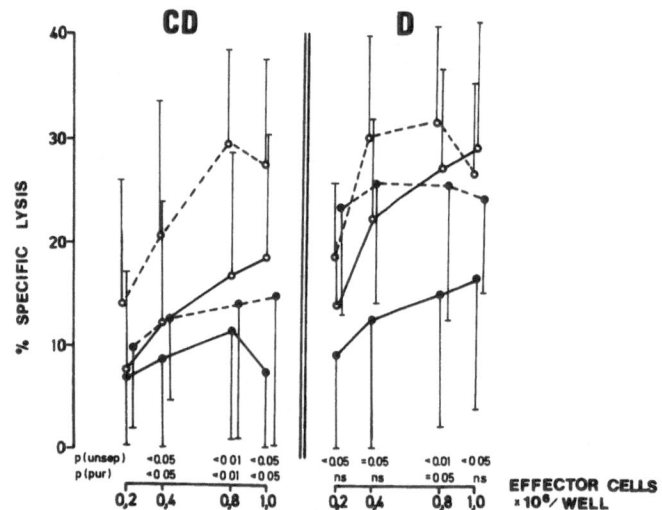

Figure 1. % specific lysis [$\bar{x} \pm 1$ SD] of unseparated [solid
         lines] and "purified" [broken lines] leucocyte
         suspensions of patients as compared with normal.
         Closed circles, patient groups as indicated. Open
         circles, corresponding normal control as indicated.

"Purification" of the leukocyte suspensions resulted in
a significant increase of the NK cell activity in all groups.
However, even after this treatment the NK cell activity was
still significantly lower in CD patients, both in CD1 and
CD2, than in corresponding normal controls [Fig.1, n=13]. In
"purified " suspensions of group D the NK cell activity was

still modestly lower than in normals [Fig. 1].

To test the effect of CD sera on the NK cell activity, effector cells [0.4×10^6/well] of two healthy donors were preincubated with a total of 23 sera of 22 CD patients, or with heat aggregated rabbit IgG [R-IgG-agg 500 µg/50 µl] for 30' at 4^OC. These effector cell preparations were simultaneously applied both in the NK cell and the ADCC assay. While R-IgG-agg lead to an approximately 90% inhibition of the ADCC, the same effector populations still exhibited more than one half of the original NK activity [Fig. 2]. Most of the CD sera "enhanced" the NK cell activity. 17 sera were tested for lymphocytotoxic antibodies against the target cells at 15^OC and 22^OC. Only 4 sera were positive [Fig. 2].

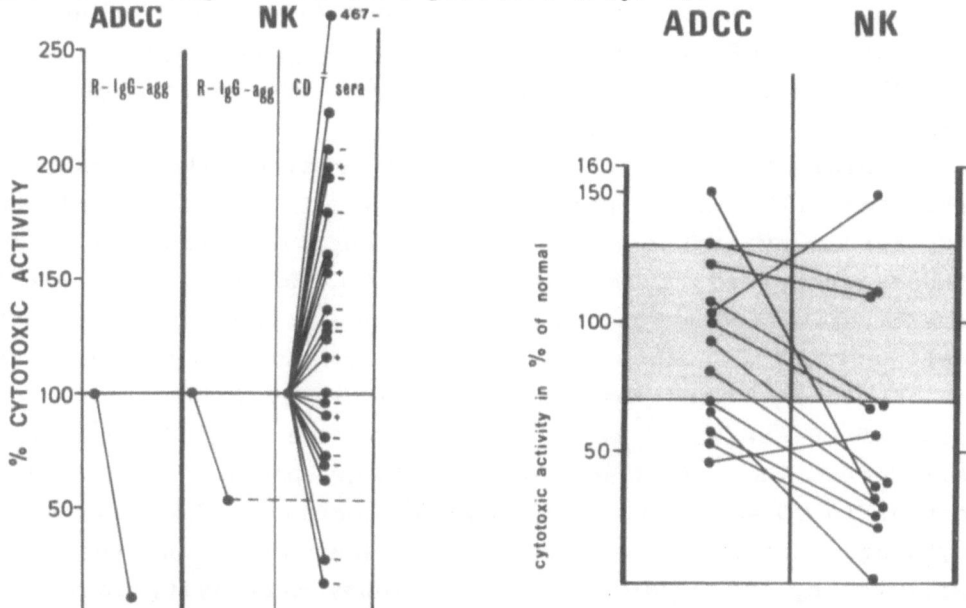

Figure 2. [left]. Influence of CD sera and R-IgG-agg on the NK cell activity of normals. For comparison the influence of R-IgG-agg on the ADCC activity is also given. CD sera positive or negative for lymphocytotoxic antibodies against the target are indicated with + and -, respectively.

Figure 3. [right]. Dissociation in the activity of the ADCC and NK cell cytotoxicity in individual CD patients.

In group CD the "% specific release" due to NK cells was below normal levels independent of the disease activity, both in unseparated and in "purified" suspensions. However, using "purified" lymphocyte suspensions from CD patients with active disease, significantly more effector cells were needed to obtain 10% specific ^{51}Cr-release than in those with quiescent or mild disease [p<0.05].

In "purified suspensions" the NK cell activity was decreased [less than 70% of the simultaneously tested corresponding normal controls] not only in those CD patients, who showed impaired ADCC activity, but also in 63.5% [5/8] of the CD patients with normal ADCC [Fig. 3].

DISCUSSION

The present work revealed an impairment of the NK cell activity in both unseparated and "purified" suspensions of both active [CDAI>150] and inactive [CDAI≤150] patients with CD. Mode and nature of this impairment are unclear at present.

Inhibition of NK cell activity by prostaglandins has been reported (11). In the present study NK cell activity could be suppressed by immune complexes to a certain extent. Both of these factors might be increased in CD. However, in view of our experiments evaluating the influence of CD sera on the NK cell activity, such serum factors seem not very likely as major cause of the impaired NK cell activity in CD. The majority of CD sera lead to an increase of the NK cell activity, similar to the effect of sera of healthy people (12). Only 3 out of 10 CD sera with such enhancing activity showed lymphocytotoxins against the target cells. However, since the sensitivity by which ADCC detects antibody reactivity is a 100 to 1000 fold greater than the sensitivity of the complement-dependent system (13), a possible role of such antibodies for this enhancement, which would than reflect an ADCC-mechanism cannot entirely be excluded.

More recently, it has been suggested that NK cell activity is regulated by levels of interferon found in vivo. Thus, depressed interferon production or decreased susceptibility of NK cells to interferon might play a role in this impairment of the NK cell activity in CD. However, sequestration of NK cells in the gut would be another possibility, although the presence of NK cells in the gut is a matter of debate (14).

This study revealed a suppressive influence of the disease activity on the NK cells in "purified" suspensions, similar to the ADCC as shown in a previous report (10). However, while inactive CD patients had a virtually normal ADCC activity in "purified" suspensions (10) the NK cell activity was significantly decreased in many CD patients with mild disease. This dissociation in the activity of the ADCC and NK cell cytotoxicity in CD is in agreement with a very recent observation of Jones et al. (15). These authors reported that CD tissue filtrates produced a strong inhibition of NK cell activity, while there was no modulation of the ADCC.

The NK cell activity is equally decreased in "virgin Crohn's" with short disease duration [group CD1] and in group CD2. This impairment, therefore, appears to be independent on disease duration and is present already at an early stage of the disease, when certain T- and B-cell parameters are unaltered (16). There was, however, also a strong tendency to an impairment of the NK cell activity in the control patients with common infectious and inflammatory bowel disease [group D]. Consequently, the decrease in the NK cell activity even in "virgin Crohns" might have to be considered as due to the disease rather than as a preexisting, possibly predisposing factor for CD. However, while NK cell impairment is transient in D patients, it seems to be chronic in CD, and even pronounced in active disease. Whether this chronic impairment may relate to the appearance of virus (1) and/or the slightly, though significantly increased propensity to high grade malignancy in CD patients (3) remains to be established.

Supported by DFG Au 35/4, 35/6 and 35/7.

REFERENCES
1. Beeken WL.(1979) Evidence of virus infection as a cause of Crohn's disease. 1. Symposium on Crohn's disease in Hemmenhofen. Z.Gastroenterol.Suppl.12:101-104

2. Harfast B, Andersson T, Perlmann P.(1978) Immunoglobulin-
   independent natural cytotoxicity of Fc receptor-bearing
   human blood lymphocytes to mumps virus infected target
   cells. J.Immunol.121:755-761
3. Gyde S, MacCartney J, Prior Waterhouse JAH, Allan RN.
   (1979) Cancer and Crohn's disease. Gut 20:A951
4. Haller O, Hansson M, Kiessling R, Wigzell M. (1977) Role
   of non-conventional natural killer cells in resistance
   against syngeneic tumor cells in vivo. Nature 270:609-611
5. Jondal M, Spina C, Targan S.(1978) Human spontaneous
   killer cells selective for tumor-derived target cells.
   Nature 272:62-64
6. Takasugi M, Ramseyer A, Takasugi J.(1977) Decline of
   natural non selective cell-mediated cytotoxicity in
   patients with tumour progression. Cancer Res. 37:413-418
7. Santoli D, Trinchieri G, Zmijewski CM, Koprowski H.
   (1976) HLA related control of spontaneous and antibody
   dependent cell-mediated cytotoxic activity in humans.
   J.Immunol. 117:765-770
8. Trinchieri G, De Marchi M, Mayr W, Savi M, Ceppellini R.
   (1973) Lymphocyte antibody lymphocytolytic interaction
   [LALI] with special emphasis on HL-A. Transplant.Proc.
   5:1631-1646
9. Auer IO, Ziemer E, Sommer H.(1980) Immune status in
   Crohn's disease. 5. Decreased in vitro natural killer
   activity in peripheral blood. Clin. Exp. Immunol. in
   press.
10. Auer IO, Ziemer E. (1980) Immune status in Crohn's dis-
    ease. 4. In vitro antibody dependent cell mediated
    cytotoxicity in the peripheral blood. Klin.Wochenschr.
    58:779-788
11. Droller MJ, Schneider MU, Perlmann P.(1978) A possible
    role of prostaglandins in the inhibition of natural and
    antibody-dependent cell-mediated cytotoxicity against
    tumour cells. Cell.Immunol.39:165-177
12. Gyorffy GY, Petranyi GY, Benczur M.(1978) The effect of
    human AB serum on the NK cell activity. 4th European
    Immunol. Meeting, Budapest
13. Dickmeiss E, Nielsen LS.(1975) Antibody-dependent lympho-
    cyte mediated cytotoxicity in an allogenic human system.
    II. Evidence for HLA-specificity. Scand.J.Immunol. 3:199
14. MacDermott RP, Jenkins KM, Franklin GD. et al.(1979)
    Antibody dependent, spontaneous, and lectin induced
    cellular cytotoxicity by human intestinal lymphocytes.
    Gastroenterology 76:1190
15. Jones MB, Gitnick G, Targan SR.(1979) Inhibition of
    spontaneous killer cell cytotoxicity by Crohn's disease
    tissue and cultures containing cytopathic agents. Gastro-
    enterology 76:1163
16. Auer IO.(1979) Immunology in Crohn's disease. 1. Sympo-
    sion on Crohn's disease in Hemmenhofen. Z.Gastroenterol.
    Suppl. 12:83-93

G25 Summary of Discussions relating to topic G24

Hodgson: What sort of cell is the NK cell you have stu-
              died?

Auer: We obtained this target cell LIK line from the
              Basel Institute of Immunology. Trinchieri, Bauman,
              DeMarchi and Tokes have shown that the effector
              cells in the ADCC and the SCMC against this target
              is a non-phagocytic, non plastic-adherent, X-ray
              sensitive cell. Studies of Santoli showed that most
              of the effector cells are non-rosetting with SBRC
              and a few cells which are rosetting with SRBC cells
              are T cells. Recently Santoli and Koprowsky showed
              that interferon increases strikingly the activity
              of the effector cells. I think that it is fair
              evidence that we are dealing with an SCMC system.

Jewell: Do you have any data on how the NK activity
              changes with the activity of disease?

Auer: NK activity is already decreased in active CD
              patients and it decreases even further with in-
              creasing disease activity.

Strober: Shorter and his colleagues demonstrated some
              years ago that there is a cell particulary asso-
              ciated with IBD which is capable of killing colon
              epithelial cell targets and one could gather from
              their papers that this cell is in fact a NK cell.
              These data would appear to contradict that but of
              course their targets were different.

Shorter: I think that is the explanation.

Thayer: In Shorter's laboratory last year we looked at NK and K cell activity using the Chang cell as a target and did not find any decrease in the IBD patients. However, many of the patients were on steroids and that may have been a factor.

Auer: We intentionally selected this LIK line because, as you saw from the data, this line has a rather low susceptibility to lysis in the SCMC assay and we felt therefore that this would increase our changes of seeing differences. I have to stress a point which was brought up by Strober that even for NK cells there is evidence arising that there might be specificity for the target. You cannot really compare results obtained with colon epithelial cells or Chang cells with that obtained with other cells.

Peña: Have you tested, if your sera containing lymphocytoxic antibodies have an effect on your system?

Auer: We tested all 17 of the 23 sera for lymphocytotoxic antibodies. 60% were positive against a panel of lymphocytes but only four against the target cell. These serum samples did not show a correlation with the SCMC activity against the LIK target but nevertheless because the sensitivity is different in the complement dependent cytotoxicity system and the ADCC, we might be dealing with the enhancing activity of CD and normal sera with an ADCC mechanism.

PROLIFERATIVE RESPONSES OF GUT MUCOSAL LYMPHOCYTES FROM CROHN'S DISEASE PATIENTS TO ENTEROBACTERIAL COMMON ANTIGEN, LIPOPOLYSACCHARIDE AND CELL WALL-DEFECTIVE BACTERIA

C. FIOCCHI, K. PARENT and P. MITCHELL

INTRODUCTION

Enterobacterial flora has long been implicated in the pathogenesis of non-specific inflammatory bowel disease[IBD]. The existence of immunological cross reactivity between human colon and the enterobacterial common antigen of Kunin [ECA] (1), as well as the detection of both cellular and humoral immunity to ECA in ulcerative colitis and Crohn's disease [CD] (2,3), have suggested that lymphoid cells sensitized to colonic and bacterial antigens may mediate IBD. Such studies have been performed using peripheral blood lymphocytes [PBL], but these may reflect little of the immunological events occurring at the level of the mucosal lesions. Since isolated, purified lymphoid cells from intestinal mucosa can now be recovered, exploration of the immunological reactivity of gut mucosal lymphocytes [GML] towards gut related antigens becomes feasible. The aim of this study was to compare the proliferation of PBL and GML from individuals with CD and colon carcinoma [CA] in response to ECA, lipopolysaccharide [LPS] and cell wall-defective variants of Pseudomonas-like [group Va] bacteria [CWDB] (4).

MATERIALS AND METHODS

Patients

Fifteen patients with CD [7 on corticosteroids] and 19 patients with CA constituted the source of both PBL and GML. Fifteen normal volunteers served as normal controls.

Lymphoid Cells

PBL, derived from heparinized blood obtained immediately after the removal of the surgical specimen, were purified

434

over a Ficoll-Hypaque gradient. GML were isolated from the
lamina propria of normal [CA] and inflamed [CD] intestinal
mucosa by using an enzymatic and sedimentation technique (5).

Effect of the enzymatic treatment on PBL

To determine whether proliferative responses of GML were
altered by the isolation process, PBL were exposed to the
same enzymatic treatment of GML and/or cultured in the cell-
free supernatants obtained from the enzymatic solutions used
to liberate autologous GML. Prior to and after such treatment, PBL were cultured in the presence of the antigens, as
described in the following paragraph.

Proliferative responses to gut related bacterial antigens

ECA was isolated from cultures of S. typhimurium as described by Suzuki et al. (6). LPS, derived from E. coli
0111:B4, was obtained from Difco. CWDB were cultured in hypertonic medium from filtered CD tissue homogenates (4); the
formalinized revertant forms were washed and sonicated until
>95% of the organisms were disrupted; the sonicated material
was spun at 25000g for 15 minutes, dialyzed against 0.05M
NH_4CO_3, lyophilized and the final solid residue was suspended
in Hanks balanced salt solution. PBL and GML [$1x10^6$/ml] were
suspended in RPMI 1640 with L-glutamine, Hepes buffer, penicillin streptomycin, gentamycin and 10% pooled human AB serum. The lymphoid cell suspensions were distributed [0.2 ml]
in wells of microtiter plates in the presence of pre-deter-
mined optimal concentrations of antigens: 1] 1/10 of the
original ECA solution; 2] 250 μg/ml of LPS; 3] 50 μg/ml of
CWDB. After 72 hr in a humidified atmosphere with 5% CO_2, the
cultures were pulsed with tritiated [^{3}H] thymidine for 6 hr,
harvested with a Mash II and the uptake was measured in a
scintillation counter as counts per minute [CPM]. Stimulation
indices [SI] were derived from the CPM of stimulated cultures
divided by the CPM of unstimulated cultures.

Analysis of data

Statistical analysis was performed by Student's t test.

RESULTS

Effect of the enzymatic treatment on PBL

The exposure of PBL to both fresh and used enzymatic solutions caused no significant changes in their uptake of ^{3}H-thymidine prior to and after stimulation by the bacterial antigens [Table 1].

Table 1. Effect of the enzymatic treatment on the spontaneous and gut related antigen-induced proliferation of PBL

Antigen	Enzymatic Treatment	CPM [±SE]	Treated Untreated
None	Yes	640 [171]	1.1
	No	614 [118]	
ECA	Yes	402 [210]	0.9
	No	446 [218]	
LPS	Yes	999 [310]	1.4
	No	575 [116]	
CWDB	Yes	2290 [746]	1.4
	No	1463 [437]	

Table 2. Proliferative responses of lymphocytes from normal, CA and CD individuals to gut related bacterial antigens

Antigen	Cells from	CPM	PBL [±SE]	SI	CPM	GML [±SE]	SI
None	Normal	761	[78]		—		
	CA	420	[93]		2049	[405]	
	CD	324	[33]		1954	[464]	
ECA	Normal	1260	[122]	1.6	—		
	CA	433	[63]	1.3	9463	[1701]	5.0
	CD	708	[281]	2.0	5730	[1026]	4.3
LPS	Normal	734	[79]	1.0	—		
	CA	402	[76]	1.3	6260	[1032]	3.1
	CD	413	[58]	0.6	15784	[2732]	6.2
CWDB	Normal	2067	[499]	2.2	—		
	CA	542	[89]	1.9	5949	[1178]	2.4
	CD	700	[131]	1.8	4499	[942]	2.7

Proliferative responses to gut related bacterial antigens

No significant differences were seen in the spontaneous replication of normal, CA and CD PBL [Table 2]. Unstimulated

CA and CD GML displayed similar values of ^{3}H-thymidine uptake and these were consistently and significantly greater [p<0.005] than those of patient matched PBL.

All three bacterial antigens were essentially not stimulatory for PBL from all sources, with exception of a mild stimulation of CD PBL by ECA and normal PBL by CWDB. In contrast, GML from both normal and inflamed mucosa were stimulated by all three antigens: all CPM derived from CA and CD GML were significantly different [p<0.005 to p<0.001] from those of patient-matched PBL.

The SI of PBL and GML in response to ECA were significantly different for CA [p<0.001], but not for CD. In response to LPS, both CA and CD displayed significantly different SI from those of PBL [p<0.025 and p<0.005 respectively]. Finally, no differences were observed between the SI of PBL and GML following exposure to CWDB.

When the proliferative responses of GML from normal mucosa were compared to those of GML from CD involved mucosa, only LPS induced a significantly different stimulation [p<0.005 for CPM and p<0.05 for SI].

No differences were observed in regard to the state of immunosuppression [steroids vs. non steroids] or the origin of the lymphoid cells [small vs. large bowel].

DISCUSSION

This study demonstrates that human intestinal mucosa contains lymphoid cells capable of recognizing and proliferating in response to at least three different gut related bacterial antigens.

With regard to ECA, it is significant that both CA and CD GML react to a similar degree. Indeed, if the immune response mounted by lymphocytes to this antigen was relevant to the inflammatory process of CD(7), such cells would not be expected to be present in the normal state. However, different suppressor cell activities, controlling the response to ECA in vivo, may exist between normal and inflammed mucosa, that are not expressed under in vitro experimental conditions.

The LPS induced reactivity of GML most likely represents an antigen recognition phenomenon, since LPS is not considered to be mitogenic for human lymphocytes. Its greater stimulatory effect on GML in CD may represent a greater degree of sensitization due to bacterial products freely transpassing a disrupted mucosal barrier. The reactivities of GML to LPS and ECA are probably unrelated. The latter is seldom completely LPS free and one could assume that GML response to ECA could be at least in part due to contaminating endotoxin. If this was the case, one would expect the response of GML to the Kunin antigen to be greater in CD than in CA and it was not.

The stimulation of GML by CWDB cannot be attributed to ECA since Pseudomonas do not possess this antigen. While these organisms cause GML to respond, they may not be unique to CD, since normal GML proliferate equally in response to them. Recent microbiological and humoral immunity studies support this concept.

CONCLUSIONS

GML represent a population of lymphoid cells suitable for the study of cell mediated immunity to enteric bacterial antigens. GML exhibit a stronger proliferation in response to ECA, LPS and CDWB than patient-matched PBL. LPS induces a greater replication of GML derived from CD involved than normal mucosa, while GML from both sources are equally stimulated by ECA and CWDB.

Our data do not support the concept that IBD, particularly CD, represents a state of hypersensitivity to the bacterial antigens evaluated in this study.

ACKNOWLEDGEMENT

The author thank Dr. E. Neter for supplying enterobacterial common antigen.

438

REFERENCES

1. Perlman P, Hammarstrom S, Lagercrantz R, Campbell D. (1967) Autoantibodies to colon in rats and human ulcerative colitis:cross reactivity with Escherichia coli 014 antigen. Proc.Soc.Exp.Biol.Med. 125:975-980

2. Thayer WR, Brown M, Sangree MH, Katz J, Herst T. (1969) Escherichia E. coli 0:14 and colon hemagglutinating antibodies in inflammatory bowel disease. Gastroenterology 57:311-318

3. Bull DM, Ignaczak TF. (1973) Enterobacterial common antigen induced lymphocyte reactivity in inflammatory bowel disease. Gastroenterology 64:43-50

4. Parent K, Mitchell P. (1978) Cell wall-defective variants of Pseudomonas-like [group Va] bacteria in Crohn's disease. Gastroenterology 75:368-372

5. Fiocchi C, Battisto JR, Farmer RG. (1979) Gut mucosal lymphocytes in inflammatory bowel disease. Isolation and preliminary functional characterization. Dig. Dis. Sci. 24:705-717

6. Suzuki T, Gorzynski EA, Neter E. (1964) Separation by ethanol of common and somatic antigens of enterobacteriaceae. J.Bacteriol. 88:1240-1243

7. Shorter RG, Huizenga KA, Spencer RJ. (1972) A working hypothesis for the etiology and pathogenesis of non specific inflammatory bowel disease. Am.J.Dig.Dis. 17:1024-1032.

HUMAN INTESTINAL MONONUCLEAR CELLS [MNC] ISOLATED FROM NORMAL
AND INFLAMMATORY BOWEL DISEASE [IBD] SPECIMENS ARE A FUNC-
TIONALLY UNIQUE LYMPHOID POPULATION

R.P. MAC DERMOTT

INTRODUCTION

The development of techniques for the isolation of MNC
from intestinal mucosa has begun to lead to the characterization of intestinal MNC. We have examined the functional
capabilities of T, B, and Fc receptor bearing intestinal MNC
from normal and IBD resected specimens using in vitro cytotoxicity, proliferation, and antibody synthesis assays.

PROCEDURE

Intestinal tissue was obtained from 84 surgically removed
specimens from patients with adenocarcinoma [40], recurrent
volvulus [2], diverticulitis [8], ulcerative colitis [UC]
[18], and Crohn's disease [CD] [16]. Intestinal MNC from the
mucosa of uninvolved bowel from the non-IBD patients and
involved bowel from the IBD patients were isolated using the
EDTA and collagenase method as described by Bull and Bookman
(1) and modified as described by MacDermott et al. (2). The
isolated intestinal MNC were evaluated using standard techniques as to presence of E rosette forming cells [T cells],
Fc receptor bearing cells, esterase staining cells [macro-
phages], and surface immunoglobulin bearing cells [B cells].
Functional capabilities were assessed in vitro by examining:
1] responsiveness to mitogenic lectins and foreign cell surface antigens in the allogeneic mixed leukocyte reaction
[MLR]; 2] cytotoxic effector capacity in antibody dependent
cellular cytotoxicity [ADCC], spontaneous cell mediated cytotoxicity [SCMC], lectin induced cellular cytotoxicity [LICC],
and cell mediated lympholysis [CML]; and 3] synthesis and
secretion of IgM, IgG, and IgA during a 12 day in vitro cul-

ture with the secreted antibodies measured using radioimmunoassay.

RESULTS

The percentage of T, B, "Null", Fc receptor bearing cells
and macrophages found in isolated intestinal MNC populations,
normal peripheral blood [PB] MNC, and PB MNC processed using
EDTA and collagenase, are presented in table 1.

Table 1. Surface characteristics of intestinal [Int] MNC

	Normal PB MNC	Processed[d] PB MNC	Control Int MNC	Crohn's Int MNC	UC Int MNC
% T [E]	57[a] [31]	63 [20]	45 [32]	33 [7]	38 [10]
% B [sIg][c]	14 [45]	10 [24]	14 [32]	23 [6]	11 [7]
% MØ[Est][c]	14 [22]	10 [15]	11 [21]	7 [5]	11 [6]
% Null[b]	15	17	30	37	40
% Fc+[EA][c]	7 [16]	5 [15]	7 [12]		6 [3]

a] Mean for number of specimens examined in parenthesis
b] Calculated value: 100 - [%T + %B + %MØ]
c] sIg=surface Ig positive; Est=esterase stain; EA=% EA rosette positive
d] Processed with EDTA and collagenase

We have previously shown (2) that isolated intestinal MNC
populations will mediate ADCC and LICC with red blood cells
as targets, but do not mediate either ADCC or SCMC with Chang
or K562 cell line cells as targets. Thus, cell surface receptors in addition to the presence of an Fc receptor may be
important in determining whether or not a target cell will be
killed in either ADCC or SCMC, and these receptors may be
absent from intestinal MNC. Lectins such as erythroaggluti-
nating phytohemagglutinin [E-PHA], concanavalin A [Con A],
wheat germ agglutinin [WGA], and pokeweed mitogen [PWM] induce normal intestinal MNC to kill colon tumor cell line
cells [Table 2]. Furthermore, interferon causes a moderate
increase in SCMC and additively increases total LICC due to
the SCMC enhancement [Table 2]. These data indicate that
exogenous agents such as lectins and interferon induce and

potentiate cytotoxic effector function by intestinal MNC toward cell line cell targets.

Intestinal MNC T cells respond to mitogenic lectins (3) and foreign cell surface determinants in the allogeneic MLR, but do not subsequently kill the sensitizing cells in CML [Table 3]. Thus, the subclass of T cells which mediates CML may either be absent from the intestine or not functional due to immunoregulatory abnormalities, while the subclass of T cells responding in MLR is both present and active (3).

Table 2. Effect of interferon [IF] on SCMC and LICC against colon tumor cell line cells by normal intestinal [Int] MNC

	SCMC		LICC		
		E-PHA [20 µg/ml][a]	Con A [10 µg/ml]	WGA [10 µg/ml]	PWM [1:100]
PB MNC [3][b]	21±5[c]	43±8	41±7	24±6	62±8
IF treated[d] PB MNC [3]	53±15	69±5	65±8	50±10	76±5
Int MNC[4]	3±0.3	29±4	27±4	10± 3	27±3
IF treated[d] Int MNC [4]	11±3	35±5	30±4	16± 4	30±4

a] Final concentration in the assay
b] Number of specimens examined
c] Mean percent cytotoxicity ± SEM
d] One million MNC pretreated 2 hours at 37° C with 100 units/cc of human fibroblast IF.

Table 3. T cell functional capabilities of intestinal [Int] MNC

	Normal PB MNC	Processed[c] PB MNC	Control Int MNC	Crohn's Int MNC	UC Int MMC
MLR	22[a] (23)	12 (14)	30 (18)	18 (4)	9 (7)
CML	23[b] (12)	25 (10)	3 (9)	6 (4)	3 (4)

a] Mean stimulation index for number of specimens in parenthesis
b] Mean percent cytotoxicity
c] Processed with EDTA and Collagenase

Finally, we have examined the synthesis and secretion of IgM, IgG, and IgA during 12 days of _in vitro_ culture (4). In contrast to normal peripheral blood MNC, which have low spontaneous antibody secretion with an increase after PWM stimulation, normal and UC intestinal MNC [Table 4] as well as UC, CD, and systemic lupus erythematosus [SLE] peripheral blood MNC [Table 5] exhibit altered spontaneous antibody secretion with moderately increased IgG and IgM and markedly increased IgA synthesis and secretion. PWM does not further enhance and in some instances suppresses antibody secretion. These alterations in antibody secretion may reflect highly stimulated population of B cells with readily activatable or PWM inducible presuppressor cells.

Table 4. Antibody synthesis and secretion by isolated intestinal MNC during 12 days _in vitro_ culture

	IgM		IgG		IgA	
	Media	PWM	Media	PWM	Media	PWM
Control PB MNC [33[a]]	312[b]	3893	472	4195	437	2443
Normal Int. MNC [7]	2208	2155	1296	1202	8515	5327
UC Int. MNC [7]	197	513	1221	2420	3086	3523
CD Int. MNC [6]	139	1167	194	926	986	2548

a] Number of specimens examined
b] Mean [geometric] nanograms antibody secreted per ml of culture supernatant [2×10^6 cells] after 12 day in vitro culture

Table 5. Antibody synthesis and secretion by peripheral blood MNC during 12 days in vitro culture

	IgM		IgG		IgA	
	Media	PWM	Media	PWM	Media	PWM
Control PB MNC [19][b]	255[a]	2766	373	4596	561	2397
UC PB MNC [4]	776	661	2155	1581	4831	2736
CD PB MNC [3]	1018	1091	730	958	2654	2421
SLE PB MNC [11]	477	355	1108	663	2907	1020

a] Number of active, untreated patients examined
b] Mean [geometric] nanograms antibody secreted per ml of culture supernatant [two million cells] after 12 day _in vitro_ culture

DISCUSSION

These studies add to the evidence of major functional differences between intestinal MNC and normal peripheral blood MNC (2,3,4). In addition, we have noted potential alteration in immunoregulatory function by peripheral blood MNC from active, untreated IBD patients which are similar to changes seen in SLE. The lack of cytotoxic effector functions in ADCC, SCMC, and CML raises the issue of what effector mechanisms mediated by intestinal MNC might be involved in the immunopathogenesis of IBD. Therefore, the inducement and modulation of cytotoxicity by exogenous agents such as lectins and interferon will be an important area for future research. Finally, investigation of IgM, IgG, and in particular IgA synthesis and secretion by IBD intestinal and peripheral blood MNC should be undertaken, with emphasis on cellular regulation mechanisms and determination of the antigens toward which the antibodies are directed.

CONCLUSIONS

The delineation of major functional dichotomies between intestinal and peripheral blood MNC (2,3,4) leads us to speculate that the immunobiology of lymphoid cells when resident in non-lymphoid tissues may be different from the immune functional capabilities of MNC in the peripheral blood or spleen. From this we conclude that it will be necessary to better understand the factors regulating the immunocompetence of the cells which comprises the intestinal immune system prior to the delineation of immunopathologic events in these tissues.

ACKNOWLEDGEMENTS

The careful work and tireless efforts of Ms. Jan Bragdon and Mr. Geoff Nash and the typing skills and patience of Ms. Pam Helms are gratefully acknowledged.

REFERENCES
1. Bull DM, Bookman MA.(1977) Isolation and functional cha-
    racterization of human int. MNC. J.Clin.Invest.59:966-974
2. MacDermott RP, Franklin GO, Jenkins KM, Kodner IJ, Nash
    GS, Weinrieb IJ. (1980) Human intestinal MNC. I. Inves-
    tigation of ADCC, LICC, and SCMC. Gastroenterology 78:47-
    56
3. MacDermott RP, Bragdon MJ, Jenkins KM, Franklin GO, Shed-
    lofsky S, Kodner IJ. (1980) Investigation of T cell
    function by isolated human int. MNC. Gastroenterology
    78:1213
4. MacDermott RP, Nash GS. (1980) In vitro synthesis and
    secretion of IgM, IgG, and IgA by isolated human int. MNC
    Clinical Research 28:280A.

G28 Summary of Discussions G26 - G27

Bienenstock: Fiocchi made the statement that his prepara-
           tions do not contain epithelial lymphocytes; what
           is the evidence for that? There are within the
           epithelium, a lymphocyte population which is almost
           exclusively a T cell population (in the mouse) and
           which has spontaneous cell cytotoxic activity as
           well a natural killer cell and T cell activity (in
           the guinea pig). The lamina propria cells below the
           epithelium do not have all those activities. There-
           fore, the statement that Fiocchi made about the
           presence or absence of epithelial lymphocytes is
           rather important in understanding and interpreting
           his results.

Fiocchi: I cannot do anything else but agree with you.
           The only thing I can add is that we have to isolate
           both populations with better methods and then com-
           pare them. There is some information from Shorter's
           group that the intra-epithelial lymphocytes are not
           only T cells but also B cells and null cells. So we
           have another reason for confusion here.

Bienenstock: I think the difficulty is that nobody really
           has a pure population of epithelial lymphocytes and
           even in the work we have done we are dealing with
           mixed populations. So I think that Shorter's re-
           sults and our results can in part be explained by
           our incompetence in not being able to obtain pure
           cell populations.

Asquith: How can you be sure that the differences be-
           tween peripheral blood and mucosal cells are not

due to the separation technique? I noticed that Fiocchi said his lymphocyte yield was very good. How do you judge that?

Fiocchi: We are sure that we have numerical loss but whether or not we have loss of particular subpopulations we cannot determine. We expressed cell recovery as the number of cells obtained per gram of tissue processed; one should be aware that this could lead to error because by the time the tissue gets to us there may be a fair amount of edema. This may explain the variation in the recovery of lymphocytes from the lamina propria. For normal tissue, we get from two to three million cells up to almost 20 million cells per gram of mucosa. On the other hand from CD mucosa we can get from 5 to 6 up to 70 million cells per gram of mucosa and from UC mucosa we can get up to 100 million cells per gram of mucosa.

Thayer: We obtained results similar to those of Mac-Dermott but we interpreted our results a little differently. We also found a very weak reactivity against the Chang cell in ADCC, but if we increase our effector to target cell ratio we can show that there does appear to be some capacity to mediate cytotoxicity. In addition, we found that if we subjected peripheral blood cells to the same treatment mucosal cells must go through during isolation the peripheral cells are reduced in their capacity to mediate cellular cytotoxicity by 50%. Therefore we believe that one of the reasons why the cytotoxicity appears depressed in the lymphoid cells in the intestine is because of the isolation technique.

MacDermott: With regard to separation techniques, the data that I showed, mitogens reactions and MLC reactivity are very much in agreement with the data of Goodacre and co-workers from Bienenstock's lab. using a mechanical separation technique. So that I think the two techniques in certain instances are comparable.

Knapp: MacDermott, does the spontaneous Ig synthesis occur only after 5 days?

MacDermott: That is correct.

Knapp: Is it not surprising that there are no plasma cells and plasmablasts in the mononuclear cell preparation obtained from the intestine?

MacDermott: Yes I would agree. The number of nanograms of immunoglobulin synthesized and secreted by peripheral blood cells during the first one day period of culture is less than 15 nanograms per 2×10^6 cells. With intestinal mononuclear cells we can see up to 300 nanograms, so there is much less than the 4000 to 6000 nanograms that are subsequently synthesized and secreted. So I agree, there is some synthesis in secretion due to plasma cells at the beginning.

Knapp: What do you regard as a suppressive effect of PWM? When you look at your figures, there is great variation and one might question if the suppression is statistically significant.

MacDermott   It is not statistically significant. It is in a suppressive direction.

Tγ CELLS AND NON-SPECIFIC CONCANAVALIN A-INDUCED SUPPRESSOR CELL ACTIVITY IN VITRO IN COLONIC INFLAMMATORY BOWEL DISEASE AND IN COLORECTAL CARCINOMA

R.G. SHORTER

INTRODUCTION

Recently, Hodgson et al. (1) concluded that nonspecific, mitogen-induced suppressor T cell activity of peripheral blood lymphocytes [PBL] in vitro was decreased in active inflammatory bowel disease [IBD] and suggested that this was important to any concept involving a pathogenetic role for the immune response. In addition, IBD is a risk factor in gastrointestinal malignancies, particularly colorectal carcinoma, and Naor (2) has reviewed the data which led to a hypothesis that suppressor cell activities, both specific and nonspecific, may be significant to the emergence and growth of some malignant tumors. Thus, we quantitated Tγ cells in isolates of PBL and in isolates of lamina proprial lymphocytes [LPL] form patients with IBD, and from patients with colorectal carcinoma, and compared the results with controls including other chronic inflammatory intestinal lesions or benign colonic tumors. Using PBL and LPL, we also assayed Concanavalin A-induced nonspecific suppressor T-cell activity on T-cell responsiveness to Con-A in vitro.

MATERIALS AND METHODS

Study groups

A] 20-25 ml venipuncture samples of heparinized blood were obtained from 25 healthy volunteers aged 21-66 yrs. [13 F; 12 M]. B] 20-25 ml samples of venous blood were taken from 5 patients [4 F; 1 M], aged 21-66 yrs. with various intestinal inflammatory conditions, namely acute or chronic diverticulitis, 2; chronic active bacterial typhlitis, 1; chronic bacterial pericolic abscess, 1; chronic Giardia Lamblia infestation, 1. C] 20-25 samples of venous blood were obtained from 18 patients with IBD [chronic ulcerative colitis [CUC], 13; Crohn's colitis, 5]. Nine were males and 9 females, aged 16 to 54 yrs. and eleven [9 CUC; 2 Crohn's disease [CD]] were receiving prednisone in daily doses of 20 mg or less. Four had severe activity [all CUC], 9 were moderately active [7 CUC; 2 CD] and 5 had mild disease [3 CUC; 2 CD]. None had extraintestinal manifestations of their disease.

Samples of therapeutically resected colon were available from 10 of these patients [8 CUC; 2 CD] of whom 5 with CUC and 1 with CD were on steroids. Of the 8 with CUC, 3 had severe activity, 2 moderate activity and 3 mild disease. The activities were moderate and mild respectively in the two with CD. In those undergoing therapeutic colonic resection, the blood samples were obtained immediately prior to surgery. D] Similar samples of blood and colonic tissues were obtained from 15 [8 M; 7 F] patients, aged 49-80 yrs. undergoing colonic resection for colorectal adenocarcinomas, the blood being collected immediately before surgery. Four tumors were Dukes' Group B_1, five B_2, and six Group C(3). E] Samples were available from six colonic specimens removed for intestinal diseases other than IBD or cancer, including chronic rectal prolapse with nonspecific chronic mucosal inflammation, 2; chronic colonic diverticulitis, 1; chronic bacterial typhlitis sequela appendicitis, 1; large, benign adenomatous colonic polyp, 2. Of these patients, 2 were male and 4 female, aged 51 yrs. to 72 yrs.

Isolation of lymphoid cells

A] Peripheral blood lymphocytes [PBL]: Macrophage-depleted isolates of PBL were obtained by the Ficoll-Hypaque method (4). Residual contamination by monocyte-macrophages was less than 1%. B] Isolation of colonic lamina proprial lymphocyte-enriched populations [LPL]: The technique has been described elsewhere (4). Contamination of the final isolates by monocyte-macrophages was less than 1%. The mean viability for 31 colonic lymphoid isolates was 90.0% ± 1.6 [SEM], estimated by trypan blue exclusion [0.1%].

Rabbit anti-ox erythrocyte IgG

Antisera to ox red blood cells [ORBC] were raised in New Zealand albino rabbits by intravenous injections of ORBC (5). The resulting IgG preparation agglutinated ORBC [1:250], gave a single band of precipitation on immunoelectrophoresis when reacted with goat anti-rabbit whole serum, and the agglutinating activity was unaltered by penicillamine reduction.

Characterization of lymphocyte isolates from peripheral blood or colon. Enumeration of B, T and null cells:

These were estimated as described previously (4).

Preparation of T-cell enriched isolates and enumeration of Tγ cells.

The methods used were described by Ferrarini et al (6). For 63 samples of PBL, the mean content of T cells in the enriched isolates was 96.7% $\pm$ 0.8 [SEM] with a mean contamination by cells of 1.9% $\pm$ 0.6. The respective values for the T-cell preparations from 31 isolates of LPL were 91.5 $\pm$ 1.1 and 3.4 $\pm$ 0.8.

The reproducibility of the methods for enumerating Tγ cells were determined by testing PBL from 4 of the healthy volunteers on five occasions over a 10-week period. In addition, aliquots of normal PBL were tested after treatment with EDTA and collagenase [EDTA-C] as used for the isolation of the LPL, or after incubation at 37° for 18 hours in TC 199 with 10% v.v. FCS.

Assay of Concanavalin-A induced non-specific suppressor T-cell activity

The technique used was that of Hodgson et al. (1). All testing was done in quadruplicate. The range of counts per minute [cpm] shown by responder cells was approximately 15,000 to 80,000.

The reproducibility of the method was determined by testing PBL from 2 healthy volunteers on three occasions. The effects of EDTA and collagenase [EDTA-C] were evaluated by testing aliquots of normal PBL treated with these agents as described for the isolation of LPL, as were those of 18 hours incubation per se. Cells from one healthy individual with a

negative value for suppressor cell activity [SCA] using untreated PBL, also were tested for the effects of EDTA-C
treatment.

Comparisons were made using the Wilcoxon Rank Sum test
and Student's t-test. A p value of 0.02 or less was demanded
for significance of difference.

RESULTS

T, B and null cells in PBL and LPL.

The percentage of T, B and null cells in PBL or LPL are
shown in table 1. The effects of EDTA-C treatment on these
estimations in normal PBL were negligible, as shown previously (4).

Table 1. Mean percentages [± one standard error] of T, B and
null cells in the isolation of peripheral blood and
colonic lymphocytes in the various study groups

Study Group	N	Peripheral blood lymphocytes T	B	null
Normal	25	68.2 + 0.7	14.8 + 0.8	17.4 + 0.6
IBD	18	62.1 + 1.3	13.8 + 0.9	20.6 + 0.9
Cancer	15	69.4 + 1.7	13.4 + 0.8	17.8 + 1.3
Others	5	65.8 + 1.5	13.8 + 2.3	20.6 + 2.1

Study Group	N	Colonic lamina proprial lymphocytes T	B	null
IBD	10	58.2 + 2.5	18.7 + 1.0	22.8 + 1.6
Cancer	15	62.4 + 2.2	20.9 + 1.8	17.1 + 2.3
Others	6	62.5 + 2.7	19.0 + 1.2	18.5 + 1.8

Tγ cells in PBL and LPL.

The reproducibility of the method with PBL and the effects of treatment with EDTA-C or incubation for 18 hours are
shown in table 2. Also shown are the effects of pretreatment
of aliquots of lymphocytes from two of the volunteers with
EDTA-C or incubation for 18 hours.

Table 2. Reproducibility of estimations of Tγ percentages in
PBL from 4 healthy volunteers tested 5 times over a
10 week period.

Subject	untreated					EDTA-C					18 hrs. incubation				
	1	2	3	4	5	1	2	3	4	5	1	2	3	4	5
SR	22	20	15	18	19										
WB	12	11	12	14	15	14	11	13	11	12	nt	nt	8	10	13
RS	13	9	13	9	9	14	8	12	8	7	nt	8	nt	9	9
MW	11	12	10	11	9										

nt: Not tested

Mean percentage of Tγ cells in PBL and LPL are shown in
table 3 and figures 1, 2, 3 and 4.

Table 3. Mean percentage [+ one standard error] of T cells
in the isolates of PBL and colonic LPL from the various study groups.

Study group	N	PBL percentage Tγ	N	LPL percentage Tγ
Normal	25	13.5 ± 1.7	–	9.4 ± 1.9
IBD	18	11.6 ± 1.7	10	9.4 ± 1.9
mild	6	18.8 ± 2.2	4	9.8 ± 3.4
moderate	8	9.8 ± 2.2	3	9.0 ± 1.2
severe	4	6.5 ± 1.3	3	9.3 ± 5.8
Cancer	15	21.7 ± 2.5	15	14.9 ± 2.2
Dukes' B_1	4	15.8 ± 4.6	4	9.3 ± 2.4
Dukes' B_1	5	20.2 ± 3.9	5	23.2 ± 4.3
Dukes' C_1	6	27.0 ± 4.0	6	12.0 ± 1.7
Others	5	12.8 ± 1.4	6	16.2 ± 2.9

Non-specific SCA

The reproducibility of measuring Concanavalin A-induced
suppressor cell activity using PBL, and the effects of EDTA-C
or incubation overnight are shown in table 4. Also shown are
the effects of pretreatment of aliquots of cells with EDTA-C
or incubation for 18 hours. Each percentage is an average of
quadruplicate assays.

Table 4. Reproducibility of Con A-induced SCA in the three separate tests of PBL from two healthy volunteers.

Subject	untreated			EDTA-C			18 hr incubation		
	1	2	3	1	2	3	1	2	3
WB	35%	27%	25%	24%	23%	13%	21%	21%	19%
MW	42%	46%	26%	33%	26%	19%	47%	31%	19%

Another individual showed 'negative' SCA on two separate tests of freshly isolates PBL [-22, -29%]. In the second test, EDTA-C treated aliquots showed SCA of -45% and those incubated for 18 hours gave a value of -47%. The viabilities of the treated cells were in excess of 90% in all instances [trypan blue, 0.1%] and the total numbers of cells did not vary in excess of ± 5% compared to the initial counts.

Percentage of Con A-induced SCA of PBL and of LPL from different patients are shown in table 5.

Table 5. Mean percentage [± one standard error] of Con A-induced SCA of PBL and colonic LPL in the various study groups.

Study group	N	PBL percentage SCA	N	LPL percentage SCA
Normal	21	28.4 ± 5.6		
IBD	15	− 1.0 ± 7.7	7	− 3.0 ± 10.9
mild	4	− 6.5 ± 10.4		
moderate	7	17.3 ± 11.4		
severe	4	− 21.3 ± 11.3		
Cancer	10	20.7 ± 11.1	11	14.8 ± 12.9
Dukes' B	6	31.8 ± 13.9	6	18.0 ± 13.0
Dukes' C	4	7.0 ± 14.5	5	12.7 ± 22.2
Others		0.8 ± 18.6	4	1.8 ± 10.5

CONCLUSION

The percentage of T_γ lymphocytes in the peripheral blood in IBD was lower than in healthy individuals, reflecting disease activity [Fig. 1].

454

This was not associated
with a change in the total number of circulating T cells and
seemed not to relate to steroid
therapy. Tγ counts in patients
with other colonic inflammatory
lesions were normal The percentage of Tγ cells in colonic
LPL from patients with IBD was
lower than that in other colo-

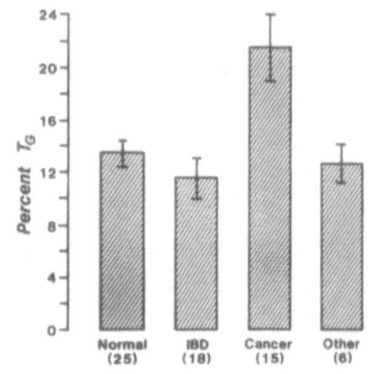

Figure 1.

nic inflammations, regardless of disease activity. The measure of Concanavalin A-induced suppressor cell activity [SCA]
in vitro of PBL from patients with IBD was lower than normal
and correlated with disease activity. However, those with
other colonic inflammatory lesions showed a trend towards
subnormal values. In contrast, Con A-induced SCA of colonic
LPL in IBD did not differ from those in the other disease
groups.

The percentage of Tγ lymphocytes in the peripheral blood
of patients with colorectal cancer was higher than normal and
correlated with the Dukes' classification, being greatest in
subgroup C [Fig. 2].

The Tγ results were different in the isolates of colonic
lymphocytes and the highest
value was found in Dukes' subgroup B_2; the Tγ percentages in
patients with B_1 or C tumors
were similar to those in the
colonic lymphocytes in IBD. The
SCA of PBl from individuals
with Dukes' C tumors was lower

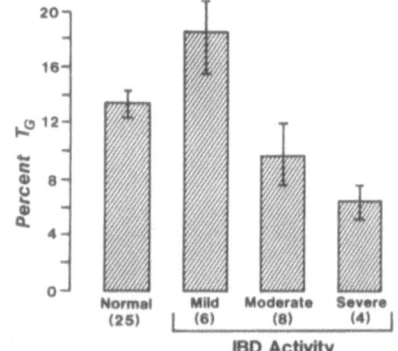

Figure 2.

than normal and similar to that in IBD. However, the SCA of
LPL in colorectal cancer did not differ from that in the
other colonic diseases.

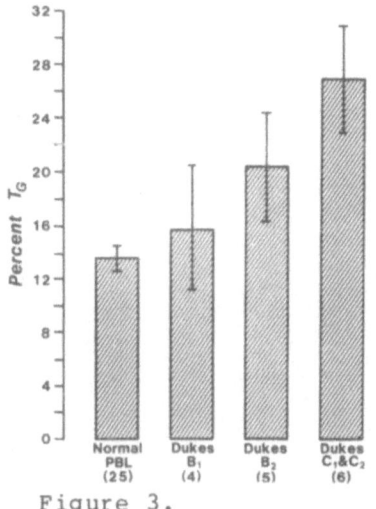

Figure 3.

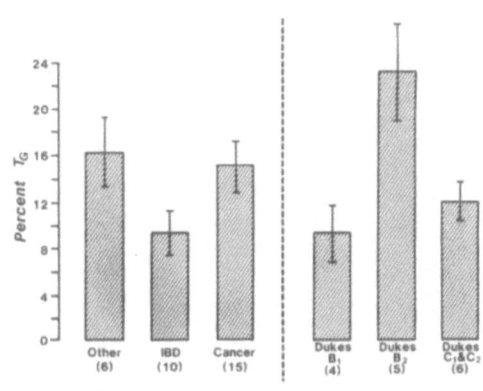

Figure 4.

The results stress the importance of studies which include observations on lymphoid cells from the disease "target organ" as well as the peripheral blood. They provide some indirect evidence to support current hypothesis involving roles for immunological mechanisms in the pathogenesis of UC and CD, and add to the limited information on Tγ cells and Con A-induced SCA in colorectal cancer.

ACKNOWLEDGEMENTS

This work was supported in part by a grant from the National Foundation for Ileitis and Colitis.

REFERENCES

1. Hodgson HJF, Wands JR, Isselbacher KJ. (1978) Decreased suppressor cell activity in inflammatory bowel disease. Clin. Exp. Immunol. 32:451-458
2. Naor D. (1979) Suppressor cells: Permitters and promoters of malignancy? Adv. Cancer Res. 29:45-125
3. Astler VB, Coller FA. (1954) The prognostic significance of direct extension of carcinoma of the colon and rectum. Ann. Surg. 139:846-852
4. Bartnik W, ReMine SG, Chiba M, Thayer WR, Shorter RG. (1980) Isolation and characterization of colonic intra-epithelial and lamina proprial lymphocytes. Gastroenterology 78:976-985
5. Mayer MM. (1961) In: Experimental Immunochemistry. Eds. Kabat EA, Mayer MM. Charles C. Thomas, Springfield, Illinois. 2nd ed. pp 326-360; 871-872
6. Ferrarini M, Moretta L, Abrile R, Durante ML. (1975) Receptors for IgG molecules on human lymphocytes forming spontaneous rosettes with sheep red cells. Eur.J.Immunol. 5:70-73

G30 Summary of Discussions relating to topic G29

Bienenstock: Mouse work suggests that T-cells derived from the bowel, have a marked tendency to go back to the bowel; in view of the compartmentalization that this infers, it should not surprise one if one found differences between peripheral blood cell function and gut cell function.

Verspaget: Has anyone looked at the tissue macrophages. According to Ward there is macrophage dysfuntion in Crohn's disease?

MacDermott: With regard to macrophages, the question is what test would be the appropriate and best test to use in seeking a macrophage dysfunction? We have isolated macrophages using our techniques of leuco-cytotoxicity. I am not sure that is the appropriate test. Perhaps MIF, perhaps a variety of other tests, are more important. One of the important things that Elson and his colleagues did was use separation technology to uncover new findings. The criticism was made that some of the findings could be due to the technology. The same criticism was made in regard to the isolation of intestinal mononuclear cells. I don't think we should be afraid of using separation techniques. These are techniques which are tremendously powerful as a means of dissecting the immune response. Instead of studying unseparated populations we are going to have to get our helper and suppressor macrophages, helper and suppressor T-cells, pre-suppressor T-cell, and look at the isolated functional capabilities with appropriate functional assays.

Verspaget: Epithelial cells are also very important, Perhaps Gebbers would like to comment on this.

Gebbers: I think our methods electron microscopy and immuno-histochemistry, is far too limited to get a real insight into the function of the epithelial cells. We have observed lesions in the dome epithelium of the Peyer's patches. Is it really the early lesion or is it a consequence of an inflammatory response of the gut? We can not decide because we do not see the sequence of events.

General Discussion and Conclusions

Reported by W. Strober

It is quite obvious that immunologic processes play a role in Crohn's disease [CD], but whether that role is helpful or harmful, primary or secondary cannot yet be decided. During this conference we learned that epithelial cell death, associated with local lymphoid infiltration, is an early pathologic feature in CD. On the one hand, it is possible that such cell death is induced by an exogenous agent, such as a virus or other organism, and this triggers a massive avalanche of lymphoid events which can be considered an essentially normal response. In this view, the immune system at best is protective to the host, and at worst causes disease only as a secondary effect. On the other hand, it is possible that while the exogenous agent is not primarily responsible for epithelial cell death it nevertheless causes a subtle alteration in the epithelial cell which then induces an essentially abnormal immune response which in turn results in epithelial cell death. In this view the interaction of the exogenous agent with intestinal cells is assumed to be a benign event in the vast majority of individuals and only causes disease in those with a genetically determined abnormality in the immune system. Immunologists are proceeding on this latter presumption and are actively searching for both non-specific defects in immune responses that alter the response to large classes of exogenous and endogenous (self) antigens, and specific defects in immune responses that relate to particular antigens.

Within the category of non-specific immune defects is the possibility that CD is due, in common with a number of other diseases, to a disorder of immunoregulation. In this regard, Knapp reported, in agreement with earlier work by Hodgson, that active CD but not inactive CD is associated with decreased suppressor T cell activity, as evidenced by the reduced ability of Con A stimulation of CD peripheral blood cells to suppress Con A stimulated proliferative responses of allogeneic cells. CD is therefore similar to SLE and several other "auto-immune states" wherein it is felt that reduced suppressor T cell activity leads to hyper-responses to antigens in general and self antigens in particular. Such a defect cannot in itself explain disease more or less limited to the GI tract, but it could help account for immunological events precipitated by more disease-specific immunologic or nonimmunologic events. Several questions regarding the existence of a defect in Con A induced suppressor T cell dysfunction in CD might be posed. Firstly, it is not clear that this defect represents decreased T cell suppression; the data is equally compatible with the concept that CD is associated with increased T cell help. Secondly, some investigators, notably Fiocchi and his colleagues, have not noted an abnormality in Con A induced suppression in CD patients. In this case the T cell function was tested in a syngeneic system and it is thus possible that the allogeneic system used by Knapp and Hodgson may have led to artifactual result. Finally the proliferative assays used in all of the studies of Con A induced T cell regulation provides no insight as to the functional effects of induced cells. What is interpreted as reduced suppression, i.e., increased proliferation of indicator cells, may actually represent a stimulation of cells destinated to subserve suppressor function.

Another kind of disordered immunoregulation has been reported in CD by Elson and his colleagues. In this case it was found that a significant proportion of CD patients contained a population of T cells which manifested increased suppressor T cell activity, as opposed to the decreased suppressor T cell activity indicated above. In the study reported, purified cells from CD patients were shown to be potent suppressors of PWM-induced Ig synthesis. However, this suppressor cell function was only manifest after the T cells

were separated from whole populations with anti-Ig columns.
It was postulated that such cells could be a secondary res-
ponse called into place to suppress local immune responses.
More interestingly, such cells could lead to local immuno-
deficiency and infection with the etiologic agent involved in
CD.

An abnormality related to a possible immunoregulatory
defect was described by two groups, Hodgson and Victorino and
Peña and colleagues. These workers found reduced numbers of T
cells bearing Fcμ receptors associated with more or less normal numbers of cells bearing Fcμ receptors. Tγ cells are
reported to mediate suppressor cell function whereas Tμ cells
are reported to mediate helper cell function. Thus, the changes found in CD patients would be most compatible with a
helper cell insufficiency, an abnormality which has not yet
been found. Thus, the quantitative abnormality in a T cell
sub-population does not yet have a functional correlate. The
area of abnormal immunoregulation is one that will receive
increased attention in the immediate future. As a preliminary
conclusion, it is likely that Con A induced suppression is a
non-specific and poorly understood test which is found to be
abnormal in a variety of disease states; this test is therefore not likely to be productive of further insight into diseases pathogenesis. In contrast, assays involving the measurement of the regulation of immune function such as polyclonal Ig synthesis or specific antibody synthesis is likely
to prove a more fruitful pathway of research.

A number of workers reported on neutrophil abnormalities
in CD. This consisted of reduced ability of neutrophils from
CD patients to migrate into skin window chambers. In two
studies, those conducted by O'Morain and Levi and Wandall and
Binder,the neutrophil migration abnormality could not be
related to the presence of serum chemotactic inhibitory factors. However, in a third study by Rhodes et al. a serum
inhibitory factor acting on C5a was found. Several of the
workers in this area feel that the neutrophil defect may be a
primary abnormality in CD because the abnormality is not

related to disease activity. However, it was pointed out by Van der Meer that circulating neutrophils consist of at least two subpopulations and it is possible that the migration abnormality could be due to compartmentalization of a sub-population that normally exhibits the most vigorous mobility.

Parallel studies of monocytes by Jewell and his collea-gues revealed several defects of circulatory monocytes. In particular these workers found increased levels of a specific lysosomal enzyme which was related to disease activity, in-crease phagocytic activity and normal chemotaxis which was not related to disease activity. These results were cited as evidence of monocyte activation perhaps mediated by circula-ting immune complexes.

The issue of whether or not CD is associated with de-creased responsiveness to PHA was addressed by Thayer. In his studies he could find no difference between CD and normal lymphocytes in PHA concentrations even when using a range of PHA concentrations. There appears to be general agreement that in patients with mild or inactive CD, i.e., those who do not exhibit nutritional deficiency and who are not on drugs which affect immune responses, one does not find reduced proliferative response. On the other hand, in patients with advanced disease one may find such abnormalities, possibly because of enteric loss of a selective population of lymphoid cells. Several papers were presented which focused on the possible immune effector mechanisms in IBD. Regarding the possibility that an ADCC mechanism may account for some of the cytotoxic effects observed in CD, Thayer reported that he could not obtain ADCC in a system containing normal lympho-cytes, IBD patient serum and target cells composed of red cells coated with germ-free rat colon antigen and several other gut-related antigens. On this basis ADCC does not ap-pear to be an important mechanism in the pathogenesis of CD. However, it is possible that this negative result could be due to the fact that antigens that are irrelevant to the disease process were used in the test systems. This concept is supported by the fact that Das has shown that UC serums contain antibodies which can cooperate with K cells to lyse certain epithelial cell line target cells. Thus, at least in UC, ADCC is a possible mechanism of tissue damage.

Continuing the discussion of effector mechanisms in CD, Auer reported that CD cells possess a decreased capacity to lyse LIK cells in a natural killer cell assay. The meaning of this finding is unclear, particularly since Stobo has reported that IBD cells have a unique capacity to kill colon epithelial cell targets in what is also a natural killer cell assay. Thus, if NK cell cytotoxicity is reduced in CD, as Auer suggest, then the defect is limited to certain kinds of target cells.

An approach to the study of CD that is being used with increasing success is that involving the study of mucosal lymphocytes. The rationale for such studies is that one is more likely to find out about immune dysfunction in CD if one goes directly to the site of tissue injury. One caveat that should be made here is that the local site of inflammation may be overwhelmed by processes that are more or less secondary to the primary disease process. Fiocchi reported on the basic method of obtaining mucosal lymphocytes. This method involves treatment of surgically obtained tissue with mucolytic agents, EDTA and collagenase. Some evidence was presented that this treatment does not adversely affect lymphoid function. Fiocchi showed that various lymphocyte stimulants such as lipopolysaccharide, enterobacterial common antigen and cell-wall defective bacteria were able to stimulate proliferation in mucosal lymphocytes whereas they were not able to stimulate peripheral lymphocytes. However, there was no essential difference between controls and CD mucosal lymphocytes, except perhaps in the case of LPS stimulations. These studies underscore the fact that mucosal lymphocytes may behave differently from peripheral lymphocytes and the responses of the former must be evaluated in CD.

MacDermott has conducted a survey of the functional capability of mucosal lymphocytes. He finds that such cells are not capable of performing cell mediated lympholysis, SCMC or

ADCC when nucleated targets are used but can mediate SCMC and ADCC when red cell targets are used. On the other hand, the cells can be stimulated with lectins to become cytotoxic. An interesting area of study was conducted by MacDermott concerning polyclonally-activated Ig syntheses by mucosal lymphocytes. In this regard, mucosal lymphocytes have high "spontaneous" Ig synthesis, i.e., synthesis not requiring the presence of mitogen. This is particularly true in the case of IgA synthesis since this immunoglobulin class is actually inhibited by the addition of mitogen. This may indicate that mucosal cells are preactivated in IBD and mitogens may activate suppressor cells such as those found by Elson and his colleagues.

Shorter has also examined mucosal lymphocyte populations and has shown that T_γ cell populations are decreased in patients with active CD compared to control cell populations. In contrast, mucosal cells from colon cancer patients had increased numbers of T_γ cells. Generally speaking, the T_γ cell levels, at least in CD patients, correlated with Con A-induced suppressor T cell activity. In the discussion of this area it became obvious that much contradictory data is presently being gathered by various investigators on mucosal lymphocytes. These undoubtably relate to technical factors in the isolation of mucosal lymphocytes and should be resolved as techniques improved.

In the other area of humoral immunity a number of reports of immune complexes in CD were presented and discussed. The chief report is that of Soltis who has carefully examined methods of measuring immune complexes and concludes that most if not all methods detect aggregated Ig as well as immune complexes. He concludes that when assay of CD serum is performed so as to exclude measurement of aggregated Ig, no circulating immune complexes are in fact found. Similar results have been obtained by several other groups. After due discussion it appeared to be a consensus that CD is not associated with immune complexes, even in those patients with extra-intestinal disease manifestations. This conclusion has considerable impact to effector mechanisms in CD since it now appears unlikely that complexes mediate activation of cytoto-xic cells such as those identified by Perlman, Shorter and many others over the last ten years. This lack of circulating complexes does not exclude the possibility that complexes are deposited at tissue sites and there activate pathologic me-chanisms. However, this remains to be proven. Jewell and his colleagues reported on C3 and Clq turnover studies in CD. These authors found that the disappearance of labelled Cl and Clq was accelerated in CD, probably indicating an increased rate of complement consumption. Interestingly, this increase in catabolism is associated with complement component seques-tration. Thus, it is likely, although not proven, that com-plement is activated and deposited at extravascular sites, presumably the GI tract. Such activation could be mediated by local immune complexes, but other mechanisms are also possi-ble.

Finally, an extensive study of lymphocytoxic antibodies was reported by Kuiper. This represents an extensive follow-up of the work of Strickland and his colleagues. In general, these workers have shown that at least half of the patients with CD and UC have lymphocytoxic antibodies which have broad specificity for both B and T cells and which lyse lymphocytes regardless of their HLA type. The origin and function of these antibodies are not known. It is possible that the anti-bodies subserve regulatory function – but no evidence on this point is at hand. It is also possible that these antibodies are recognizing exogenous antigens present in the surface of cells, such as viral antigens. As such the antibodies can be considered footprints of a subtle viral infection. Future research into the nature of the anti-lymphocyte antibodies will involve the deliniation of the antigens with which they react and whether or not they can effect T cell regulatory function as they apparently do in SLE.

In summary, the immunologic study of CD is an exceedingly active area that holds considerable promise of providing important insights into disease pathogenesis.

SECTION H

CERTAIN TOPICS OF THE TREATMENT

Section Editor: S.C. Truelove

TREATMENT OF ACTIVE CROHN'S DISEASE WITH METRONIDAZOLE OR
SULFASALAZINE. A PRELIMINARY REPORT OF A DOUBLE BLIND CON-
TROLLED TRIAL [CCDSS]

G. JÄRNEROT, B. URSING, T. ALM, F. BÁRÁNY, I. BERGELIN
K. GANROT-NORLIN, U. KRAUSE, AUD KROOK AND A. ROSEN

INTRODUCTION

In 1975 Ursing and Kamme (1) reported in an uncontrolled
study, that metronidazole [M] had a therapeutic effect on
Crohn's disease. In two small studies this finding has both
been disputed (2) and confirmed (3). As the need for better
medical treatment of this disease is great a multicenter
trial was set up and named: Cooperative Crohn's Disease Study
in Sweden [CCDSS]. The aim of the study was to investigate
the clinical efficiency of treatment with metronidazole in
active Crohn's disease in comparison to treatment with sulfasalazine [S], that is to test the null hypothesis that
metronidazole is not more effective than sulfasalazine.

PROCEDURE

Only patients with active Crohn's disease were included
in the study. Criteria for activity were a Crohn's disease
activity index [CDAI] > 200 and a serum orosomucoid concentration of $\geqslant$ 1.55 g/l, where the upper reference value is
1.05. The lower limit of CDAI for entrance to the study was
later reduced to 150. However, only four patients were included with CDAI < 200. The CDAI was slightly modified in
comparison to the one used in the National Cooperative
Crohn's Disease Study (4).

Using a double dummy design the patients were randomized
to metronidazole [400 mg twice daily] or sulfasalazine [1.5 g
twice daily] with cross over after 4 months of treatment.
Stratification was based on the localization of the lesion in

the gut, earlier operation and the level of CDAI.

The therapeutic effect on CDAI and laboratory values were evaluated monthly as well as side effects. Radiological examinations were obtained at the start and the end of the first 4 months period. All X-ray films were evaluated by a single observer before the code was broken. Sigmoidoscopy was performed on three occasions.

After 4 months cross over was done in order to test both drugs in all patients. This report deals solely with the preliminary results from the first 4 months period. Six gastroenterological units were involved in the study which comprised 78 patients. Forty patients were randomized to start with metronidazole and 38 with sulfasalazine treatment. Ten patients who previously had had bowel resection and 36 patients earlier not treated medically or surgically were equally distributed in the two treatment groups.

Patients who dropped out or had an early cross over were judged by the study group to be treatment failures or treatment failures questionable before the code was broken.

Standard statistical methods were used. In order to evaluate the effect of the two drugs in all 78 patients included in the study the Wilcoxon Rank Sum test was used.

RESULTS

Twenty-eight patients in each group completed the first 4 months treatment period. Thirteen patients dropped out, 4 as treatment failures [2M, 2S] and 9 as questionable treatment failures [6M, 3S]. Eight of them belonged to the metronidazole group and five to the sulfasalazine group. Nine patients had an early cross over. Seven of these nine patients were judged to be questionable treatment failures [3M, 4S] and two as questionable treatment failures [1M, 1S]. No patient was removed from the study because of drug toxicity.

For the 56 patients who completed the first 4 months period the mean CDAI was reduced significantly [p<0.001] by both drugs without any difference between the drugs. Neither did Wilcoxon Rank Sum test show any difference in the clinical outcome [CDAI] between the two drugs when all 78 patients were analyzed.

The mean serum orosomucoid level in the 56 patients completing the 4 months period was also significantly reduced by both drugs [p<0.001] but the reduction was more pronounced for metronidazole than for sulfasalazine with statistically significant difference between the drugs [p<0.01]. When all 78 patients were analyzed by Wilcoxon Rank Sum test there still existed a difference between the drugs [p<0.05] in favour of metronidazole.

The mean ESR was reduced to the same extent by both drugs [p<0.001]. The mean hemoglobin concentration increased significantly during treatment with metronidazole [p<0.001] but not during sulfasalazine treatment.

The radiological small bowel lesions were not improved by any of the drugs but the colonic changes were significantly more often improved in the metronidazole group. Eight of 17 in this group improved in comparison to one out of 13 in the sulfasalazine group [p<0.05].

DISCUSSION

We did not include a placebo group in this study as it has been shown earlier that sulfasalazine was better than placebo in the treatment of Crohn's disease (5). This has later been confirmed by a report published after the design of our study (6). The results of the present study show that the effect of metronidazole or sulfasalazine on active Crohn's disease is very similar. The laboratory indices of inflammation and the hemoglobin levels are normalized faster and more completely with metronidazole. However, the clinical effect as measured by CDAI did not differ. This study shows that both drugs are useful in active Crohn's disease and no one is superior to the other.

As the etiology of Crohn's disease is unknown we do not know how these drugs act. Both drugs have antibacterial properties and especially metronidazole is very effective against anaerobic bacteria. A previous uncontrolled study (7) showed a good correlation between the clinical effect of metronidazole on Crohn's disease and the reduction of Bacteroides species in the faecal microflora. This result has recently been confirmed in a controlled study (8). However, if the anaerobic gut bacteria play a primary or a secondary role in the pathogenesis of Crohn's disease is unknown. It is possible that metronidazole affects a secondary superinfection imposed on an already diseased bowel. If so, treatment of the superinfection is of benefit to the patient and metronidazole appears to be an alternative treatment.

CONCLUSIONS

The preliminary results of a double blind controlled trial show that the effect of metronidazole or sulfasalazine on active Crohn's disease is very similar. The laboratory indices of inflammation and the hemoglobin levels are normalized faster and more completely with metronidazole. However, the clinical effect as measured by CDAI did not differ. It can be concluded that both drugs are active in Crohn's disease and none of them is superior to the other.

ACKNOWLEDGEMENTS

We wish to express our gratitude to Dr. C. Johansson, Dept. of Internal Medicine, Karolinska Sjukhuset, Stockholm and to Dr. A. Walan, Dept. of Internal Medicine, University Hospital, Linkoping for their help during the early part of the study.

REFERENCES
1. Ursing B, Kamme C. (1975) Metronidazole for Crohn's disease. Lancet 1:775-777
2. Allan R, Cooke WT. (1977) Evaluation of metronidazole in the management of Crohn's disease. Gut 18:A422
3. Blichfeldt P, Blomhoff JP, Myhre E, Gjone E. (1978) Metronidazole in Crohn's disease. A double blind cross-over clinical trial. Scand.J.Gastroenterol. 13:123-127
4. Best W, Becktel JM, Singleton JW, Kern F, Jr. (1976) Development of a Crohn's Disease Activity Index. Gastroenterology 70:439-444

5. Anthonisen P, Bárány F, Folkenborg O, Holtz A, Jarnum S, Kristensen M, Riis P, Walan A, Worning H. (1974) The clinical effect of salazosulphapyridine in Crohn's disease. A controlled double-blind study. Scand.J.Gastroenterol. 9:549-554
6. Summers RW, Switz DM, Sessions JT, Jr. Becktel JM, Best WR, Kern F, Jr., Singleton JW. (1979) National Cooperative Crohn's Disease Study: Results of drug treatment. Gastroenterology 77:829-842
7. Krook A, Danielsson D, Kjellander J and Järnerot G.(1979) Changes in the fecal flora of patients with Crohn's disease during treatment with metronidazole. A preliminary report. Scand.J.Gastroenterol. 14:705-710
8. Krook A, Järnerot G, Danielsson D. In preparation.

EFFECT OF SULPHASALAZINE IN PATIENTS WITH ACTIVE CROHN'S
DISEASE. A CONTROLLED DOUBLE-BLIND TRIAL

P.A.M. VAN HEES, G. TEN VELDE, R. VAN HOGEZAND, W.DRIESSEN, J
BAKKER, H.J.J. VAN LIER, Ph. VAN ELTEREN and J.H.M. VAN
TONGEREN

INTRODUCTION

Sulphasalazine [SASP] is widely used in the medical
treatment of Crohn's disease but until recently its efficacy
has not been studied by controlled trials. Therefore, we
started a few years ago a study to evaluate the efficacy of
SASP in the treatment of patients with active Crohn's disease.

METHODS

The response of active Crohn's disease to SASP was studied in a placebo-controlled trial. A nine-item index of inflammatory activity [AI] was used as the primary measure of
response (1). The principal variables in this index are serum
albumin, ESR and body weight. In healthy subjects the AI is
less than 110. From October 1977 to August 1979 all patients
with established Crohn's disease, referred to one of the two
hospitals and the patients who were being followed and in
whom a recurrence or a relapse of Crohn's disease was diagnosed, were examined for their eligibility for the trial. Of
the 68 patients seen during this period 41 patients were
excluded; 18 patients because of a low AI [<140]; 18 patients
were in need of surgery because of complications of Crohn's
disease and 5 patients were excluded for other reasons.

Twenty-seven patients fulfilled all intake criteria and
were randomized for the study. One patient dropped out early
because of drug toxicity. Twenty-six patients with active
Crohn's [AI>140] have been followed for 6 months after random
allocation to SASP [4-6 g per day] or placebo at bi-weekly

intervals for 8 weeks, thereafter every 4 weeks. Patients and evaluating physicians remained blind to the nature of the regimen. Compliance to therapy was assessed by determining serum SP levels at each visit. The patients in the SASP- and placebo-group were comparable in all aspects. The AI [mean $\pm$ SD] before therapy was 185 $\pm$ 30 and 165 $\pm$ 22, respectively. Response to therapy was defined as a decrease of the AI with at least 25% at the end of the trial period, compared to the initial value.

RESULTS

Results were assessed using the Fisher exact test and are shown in the table.

Therapy	patients	response		significance
	(n)	(n)	%	p
SASP	13	8	61.5	
placebo	13	1	7.6	0.0056

In the 8 patients in the SASP group with a favourable response the mean fall in AI was 37%. This fall was reached 4 to 12 weeks after start of the therapy and could be maintained during the remainder of the 26 weeks follow-up period. In 8 patients of the SASP group the dose of the drug had to be reduced to 4 g per day because of side effects; 5 of them showed a favourable response to therapy.

CONCLUSIONS

From the results of this study it can be concluded that SASP [4-6 g per day] is superior to placebo in the treatment of patients with active Crohn's disease.

REFERENCE

1. Hees van PAM, Elteren van PH, Lier van HJJ, Tongeren van JHM. (1980) An index of inflammatory activity in patients with Crohn's disease. Gut 21:279-286

H3 Summary of Discussions relating to topics H1 to H2

Gilat: The international cooperative study from the USA found that sulphasalazine was effective for colonic disease but ineffective for small bowel disease.

v. Tongeren: We found that CD patients confined to the ileum also showed a good response to sulphasalazine. The numbers are small but five of the seven patients with ileitis responded very well.

Das: What is the mode of action of sulphasalazine in small bowel disease? As shown by your group and Truelove's group from the local instillation studies it is thought that 5-amino-salicylic acid is the active moiety of sulphasalazine. However, this metabolite is not released in the small intestine.

v. Tongeren: The splitting of sulphasalazine by bacteria occurs mainly in the colon but also in the small bowel, especially if the small bowel is affected by CD. There is bacterial overgrowth in the distal part of the ileum.

Booth: Levi has observed transient sterility in the male in patients treated with sulphasalazine and has been collecting other cases from centres throughout Great Britain. What is the experience in other countries?

Järnerot: I have reported one case of male infertility myself in the Swedish Medical Journal and I think that probable it is much more common that suspected.

Korelitz: Järnerot, you did not mention anything about toxicity of the metronidazole.

Järnerot: We never saw any serious side-effects, such as neuropathy.

Jeejeebhoy: It appears to me that metronidazole was better than sulphasalazine in suppressing inflammation, as judged by the orosomucoid and haemoglobin levels.

Thayer: Many physicians in the USA are using metronidazole to treat fistulae, especially perianal fistulae.

Järnerot: I can not tell you the results obtained in our cooperative study because they have not yet been analysed in detail. Our opinion based on the patients who were treated openly with metronidazole is that perianal fistulae frequently closed. It seems to be a good treatment for perianal CD.

SUCCESSFUL TREATMENT OF CROHN'S DISEASE WITH AN IMMUNOSUPPRESSIVE DRUG [6-MERCAPTOPURINE]

B.I. KORELITZ

INTRODUCTION

It was inevitable in the days when all diseases of unknown cause were being considered as possible autoimmune phenomena that an appropriate form of treatment of inflammatory bowel disease should be sought (1). Subsequently both Crohn's disease and ulcerative colitis have been shown to be associated with abnormalities of the immune system, humoral and cell mediated.

Influenced by early reports of success in the treatment of inflammatory bowel disease with immunosuppressive drugs (1-3), my colleagues and I treated 14 ulcerative colitis patients with 6-mercaptopurine [6-MP] when they were considered to have failed to respond to treatment with adrenal steroids and sulphasalazine but did not have absolute indications for surgical intervention. When 11 out of 14 improved, we concluded that this drug had a sustaining or supplementary role to decrease the frequency and severity of recurrences. At the time when the series was increased to 25 patients and reported, 15 patients were completely well and eight had improved, while two had required surgery (4). Toxicity was minimal and the drug could be used for long periods.

Most impressive were the successes in children. In six the response was excellent, nine did well without steroids for seven to 43 months, and eight grew and developed while receiving the 6-MP, including five with earlier growth retardation (5).

The time had come for double blind studies. Efforts were then directed towards Crohn's disease rather than ulcerative colitis since its course was often unrelenting, the involvement was often extensive and the disease recurred after surgical resection. Furthermore there was less enthusiasm for trials of drugs then considered carcinogenic for a disease like ulcerative colitis that was in itself potentially carcinogenic and could be cured by total proctocolectomy.

6-MP was favoured over azathioprine because patients were co-managed with hematologists who had already acquired a large experience in its use in the treatment of leukemia, because there had been no cases of complicating carcinoma or lymphoma reported, and because we had gained experience with its use in ulcerative colitis.

MATERIALS AND METHODS

Eleven years ago my colleagues and I initiated a longterm double blind randomized study to determine the effectiveness of 6-MP vs. placebo in patients chronically ill with Crohn's disease (6). Eighty-three out of 700 patients seen in private practice fulfilled the criteria; all were considered failures with sulphasalazine and/or steroids, the latter having been used many times and for long periods. Forty-three of the 83 patients had already had one or more bowel resections and suffered with recurrent Crohn's disease, some with complications. The patients were followed at a minimum of three month intervals and activity changes were recorded. These included well-being, abdominal pain, fever, number and consistency of stools, activity of fistulae and abscesses, evidence of an abdominal mass or bowel obstruction and anemia. The steroid dosage and the presence or absence of cushingoid features were monitored; the opportunity to reduce or terminate steroid therapy was a criterion for the success of 6-MP therapy. Since all design criteria were not present in all patients, specific treatment goals were established in each case. For one it was prevention of small bowel obstruction, for another elimination of a right lower quadrant mass or fistula, and for a third it was elimination of steroids. Usually there was more than one goal for each patient.

Seventy-two patients completed at least the first year of the study; 36 received 6-MP and 36 the placebo. Of the 36 receiving 6-MP, 26 [72 per cent] improved, whereas, of the 36 receiving placebo, only five [14 per cent] improved; these differences are very highly significant [Table 1]. Thirty-nine completed the study with crossover. Twenty-nine improved in one of the two years; 26 were taking 6-MP and three placebo. The proportion who improved with 6-MP was 66.7 per cent [26/39] whereas the proportion who improved with placebo was 7.7 per cent [3/39]. This combination of results was of still higher significance statistically [Table 2].

Table 1. Combined first year experience in Crohn's disease patients receiving immunosuppressives.

	Improved	Not improved	Total
6-MP	26*	10	36
Placebo	5*	31	36

*p<0.001

Table 2. Results in patients completing Crohn's disease immunosuppressive study with crossover

	Improved	Not improved	Total
6-MP	26*	13	39
Placebo	3*	36	39

*p<0.0001

In regard to specific goals, the following observations were made. Steroids could be discontinued with a coincident improvement in 53 per cent during the year the patient received 6-MP, and could be significantly reduced, but not stopped in another 22 per cent. Fistulae were totally closed in 31 per cent [nine patients] of those receiving 6-MP and were partially healed in another seven. The types of fistula which responded best to 6-MP were the abdominal wall and the internal [entero-enteric], but there was a 50 per cent response rate in the perirectal and rectovaginal fistulae as well. There were instances of clear cut response to 6-MP with resolution of abdominal mass, improvement in malabsorption and relief from recurrent small bowel obstruction, although this last group in general seemed the least likely to respond. Those patients with colonic involvement [colitis and ileocolitis] fared better than those where the disease was limited to the small bowel. Those treated prior to any surgery had an advantage over those who had already undergone one or more resections.

The mean time of response to 6-MP was 3.1 months with a range of two weeks to nine months. Though 10 per cent responded in one month or less and 68 per cent had responded by three months, some of the patients who ultimately responded the best of all did not begin to show improvement until as many as 10 months had passed.

The mean initial dose of 6-MP has been 1.5 mg/kg, rounded off to the nearest 50 mg. A complete blood count and platelet count are done weekly until they are stable and then at one to four week intervals depending on the consistency of findings. The hematological objective of dose adjustment was to maintain the white blood count at 5,000 and not to permit it to fall below 4,500. If the patient should develop fever, a rash, an upper respiratory infection or some other intercurrent illness, the 6-MP is stopped temporarily and later cautiously reintroduced. The average initial dose has been 50 mg b.i.d. In most instances the maintenance dose has been the same as the initial dose; in a very few it has been increased, and in more it has been reduced because of leucopenia, to a dose such as alternating 50 mg on one day with 100 mg the following day, or as little as 50 mg twice a week.

Almost all patients receiving 6-MP develop mild leucopenia at some time. This is a usual and acceptable finding. In over 150 patients treated with 6-MP, only three developed significant bone marrow depression; one developed a gram-negative septicemia, but in all three the bone marrow returned to normal when the 6-MP was stopped. One patient receiving 6-MP and another receiving azathioprine developed pancreatitis; these also resolved without sequelae. Nausea was often seen early in the course of treatment with 6-MP, but usually disappeared within one month. In only one patient did the drug have to be stopped because of intractable nausea. Two patients developed fever during the first three weeks of 6-MP therapy; in each case they also became febrile when azathioprine was substituted. One instance each of hepatitis and fever of unknown origin occurred during the course of treatment with 6-MP; both were self-terminating. One neoplasm, an islet cell carcinoma of the pancreas, was found incidentally during abdominal surgery in one patient who had received 6-MP for seven months six years before. There have been no deaths in patients who have received 6-MP.

DISCUSSION

Since 6-MP is effective in a large percentage of patients with Crohn's disease, the question logically arises as to how long the drug should be continued, when should it be stopped, and, if stopped, will it again be effective in the event of relapse. Preliminary data are available on 52 patients after improvement on 6-MP during the double blind study as well as results of restarting the drug in 16 after relapse (7). Of the 20 who continued the 6-MP, the improvement was maintained or even increased in 19 after 18 to 77 months [mean 37 months]. [O'Donoghue et al. (8) have conducted a double blind withdrawal trial proving that azathioprine was successful in maintaining remissions in Crohn's disease]. Of the 32 who stopped taking 6-MP, relapse took place in 26, but in only half of these did the recurrent symptoms appear within six months. In 16 patients in whom the 6-MP was restarted after relapse, not only did the Crohn's disease improve in all instances, but the mean time of response was significantly less for the second course of therapy than for the first [mean 1.5 months as compared to 3.5 months].

The differences between the results of this study and the

National Cooperative Crohn's Disease Study [NCCDS] (9) warrant comment since we conclude that the immunosuppressive
drug 6-MP, is highly effective, in contrast with another,
azathioprine, which was reported to be ineffective. Two major
differences in study design provide the most likely explanation: 1] In the NCCDS the duration of treatment evaluation
was 17 weeks. Since 6-MP [and presumably azathioprine also]
is a slow-acting drug and the response may be late, many successful responses would be missed by premature termination of
the drug. 2] In the NCCDS all other drugs had to be stopped
at the time of randomization to the treatment drug. If the
patient's disease was controlled or modified by prednisone
and this drug was suddenly withdrawn, these circumstances
would favor a recurrence. This is particularly so when it is
unsuspected that the azathioprine could not, for some time to
come, substitute for the prednisone in maintaining some modification of the course of the Crohn's disease existing at the
start of the study. In the Lenox Hill-Mount Sinai study when
the patient was receiving steroids at the onset, that drug
was continued and its reduction was monitored as one of the
criteria of response. This is more in keeping with the natural course of the disease and the way that it is managed in
private practice. Though probably not of similar importance
to the two differences outlined above, it must also be considered that 6-MP and azathioprine are not the same drug. In
vivo, azathioprine is metabolized to 6-MP, which might be the
more effective agent. A significant portion of the azathioprine might also be sacrificed during the digestive and metabolic processes.

The reluctance of physicians who manage inflammatory
bowel disease with use of immunosuppressive drugs has been
due mainly to fear of a carcinogenic effect. Many years have
now passed and no reasonable proof of carcinogenic complications in non-transplant cases has been reported (10). Malignancies have been reported in only 11 out of more than 20,000
patients with rheumatoid arthritis treated with immunosuppressive drugs. Similarly malignancies occurring in patients

with inflammatory bowel disease receiving or having received azathioprine or 6-Mercaptopurine have been rare. Furthermore, no teratogenic effect of immunosuppressive drugs has been demonstrated. The question has also arisen as to whether "immunosuppressive" drugs really work through immunosuppression as opposed to an anti-inflammatory or other mechanism. Theoretically the main risk concerning long-term therapy should be invasion by opportunistic organisms in the chronically immunosuppressed patient. Clinically, this too has not proven to be a significant problem.

CONCLUSIONS

6-MP is effective in the treatment of Crohn's disease for long periods of time and it is reasonably safe, particularly when considering the chronic unrelenting course in so many young people. Though a relapse may be expected after cessation of the drug, it may not occur for a long time; it may occur in a milder form not requiring reintroduction of 6-MP, and if 6-MP is again necessary it is likely to be effective. 6-MP should be used in the treatment of Crohn's disease when sulphasalazine does not prevent relapse, when steroids cannot be reduced or stopped, and when steroids must be frequently reintroduced. It should be used ideally before complications ensue. Perhaps when we feel more comfortable with its use it might be justified even earlier in the course, when the disease is still considered mild.

REFERENCES
1. Bean RHP. (1962) The treatment of chronic ulcerative colitis with 6-mercaptopurine. Med.J.Austral. 2:592-593
2. Brooke BN, Jarett SL, Davison OW. (1970) Further experience with azathioprine for Crohn's disease. Lancet 2:1050-1053
3. Sachar DB, Present DH. (1978) Immunotherapy in inflammatory bowel disease. Med.Clin.N.A. 62:173-183
4. Korelitz BI, Glass JL, Wisch N. (1973) Long-term immunosuppressive therapy of ulcerative colitis. Am.J.Dig.Dis. 18:317-322
5. Korelitz BI, Glass JL, Wisch N. (1977) Long-term observation of children with ulcerative colitis treated with an immunosuppressive drug [6-mercaptopurine]. Gastroenterology 72:A-60, 1083

6. Present DH, Korelitz BI, Wisch N, Glass JL, Sachar DB, Pasternack BS. (1980) Treatment of Crohn's disease with 6-mercaptopurine. New.Engl.J.Med. 302:981-987
7. Korelitz BI, Wisch N, Glass JL, Present DH. (1978) Long-term response of Crohn's disease to treatment with 6-mercaptopurine. Gastroenterology 74:1130[abs]
8. O'Donoghue DP, Dawson AM, Powell-Tuck J, Brown RL, Lennard-Jones JE. (1978) Double-blind withdrawal trial of azathioprine as maintenance treatment for Crohn's disease. Lancet 2:955-957
9. Summers RW, Switz DM, Sessions JT Jr, Becktel JM, Best WR, Kern F.Jr.(1979) National Cooperative Crohn's Disease Study: results of drug treatment. Gastroenterology 77:847-869
10. Penn I. (1978) Malignancies associated with immunosuppressive or cytotoxic therapy. Surgery 83:492-502

SUPEROXIDE DISMUTASE AND D-PENICILLAMINE IN THE TREATMENT OF CROHN'S DISEASE

J. EMERIT and A.M. MICHELSON

INTRODUCTION

Chromosomal instability is a characteristic of Crohn's ileocolitis and other autoimmune diseases (1). Recent work of Emerit and Michelson (2) suggests the role of $O_2^-\cdot$ radical and OH$\cdot$ radical at the origin of chromosomal breakage. It appeared logical to examine the use of superoxide dismutase [SOD] for treatment of Crohn's disease. During three years we have treated patients with Crohn's disease with D-Penicillamine [DPcA] (3) and reduction of chromosomal instability was observed concommitant with clinical improvement (4). Recently Weser (5) suggested that DPcA mimics the action of SOD in dismutating $O_2^-\cdot$ radical after formation of a complex with copper. We like to present the clinical results obtained with these two superoxide dismutating agents so far.

MATERIAL AND METHODS

DPcA [low doses ranging from 300 to 600 mg/day] was used as the only treatment for Crohn's disease for the past three years in 10 patients. [see Table 1]. The therapeutic efficiency has been judged when ever possible on the skin lesions, the radiologic features, the anal and/or rectal lesions.

Also, a double blind multicentric trial was initiated 18 months ago using the Best Index activity [CDAI] (6). Patients with a CDAI between 150 to 450 were candidates for entry into the trial. The duration of this trial was two months and the CDAI was evaluated every fourteen days during this period. DPcA was given at a dose of 600 mg each day. At the end of may 1980, 17 patients from 6 centres have been enrolled in this study.

Table 1. Patients treated with DPcA only. Uncontrolled study.

	Sex	Age/ yrs	Characteristic and duration of disease prior to therapy	Surgical procedures	Duration of therapy and results	Relapses under therapy
1	F	41	9 years pancolitis	1967 left colectomy, 1974 total colectomy	3 years, good	Yes
2	M	30	12 years pancolitis;spondylartritis	none	2 years, good	Yes
3	M	36	1 year right colitis	none	16 months, good	Yes
4	M	35	3 months rectal involvement	none	12 months, good	No
5	M	42	6 years ileitis	Appendicectomy 1972	21 months, good	No
6	F	35	3 years pancolitis	none	26 months, good	No
7	F	42	16 years ileocolitis	total colectomy 1966 ileectomy 1979	12 years, good	No
8	F	28	6 months rectal and sigmoid involvement	none	6 months, good	No
9	F	14	9 years pancolitis	1976 total colectomy with ileorectal anastomosis	12 months, good	Yes
10	M	25	11 years ileocolitis	right colectomy 1972 ileotransversostomy 1979	6 months, good	No

In each patient under DPcA, hematocrit, white cell count, platelet count and test for proteinuria were performed, each fourteen days, and adverse reaction recorded.

Bovine Cu SOD was used first as a local treatment for two cases of skin lesions. The good tolerance of the drug subcutaneously administrated in terminal patients with advanced cancer or important radionecrosis allowed us to use SOD in three patients with Crohn's disease, selected on the basis of aviability and willingness to participate in an uncontrolled study.

RESULTS

The double blind study suggest that the DPcA is more active than placebo. Five of 8 patients treated with DPcA had a regression of Best Index of 100 or more, 1 of 9 patients with placebo had this result [p<0.05].

The uncontrolled study of our ten cases suggest that DPcA is active on the fibrosis shown in skin lesions and in X-ray pictures of the small bowel or barium enema. During DPcA therapy the relapses were less severe and marked by micro-ulcerations in skin lesions and barium enema. In our patients despite of these slight relapses DPcA therapy was beneficial.

During these two studies with DPcA one slight proteinuria was observed. The DPcA therapy of another patient of the double blind trial was interrupted after six months because of a platelet count's decrease, despite of a very good clinical success.

Bovine Cu SOD as local treatment gave dramatic results in treatment of ulcerations developing under D-Penicillamine therapy.

Subcutaneous injection of this pure enzyme encapsulated in liposomes gave an impressive result in a 26 years old man with a severe Crohn's disease. The first clinical diagnosis was lymphoma because of an ureteral bladder and rectal involvement. At the first laparotomy the fibrosis was so important that surgical procedures were not possible. The histological picture of the lymph nodes suggested tuberculosis or

Crohn's disease. After 4 months of SOD treatment the ureteral lesion regressed and ileectomy could be performed. In another patient subcutaneous injections of SOD, cured micro-ulcerations which developed during DPcA therapy after discontinuation of DPcA.

In a patient with micro-ulcerations developing during DPcA therapy, subcutaneous SOD seemed without action, but good results were rapidly obtained when metrodinazole was used in addition of SOD.

DISCUSSION AND CONCLUSIONS

This study suggest that SOD and DPcA are effective in the treatment of Crohn's disease but these results are clearly preliminary and must be confirmed by controlled trials. If the superoxide dismutating agents demonstrate to be efficient in the control of Crohn's disease, it may be of value for understanding the etiology of this disease.

REFERENCES
1. Emerit I, Michelson AM. Chromosome instability in man and murine autoimmune diseases. Anticlastogenic effect of superoxide dismutase. Acta Physiol.Scand. in press
2. Emerit I, Michelson AM. (1979) Chromosomal breakage, free radicals and superoxide dismutase in collagen diseases. Abst. 6th Int. Congress for Radiation Research, Tokyo
3. Emerit J, Emerit I, Levy E, Loygue J. (1978) La D-Penicillamine est-elle efficace dans la maladie de Crohn. Gast.Clin.Biol. 1:114
4. Emerit I, Emerit J, Levy A, Keck M. (1979) Chromosomal breakage in Crohn's disease: anticlastogenic effect of D-Penicillamine and L-Cysteine. Hum.Genet. 50:51-57
5. Lengferlder C, Fuchs C, Younes M, Weser U. (1979) Functional aspects of the superoxide dismutative action of Cu Penicillamine. Biochem.Biophys. Acta 567:492-502
6. Best WR, Becktel JM, Singleton JW, Kern F, Jr. (1976) Development of a Crohn's disease activity Index [NCCDS]. Gastroenterology 70:439-444

H6 Summary of Discussions relating to topics H4 and H5

Asquith: Korelitz, you have previously suggested that the closure of enterocutaneous abdominal fistulae correlates reasonably well with the presence or absence of the stenotic segment distal to internal opening of the fistula. In view of your success with 6-MP did you look at this particular point?

Korelitz: The stenotic segment in CD is similar to pyloric stenosis. Some of it is due to inflammation and some of it is due to scarring. If the fistula can be closed it usually means that the stenotic segment was mainly caused by inflammation.

Hodgson: How many patients in either group were submitted to surgery during the course of follow-up?

Korelitz: There were only three patients who came to surgery out of the total of 83. Some others have come to surgery since that time.

Best: I agree that patients who had been on steroids and were withdrawn early in our study did tend to do worse. We also did see a trend towards a late effect with the immunosuppressive drug. However, they never reached the level of statistical significance so that the question of the length at which the higher dose was used may have been a factor. One of the problems in comparing the two studies arises from your method of selecting specific therapeutic goals for individuals. Did you have some relatively rigid criteria for what presentation of a patient would lead to what therapeutic goal? How objective were these goals and were you blind in your evaluation of the patients?

Korelitz: The criteria for the double-blindness are outlined in our article. By doing it the way we did, we made the observation that 6-MP is a slow-acting drug and that it is necessary to treat sick patients with steroids first in order to buy some time for the immunosuppressive drug to take over.

Jeejeebhoy: The effects that you observed may in fact due to a combination of steroids and 6-mercaptopurine.

Korelitz: My own opinion is that the steroids are merely buying time and the good results are not due to a synergistic action of the two drugs. The forms of therapy used by Emerit are completely new to me. Are they available internationally?

Emerit: D.penicillamine is available in all countries. Superoxide dismutase is not generally available but one can ask for it from Michelson.

Hodgson: Can I ask Emerit about the cellular distribution of the superoxide dismutase in the tissue?

Emerit: We suppose that, when given in liposomes, the superoxide dismutase goes into the cell because liposomes are phospholipids and the membrane of cells are also phopholipids. Michelson has carried out EM scanning of red blood cells and has found that liposomes enter the cells.

TOTAL PARENTERAL NUTRITION [TPN] IN THE PRIMARY MANAGEMENT OF CROHN'S DISEASE

G.R. GREENBERG and K.N. JEEJEEBHOY

INTRODUCTION

In the absence of a known aetiology, the treatment of Crohn's disease is necessarily supportive and non-specific. Where complications of the disease occur, or when remission cannot otherwise be achieved, intestinal resection is currently considered the treatment of choice. There is, however, a significant recurrence rate after surgery. Indeed, Greenstein et al. (1) noted that with each successive operation, the chance of reoperation rises, and recurrences may develop faster. Therefore, any self-limiting form of therapy which would induce a clinical remission without requiring intestinal resection might be considered a therapeutic advance.

To meet this aim, total parenteral nutrition [TPN] with bowel rest has been advocated for many types of inflammatory bowel disease [IBD] including Crohn's disease(2-5). Proponents of its use suggest that by eliminating oral feedings, and hence the stimuli of intraluminal digestion, acute inflammation may gradually resolve. Simultaneously, because all nutritional requirements are met intravenously, protein anabolism with weight gain can be achieved. That TPN provides important adjunctive nutritional support to patients with IBD is well recognised. Its value as primary therapy in promoting a remission, particularly in Crohn's disease is, however, controversial (6). We therefore undertook a prospective study with two years' follow-up to assess the role of TPN as primary medical therapy in active Crohn's disease. Prior to TPN, all patients had received optimal conventional medical management and frequently the treatment of choice would have been considered to be surgical resection.

MATERIALS AND METHODS

Patients. Forty-three consecutive patients with a mean age of 33 years [range 15-58] and clinical and radiological evidence of active Crohn's disease were referred to the Gastrointestinal Unit of the Toronto General Hospital for TPN and bowel rest. Prior to TPN, 34 of 43 patients were hypoalbuminic [<35g/l]. The major indications for TPN included: acute inflammatory mass in 14 patients, subacute obstruction in four, extensive small bowel disease in 11, and fistulous disease in 14. Of the group with fistulae, 12 were enterocutaneous [seven small bowel and five large bowel] and two were enterovesicular. At the time of referral, 20 patients were receiving prednisone, which was reduced to 15 mg per day, and continued during TPN. In an additional four patients, prednisone [15 mg per day] was started after seven days of TPN alone, because of clinical signs of continuing disease activity [tender mass, fever, etc.].

Nutrient input. The mean period of TPN was 25 days. Details of the nutrient input and methods of delivery have been published previously (7,8). Briefly, three systems of TPN were used. The first [29 patients], requiring central venous infusion, provided 50% of non-protein calories as glucose and 50% as lipid [Intralipid[R]]. The second system [4 patients] provided 83% of non-protein calories as lipid [Intralipid[R]] and therefore was amenable to peripheral infusion. All these patients received 1 g/kg per day ideal body weight [IBW] of protein either as casein hydrolysate [Amigen[R]] or as a defined aminoacid mixture [Travasol[R]], and 40 Kcal per kilogram per day [IBW] of non-protein calories. This protein-calorie input has previously been shown to induce positive nitrogen balance and weight gain in a comparably stressed group of patients (8). In a further 10 patients, within 10% IBW, less than this optimum non-protein caloric requirement was given, although a mean protein input of 1.7 g/kg/day was sufficient in all cases to achieve positive nitrogen balance. Vitamins, electrolytes and trace elements were also provided to meet individual patient requirements.

Analytical methods. Albumin and total protein were measured in the routine biochemical laboratory with standard automated techniques. Total nitrogen in urine, stool and drainage was determined by a micro Kjeldahl technique described previously (8)

RESULTS

Clinical results. The mean weight gain observed in the 43 patients was 1.1 kg per week [range -0.5 to 3.5]. Of the 10 patients receiving less than optimal non-protein calories, six lost weight. The mean rise in serum albumin was 4 g/l [range 0 to 22]. Nitrogen balance determined in 26 patients was overall positive with a mean of 2.4 g/day [range 0.8 to 3.5].

Clinical remissions. A remission was defined as relief of diarrhoea and abdominal pain, closure of fistula where present, and improved well-being for at least three months after discharge from hospital. The results are summarized in table 1. In the four groups of patients studied, 33 out of the total 43 had a remission [77%]. Differences were, however, noted between groups.

Table 1. Clinical remission in disease activity after TPN, with or without corticosteroids

	Corticosteroids			
	None	Prior and continued	Started with TPN	Total number of remissions
Fistulae	1/7	6/6	0/1	7/14 [50%]
Abdominal mass	8/8	5/6		13/14 [93%]
Intestinal obstruction	1/1	2/3		3/4 [75%]
Severe active disease	3/3	4/5	3/3	10/11 [91%]

Where fistulous disease was the major indication, the clinical remission rate [including fistula closure] was only 50 percent. However, whereas one of six with enterocutaneous fistulae remitted with TPN alone, six of six patients on the combination of TPN and prednisone closed their fistulae and went into clinical remission. Enterovesicular fistulae in two patients did not close regardless of the addition of predni-sone. In the other three groups, the clinical remission rate was not influenced by prednisone. In the 10 patients recei-ving less than ideal non-protein calories, nine demonstrated a clinical remission.

Follow-up at two years. The results are summarized in table 2. In 42 of 43 patients follow-up for two years was available, to assess the relatively long-term effect of TPN. The group on prednisone either had this drug kept at a main-tenance dose of 15 mg/day, or were completely tapered off. Prednisone [15 mg/day] was added to one patient during the course of this follow-up period. In 10 patients, however, the operative specimens grossly and microscopically showed only minimal evidence of active Crohn's disease in four, while in three the disease was characterized by fibrosis without an acute inflammatory component.

After two years of follow-up, therefore, 29 patients have continued in medical remission [67%].

Table 2. Results of two year follow-up

	Surgical resection				Continued
	Immediate	Within 1 year	Pathology minimal	inactive	medical remission
Fistulae					
a] enterocutaneous					
small bowel	3		1	1	4
large bowel	2		1	1	3 [50%]
b] enterovesicular	2				0
Abdominal mass	1	3	2	1	9 [69%]
Intestinal obstruction	1				3 [75%]
Severe active disease	1				10 [91%]
Total	10	3	4	3	29 [67%]

DISCUSSION

This prospective study was designed to assess, over a two-year period the role of total parenteral nutrition with bowel rest as primary medical therapy in the management of Crohn's disease. Our results demonstrate that immediately after TPN a clinical remission was achieved in 77% of patients otherwise considered failures of medical management. This figure compares favourably with data reported previously (4,5). A two year follow-up was available for 42 of our patients, during which time 13 had required surgery. Therefore, 67% remained well, and in clinical remission after two years. Our study further allowed for the assessment of two factors considered previously to alter in a positive fashion the course of patients with Crohn's disease. These included prednisone administration and high caloric input with weight gain.

A multi-centre controlled trial has reported that prednisone can induce a remission in active Crohn's disease (9). It might be anticipated, therefore, that in combination with TPN, prednisone would improve the remission rate over that observed with TPN alone. Our data would support such a conclusion for only one of the four groups of patients studied. Those presenting with an acute inflammatory mass, subacute obstruction, and severe active disease demonstrated the best response to TPN. The addition of prednisone in these groups did not improve the remission rate over those patients receiving TPN alone.

In contrast, a rather different pattern was observed in the group with enterocutaneous fistulae, where the 50% remission rate was almost exclusively accounted for by those patients receiving the combination of TPN and prednisone. In agreement with experience of others (4) our studies demonstrate that with TPN alone, Crohn's fistulae frequently became quiescent, but generally did not completely close. This complication has therefore been considered a specific indication for surgery. Data on a combined approach has not, however, been reported. Thus, on the basis of our beneficial results, a re-evaluation of TPN and prednisone now seems warranted with selected cases of Crohn's fistulous disease before surgery is undertaken.

The mechanism by which TPN contributes to a clinical remission in patients with inflammatory bowel disease remains obscure. High caloric input with weight gain has been emphasised as one important factor. Because some of our patients in acute relapse were within 10 percent ideal body weight, we evaluated the relative contribution of a high caloric input by maintaining positive nitrogen balance in the absence of an exogenous source of non-protein calories. This "protein-sparing" therapy (10) allows for endogenous fat mobilization as a source of energy, but requires 1.7-2.0 g/kg of protein daily to achieve positive nitrogen balance (7). Ten of our patients received this regimen and all were maintained in positive nitrogen balance. Notwithstanding weight loss in six, nine of the 10 had a clinical remission, suggesting that a high exogenous calorie input, in itself, is not a primary factor accounting for the observed improvement in all the patients. Others have speculated that hypertonic glucose may contribute, in part, to a remission by exerting a relaxant effect on an inflamed, spastic bowel (3). In our study, comparable results were achieved with TPN providing 83% of non-protein calories as lipid, demonstrated previously to produce a plasma substrate and hormone profile consistent with fat providing the major source of energy (8). Any hypothesis therefore which specifically invokes glucose also seems unlikely. One common denominator in all our patients, however, was the absence of oral intake, and this intralumenal starvation must affect digestive secretory processes, gastrointestinal hormones and, perhaps, intestinal motility. Further studies in these areas may elucidate some of the mechanisms responsible for the observed improvement.

CONCLUSIONS

TPN and bowel rest provides an important therapeutic tool in the primary management of Crohn's disease. Where facilities limit the use of a TPN regimen requiring central venous infusion, a peripheral lipid system is clinically and metabo-lically just as efficacious (8). Perhaps the ultimate triumph of TPN is demonstrated in patients where multiple resections combined with active Crohn's disease preclude adequate nutri-tion orally. Here a permanent TPN programme at home has now been shown to maintain a remission and allow complete social rehabilitation (11).

REFERENCES
1. Greenstein AJ, Sachar DB, Pasternack BS, Janowitz HD. (1975) Reoperation and recurrence in Crohn's colitis and ileocolitis: crude and cumulative rates. New Engl.J.Med. 293:685-690
2. Steiger E, Wilmore DW, Dudrick SJ. (1969) Total intra-venous nutrition in the management of inflammatory dis-ease of the intestine. Fed.Proc. 28:808
3. Fischer JE, Foster GS, Abel RM, Abbott WM, Ryan JA. (1973) Hyperalimentation as primary therapy for inflamma-tory bowel disease. Am.J.Surg. 125:165-175
4. Fazio VW, Kodner I, Jagelman DG, Turnball RB, Weakly FL. (1976) Inflammatory disease of the bowel: Parenteral nutrition as primary or adjunctive treatment. Dis.colon rectum 19:574-578
5. Reilly J, Ryan JA, Strole W, Fischer JE. (1976) Hyper-alimentation in inflammatory bowel disease. Am.J.Surg. 131:192-200
6. Alexander-Williams J. (1976) Inflammatory disease of the bowel. The risk of cancer. Dis.colon rectum 19:579-581
7. Greenberg GR, Marliss EB, Anderson GH, Langer B, Spence W, Tovee EB, Jeejeebhoy KN. (1976) Protein-sparing the-rapy in postoperative patients: effects of added hypo-caloric glucose or lipid. New Engl.J.Med.294:1411-1426
8. Jeejeebhoy KN, Anderson GH, Nakooda AF, Greenberg GR, Danderson I, Marliss EB. (1976a) Metabolic studies in total parenteral nutrition with lipid in man: comparison with glucose. J. Clin.Invest. 57:125-136
9. The national co-operative Crohn's disease study [NCCDS]. (1977): Preliminary results of Part I. Gastroenterology 70:A-80/938
10. Blackburn GL, Flatt JP, Clowes GHA, O'Donnell TE. (1973) Peripheral intravenous feeding with isotonic amino acid solutions. Am.J.Surg. 125:447-453
11. Jeejeebhoy KN, Langer B, Tsallas G, Chu RC, Kuksis A, Anderson GH. (1976) Total parenteral nutrition at home: studies in patients surviving 4 months to 5 years. Gas-troenterology 71:943-953

TOTAL PARENTERAL NUTRITION [TPN] IN CROHN'S DISEASE; A CLINI-
CAL EVALUATION

L.P. BOS, M. NUBÉ and IRENE T. WETERMAN

INTRODUCTION

Loss of weight and nutritional depletion are prominent
features in patients with active Crohn's disease [CD]. Res-
triction of oral intake has long been used empirically in the
treatment of these patients. Total bowel rest and adequate
nutrition were however incompatible until the introduction of
TPN. It would seem reasonable to expect that TPN would be of
benefit to these patients. Indeed, in the last decade several
reports have been made about favourable results with TPN in
the treatment of patients with CD, especially when used as a
primary treatment in active disease (1). This study covers
our results during a 4 year period using TPN in the treatment
of patients with CD.

MATERIALS AND METHODS

Within a period of 4 years [1975-1979] 118 patients suffering from CD were treated with TPN. They received in total
144 courses with a mean duration of 34.1 days. The indications to use TPN in these patients are given in table 1.

Table 1. Indications for 144 courses of TPN in 118 patients
with CD treated during 4 years [1975-1979]

Main indications	N^+
Pre-operative management	46
Management of active disease	74
Management of complications	46
Miscellaneous	6

+ Including 22 cases with two indications and 3 with
three indications.

Within the three main groups shown in table 1 a further selection was made based on localization and clinical picture to have a more homogeneous group in each category. An extra care was taken that within these categories all patients were included into the present study.

Group 1: Pre-operative management

Thirty patients with ileo-caecal CD with a mass and obstruction and or fistulas, for which the decision to operate on them had already been made before the start of treatment, were studied. The purpose to feed these patients parenterally was to replete them nutritionally and to decrease local and systematic disease activity in the hope for less extended resections and less post-operative complications. In this group in about half the cases TPN was used without any previous medical treatment. The mean preoperative treatment period has been 24 days. At the start and immediately pre-operative the following parameters were collected: serum albumin, body weight, ESR, WBC, Hb and platelet count.

Group 2: Management of active disease

The histories of 32 patients with active CD of the colon only, and of 27 with extensive ileo-colitis were studied. With this indication TPN was practically never used as a primary treatment but almost always when sulphasalazine and corticosteroids had failed to achieve a remission. The mean length of the disease history in this group was 7 years. The clinical effect of treatment was judged here on the shortterm and during follow-up. The short term effect was judged as bad when surgical treatment had been applied during the same admission. Results were rated fair when despite improvement, symptoms of diarrhoea, abdominal cramps, pain etc. had not subsided and several objective criteria such as ESR, Hb, WBC, band forms, platelet counts, total serum protein, albumin, body temperature and the findings at endoscopy did not indicate considerable improvement. The results were considered good when clinical remission had been achieved. Long-term clinical results were assessed after a mean follow-up of 3 years, on the basis of the patients condition. Results were rated good when neither symptomatic nor objective signs of active disease were found. The results were considered bad when the patients were not able to live a normal life and objective signs of active disease were present, and when the patients were continuously in need of immuno-suppressive drugs to control disease activity. The patient's clinical condition was rated fair when one or more relapses readily controlled by medical treatment occured during follow-up or when disease activity interfered to some extent with their normal daily activities.

Group 3: Management of complications

We confined the study to our patients with fistula problems. In total we cared for 33 patients with fistula problems of which 12 enterocutaneous, 10 internal and 11 perianal fistulas.

Finally a small prospective comparative clinical trial was carried out on patients with moderately active CD of the colon only, as judged by the Crohn's disease activity index [CDAI] (2), in which besides sulphasalazine and corticosteroids either TPN or a liquid formula diet was given for exactly 21 days, when again the activity index was calculated. Fourteen patients entered and completed this trial.

RESULTS

In table 2 the six parameters collected at the start of treatment and immediately pre-operative, representing the state of nutritional and general signs of inflammatory activity, in the ileo-caecal Crohn's disease group are summarized. As can be seen in the table the state of nutrition improved and the general signs of inflammatory activity decreased. Local signs of inflammation improved too, which was reflected by a decrease in the size of the palpable masses, although this was not substantiated.

In table 3 the results are summarized concerning the management of active disease using TPN in combination with sulphasalazine and corticosteroid treatment.

Table 2. Patients with ileo-caecal Crohn's disease [n=30].
         Mean values and standard deviation of six parameters
         at the start of TPN and immediately before surgery

Parameter		normal values	before TPN	pre-operative	p-values
Serum					
albumin	[g/l]	40-50	35.6± 6.0	38.4± 5.3	<0.05
body weight	[kg]		57.8±13.1	58.5±12.2	ns*
ESR	[mm]		43.0±26.6	26.7±26.1	<0.05
leucocytes	[10^9/l]	4.5-11.0	8.4± 2.3	7.1± 3.2	<0.05
haemoglobin	[mmol/l]	8.0-10.5	7.5± 1.0	7.8± 0.9	ns*
platelets	[10^9/l]	150-350	368±105	261.5±71	<0.0005

*ns= not significant

As can be seen in table 3 in 47.5 percent surgery could
be avoided in this group which remained so in the follow-up
period of three years, although in six of the 18 initially
good responders the clinical condition changed from good to
fair.

Table 3. Short-term and intermediate-term clinical results in
         patients with active disease of the colon or exten-
         sive ileo-colitis [n=59]

Short-term results n = 59	Good 18*		Fair 10	Bad 31+
Clinical condition during follow-up n = 27	Good 11/18	Fair 6/18	Fair 10	
Mean duration of follow-up [months]	35.6		35.9	

* One patient lost from follow-up
+ Two patients died of complications associated with CD

In an attempt to predict the outcome of this treatment
several parameters [serum albumin, body weight, peak daily
temperature, ESR, WBC, Hb, platelet count, faecal weight and
endoscopy scores] were collected at the start and also after
three weeks of treatment which was continued for an average
of 33 days in this group. At the start no relevant differences could be observed between the treatment failures and

the so-called good responders. After three weeks of treatment Hb-levels had decreased significantly in the treatment failures. Findings at endoscopy improved in both groups although much more marked in the good responders.

Table 4 summarises the results we had using TPN in the treatment of patients with CD and fistula problems. The results show that TPN alone is of limited value. Only a 15 percent closure rate was observed. The 3 enterocutaneous fistulas which did close developed after recent excisional surgery and originated from the internal anastomosis. When surgical treatment followed TPN a 61% of all fistulas closed [see table 5].

Table 4. Results concerning fistula closure in CD patients given TPN only

TPN alone

Localization of fistula	n	closed n (%)	improved n (%)	failure n (%)
Enterocutaneous	12	3 (25)	3 (25)	6 (50)
Internal	10	2 (20)	2 (20)	6 (60)
Perianal	11	0 (0)	8 (72.7)	3 (27.3)
Total	33	5 (15.2)	13 (39.4)	15 (45.5)

Table 5. Results concerning fistula closure in CD patients after TPN and surgical treatment

Localization of fistula	n	closed n (%)	improved n (%)	failure n (%)
Enterocutaneous	12	7 (58.3)	1 (8.3)	4 (33.3)
Internal	10	10 (100)	0 (0)	0 (0)
Perianal	11	3 (27.3)	8 (72.7)	0 (0)
Total	33	20 (60.6)	9 (27.3)	4 (12.1)

Table 6 summarises the results of the comparative trial using TPN or a liquid formula diet besides sulphasalazine and steroids in a group of 14 patients with moderately active CD of the colon only, using the CDAI (2). No difference in disease activity was noted between the two groups neither at the start nor after three weeks of treatment. In both groups the disease activity decreased in a significant way.

Table 6. Results of TPN or LFD as part of conservative treatment in moderately active CD of the colon, assessed on the basis of the Crohn's disease activity index [CDAI]

	CDAI at the start of treatment	CDAI after 3 weeks	p-value
TPN group n = 6	317 ± 55.5	134 ± 76.5	<0.001
LFD group n = 8	294 ± 83.2	141 ± 92.7	<0.001
p-value	ns*	ns	

* ns= not significant

DISCUSSION AND CONCLUSIONS

In this predominant retrospective study an attempt was made to evaluate the contribution of TPN in the treatment of patients suffering from CD. For this, the histories were studied of distinct groups of patients out of each of the three main indications to use TPN [pre-operative management, management of active disease and management of complications].

Concerning the pre-operative use of TPN in patients with ileo-caecal CD [group 1] it was noticed that the disease activity decreased and the nutritional state of the patients improved. Because this had not been a prospective controlled study we were not able to determine whether there has been a reduction in the extent of the resections which were carried out and of the number of post-operative complications or not. In these series 5 postoperative complications were noticed: anastomotic leakage in one, three times wound infections and one intra-abdominal hemorrhage. On this point we like to refer the work of Bosetti et al. (3), and of Collins et al. (4) who showed a more quickly and less complicated wound healing after major surgery in inflammatory bowel disease patients. On the basis of these studies we consider the pre-

operative use of TPN in CD patients a useful matter. Furthermore TPN provides time for a proper diagnostic work-up of
these patients to collect data on the basis of which important decisions are made about e.g. the type and extend of the
operation. We found this an important advantage.

With regard to the use of TPN in the management of active
disease [group 2] in order to achieve a remission we were
often impressed by the immediate symptomatic relief of
putting the bowel at rest by means of an intraveneous drip.
It has been our attitude to use TPN not as a primary form of
treatment but only when sulphasalazine and corticosteroids
had failed. The mean pre-treatment disease history in this
group of patients with severe active disease has been 7
years. These factors all were considered infavourable regarding the outcome of treatment by Dudrick et al. (1). It is
therefore not surprising that only in half the cases we suc-
ceeded in achieving a remission. In less active disease [and
or when used as a primary form of treatment] like in our
small prospective comparative trial better results are obtained. These are then in accordance with the 80 per cent
response rate calculated by Driscoll and Rosenberg in their
review (5). However, in these circumstances a liquid formula
diet proved to be as effective as TPN. A similar comparative
trial in severe active disease is needed now. Unfortunately
the outcome of treatment with TPN could not be predicted. For
this reason a therapeutic trial is frequently worthwhile
especially in cases of extensive small bowel disease.

Concerning "management of complications" [group 3] this
study has been confined to patients with fistulas. The results in terms of the fistula closure rate using TPN alone
has been disappointing [15 per cent closure rate]. However,
when TPN is followed by a planned surgical attempt for final
fistula closure the results can be considered good [61%]. In
our view the use of TPN in the treatment of CD patients with
fistulas must be considered as an integrated part of surgery.
In our experience fistulas arising from active diseased bowel
do close only in exceptional cases. The rule that the more

distal a fistula arises from the gut the less can be expected
from TPN seems to be confirmed in our material by the results
of the perianal fistula closure rates.

REFERENCES
1. Dudrick SJ, MacFadyen BV Jr., Daly JM. (1976) Management
    of inflammatory bowel disease with parenteral hyperali-
    mentation. In: Gastrointestinal Emergencies. Eds: Clear-
    field HR and Dinoso Jr. VP. Grune and Stratton, New York.
    pp 193-199
2. Best WR, Becktel JM, Singleton JW, Kern F Jr. (1976)
    Development of a Crohn's disease activity index. National
    cooperative Crohn's disease study. Gastroenterology
    70:439-444
3. Bozetti F, Terno G, Logoni C. (1975) Parenteral hyperali-
    mentation and wound healing. Surg.Gynecol.Obstet.
    141:712-714
4. Collins JP, Oxby CB, Hill GL. (1978) Intravenous amino-
    acids and intravenous hyperalimentation as protein spa-
    ring therapy after major surgery. A controlled clinical
    trial. Lancet 1: 788-791
5. Driscoll RH Jr., Rosenberg JH. (1978) Total parenteral
    Nutrition in inflammatory bowel disease. Med.Clin.
    North.Am. 62:185-201

ELEMENTAL DIETS IN THE TREATMENT OF ACUTE CROHN'S DISEASE

C.O'MORAIN and A.J. LEVI

INTRODUCTION

Many different therapies have been advocated in the treatment of acute Crohn's disease including antibiotics, azathioprine, salazopyrine and steroids often without controlled trials to support their efficacy. Recently the importance of nutritional support in Crohn's disease has been emphasised. Patients with this condition are often in negative nitrogen balance as a result of anorexia and reduced protein intake, diminished absorption by the small intestine, losses by exudation from inflamed mucosa and systemic effects of chronic inflammation. In an attempt to reverse this metabolic inbalance total parenteral nutrition (1-6) and elemental diets (7-15) have been used. This form of therapy has been used when other treatment fails and prior to operative intervention. It has been found that as the negative nitrogen balance is reversed the indications for surgery often recedes. T.P.N. requires careful monitoring and serious complications have been reported. An elemental diet offers nutritional support in a simple safe non-toxic and easy to administer method.

PATIENTS

Thirty two exacerbations of Crohn's disease in 27 patients requiring hospitalisation were treated. All exacerbations were characterised by abdominal pain and diarrhoea. Weight loss more than two kilograms in the previous month occurred with twenty exacerbations. Eleven patients had a pyrexia greater than $38^{o}C$ for a week or more. Twenty four had an E.S.R. greater than 20 mm/hr. Twenty had a haemoglobin less than 12.5 g/100 ml and 18 had a serum albumin less than 35 g/l. In addition to acute activity of their Crohn's disease, six young patients had growth failure, three had clinically evident sub-acute obstruction. One patient had an abdominal wall fistula and another presented with rectal bleeding. Four patients had a sera negative peripheral arthropathy.

TREATMENT

The patient was started on an elemental diet after an initial in-patient assessment. All food except for tea and coffee without milk, boiled sweets and clear minerals were withdrawn and replace with an elemental diet [Vivonex] supplying 50-75 Kcal/kg body weight and 8-12 g of nitrogen/day.

The concentration of the diet was gradually increased over a period of three days increasing its strength successive to avoid complications such as abdominal colic and diarrhoea attributable to its hyperosmolar content. After four weeks on the elemental diet solid food was gradually reintroduced over a period of three days. The diet was initiated in hospital but the patients were allowed to go home once they had been accustomed to the diet and had chronically improved which was generally after 7-14 days.

The diet was well tolerated in all of the patients except for two who found the diet impalatable. A third patient was withdrawn from the trial for surgical resection of a chronic ileal obstruction. Of the twenty four patients [twenty since exacerbations as five were treated twice] who remained within the trial eight received no other therapy, three had steroids [Prednisone 30 mg/day for two weeks reducing to a maintainance dose of 10 mg/day] and nine had intermittent levamisole [2 mg/kg/day for 3 days every 14 days] introduced from the third week onwards. Four continued on their pre-trial drugs on which they relapsed [two were on steroids and one each on azathioprine and salazopyrine].

The patients were followed up weekly for four weeks and then at monthly intervals.

RESULTS

In all twenty nine of the acute episodes in which the four week course on the elemental diet was completed the patients showed marked clinical improvement. There was a dramatic and sustained improvement in all indices of disease activity monitored except for slight loss of weight in the first two weeks.

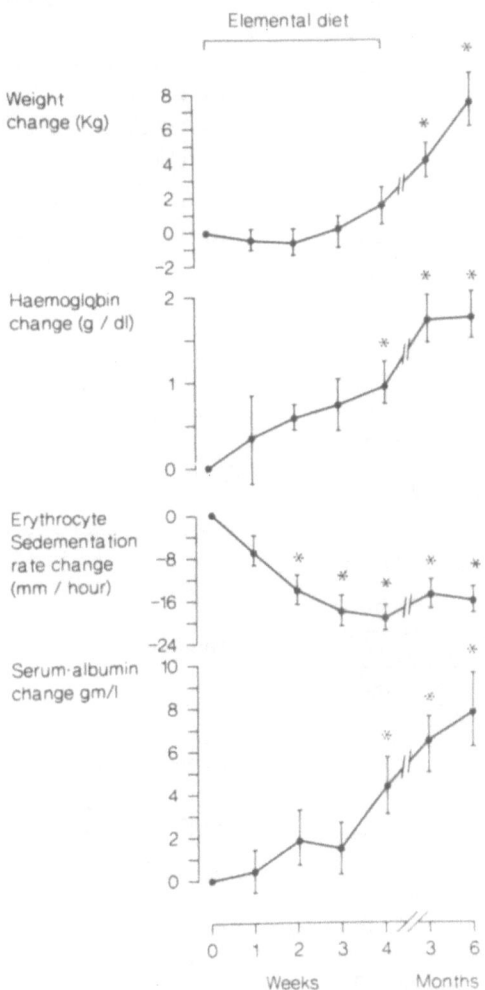

Figure 1. Effect of treatment on various indices of disease activity. [mean + SEM]
* Significance of difference from initial results P < 0.05.

510

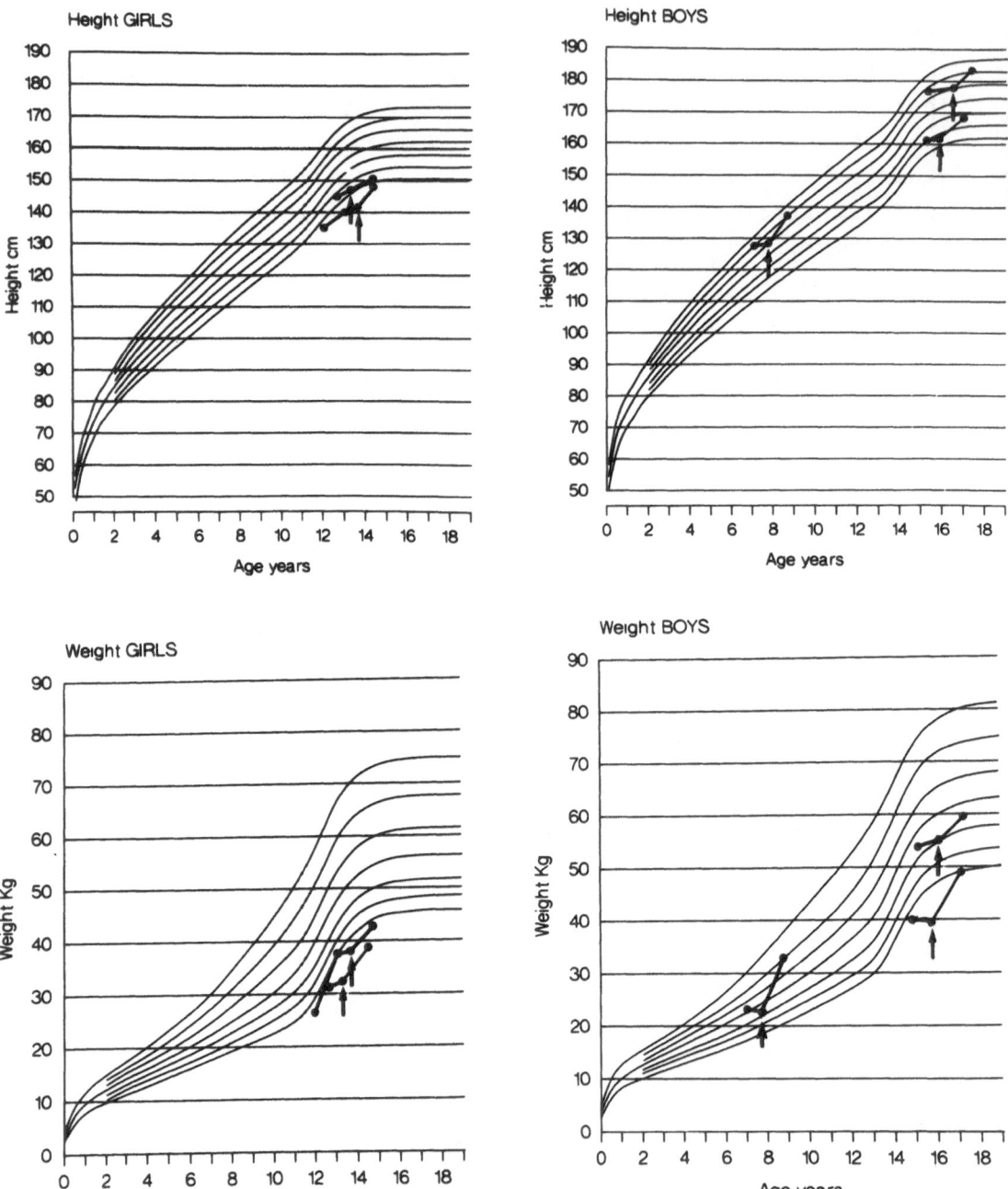

Figure 2. Height and weight rate in three boys and two girls
assessed on Tanner's tables.

There was a mean fall in the E.S.R. of 24 mm/hour, an increase in both the serum albumin of 4.3 g/1 and the haemoglobin of 1.2 g [excluding patients tranfused] Fig. 1.

Six months after the elemental diet therapy eighteen of the twenty four patients remained clinically in remission. All of these had gained weight [mean 6.1 Kg SE 1.3 Kg] and the serum albumin rose in all [mean 8.0 SE 1.76]. Of the six patients who had relapsed three require bowel resection, one was treated by increasing prednisone dosage and two patients were restudied a second time on the elemental diet.

Growth rate as assessed on Tanner Tables (18) was maintained or exceeded in five young patients [three boys, two girls] who had previously deficient growth [Fig. 2]. Two of these had concurrent prednisone therapy.

DISCUSSION

The role of elemental diets in the treatment of Crohn patients is not fully established. Previous reports are few and only small numbers of patients have been treated, and often as a last resort prior to surgical intervention. In this series all of the patients who completed the diet treatment were considered to be in clinical remission at four weeks. There was an initial loss of weight, probably due to the low residue and the gradual build up of calorie intake. At the end of the treatment period the patients nutritional status had improved as evidenced by a rise in serum albumin and weight gain. At six months six of the patients had relapsed. Three of the patients who had symptoms of sub-acute obstruction prior to the diet therapy all eventually required surgery. The diet, although unpalatable, was tolerated orally in all but two of our patients. With encouragement the patients adapt to the diet particularly when they note an improvement in their symptoms.

Total parenteral nutrition has induced [recently been reported] remission in adolescents with Crohn's disease and resumption of skeletal growth (16, 17).

An elemental diet may be as equally effective in growth

failure and avoid the potential hazards of T.P.N. Five of our patients maintained and improved their centiles for both height and weight when plotted on Tanner tables.

These findings suggest that an elemental diet is an effective therapy in acute Crohn's disease. Why this should be so is unclear. We suggest the diet may be effective because it [a] provides nutritional support, [b] is hypoallergic as it contains no whole protein [c] may act as a medical bypass from the affected area as the diet requires minimal digestion and reduces gastrointestinal secretions [d] may alter bowel flora. In addition the patients general well-being is improved by the supply of adequate calories and essential food stuffs in a form easily available without further digestion, given in a safe, simple and non-toxic way.

Acknowledgements

C. O'Morain was the recipient of an Eaton Fellowship. The authors are grateful to Miss P. Hulme and her colleagues in the Department of Dietetics for their continued help in these studies.

REFERENCES
1. Fischer JE, Foster GS, Abel RM, Abbott WM, Ryan JA.(1973) Hyperalimentation as primary therapy for inflammatory bowel disease. Am. J. Surg. 125:165-175
2. Anderson DL, Boyce HW. (1973) Use of parenteral nutrition in treatment of advanced regional enteritis. Am. J. Dig. Dis. 18:633-640
3. Vogel CM, Corwin TR, Bane AE. (1974) Intravenous hyperalimentation in the treatment of inflammatory diseases of the bowel. Arch. Surg. 180:460-467
4. Reilly J, Ryan J, Strole W, Fischer J. (1976) Total parenteral nutrition and inflammatory bowel disease. Acta Chir. Scand. 142 supp. 466: 92-93.
5. Milewski P, Irving M. (1979) The place of parenteral nutrition in Crohn's disease. Abstract D6, European Congress on Parenteral and Enteral Nutrition, Stockholm
6. Paris JC, Houcke PL, Roger J, Blais J. (1979) Parenteral exclusive nutrition in treatment of Crohn's acute manifestations. Abstract L77, European Congress on Parenteral and Enteral Nutrition, Stockholm
7. Stephens RV, Randall HT. (1969) Use of a concentrated balanced liquid elemental diet for nutritional management of catabolic states. Ann. Surg. 170:642-667

8. Bury KD, Stephens RV, Randall HT. (1971) Use of a chemi-
   cally defined, liquid elemental diet for nutritional
   management of fistulas of the alimentary tract. Am. J.
   Surg. 121:174-183
9. Voitk AJ, Echave V, Feller JH, Brown RA, Gurd FN. (1973)
   Experience with an elemental diet in the treatment of
   inflammatory bowel disease. Is this primary therapy?
   Arch. Surg. 107:329-333
10. Rocchio MA, Mo Cha CJ, Haas KF, Randall HT. (1974) Use of
    chemically defined diets in the management of patients
    with acute inflammatory bowel disease. Am. J. Surg. 127:
    469-475
11. Giorgini GL, Stephens RV, Thayer WR. (1973) The use of
    "medical by-pass" in the therapy of Crohn's disease:
    report of a case. Am. J. Dig. Dis. 18:153-157
12. Good A, Hawkins ST, Feggetter JG, Johnston ID. (1976) Use
    of an elemental diet for long term nutritional support in
    Crohn's disease. Lancet 1:122-124
13. Segal AW, Levi AJ, Loewi G. (1977) Levamisole in the
    treatment of Crohn's disease. Lancet, 2:382-384
14. Hall M Jr., Russell RI. (1979) Elemental diets in the
    management of complicated Crohn's disease. Abstract P77
    1st European Congress on Parenteral and Enteral Nutri-
    tion, Stockholm
15. Axelsson CK, Jarnum S. (1977) Assessment of the thera-
    peutic value of an elemental diet in chronic inflammatory
    bowel disease. Scand. J. Gastroenterol. 12:89-95
16. Kells DJ, Grant RJ, Shen G, Watkins JB, Werlin SL, Baehme
    G. (1979) Nutritional basis of growth failure in children
    and adolescents with Crohn's disease. Gastroenterology
    76: 720-727
17. Layden T, Rosenberg J, Nemchausky B, Elson C, Rosenberg
    IH. (1976) Reversal of growth arrest in adolescents with
    Crohn's disease after parenteral alimentation. Gastroen-
    terology 70:1017-1021
18. Tanner JM, Whitehouse RH, Marshall WA, Carter BS. (1975)
    Prediction of adult height from height, bone age, and
    occurrence of menarche, at ages 4 to 16 with allowance
    for midparent height. Arch. Dis. Childh. 50:14-26

H10 Summary of Discussions relating to topics H7 to H9

Gilat: An elemental diet may be good but the problem is palatability. What did you do to make it palatable?

O'Morain: We have a very active dietetic department and an enthusiastic nursing staff and they play an important role in the success of this therapy. None of our patients required tube feeding and all of them were able to tolerate it orally. I think another secret of our success was that we introduced it gradually. Before its introduction we gave the patient a tasting session of the various flavours available and allowed the patient to make his own choice.

Asquith: In one of your initial reports you have had two patients with polyarthritis to whom you had given an elemental diet and levamisole and you thought that the elemental diet had influenced the response to levamisole.

O'Morain: We are disappointed with levamisole in the long-term treatment for Crohn's disease.

Buchmann: Does TPN bring the patient to a point where surgery is no longer necessary?

Bos: Our policy was to carry out a resection once a considerable inflammatory mass was present in order to prevent complications and exacerbation of the disease in that part. This policy was based on the retrospective study carried out by Weterman a few years earlier.

Hodgson: The Leiden group have compared TPN with a simple nutrition supplement with a liquid formula and there does not appear to be any difference. We need more such trials of nutritional therapy.

v. Tongeren: Jeejeebhoy showed some improvements in radiological signs in his patients treated by TPN. Can he comment on the cause of this improvement.

Jeejeebhoy: Most of our patients when they are put on total parenteral nutrition have a wide separation of intestinal loops due to inflammatory reaction around the bowel and this often shows dramatic improvement, so I think that there is no question that the socalled peri-bowel inflammation seems to get better. Also, in a few patients studied by colonoscopy before and after TPN, it is clear that the colonoscopic appearances became much better.

A STUDY OF DIFFERENT FACTORS TO PREDICT THE OUTCOME OF
ILEORECTAL ANASTOMOSIS IN COLONIC CROHN'S DISEASE

P. BUCHMANN and IRENE T. WETERMAN

INTRODUCTION

There is still disagreement about the place of ileorectal
anastomosis in Crohn's disease of the colon. In a recent
retrospective study of two different centra (1) it was found
that quite a proportion of patients with Crohn's disease had
a succesful functioning ileorectal anastomosis after a mean
period of follow-up of 7.6 years [6 months - 20 years]. It is
possible that some of the following factors might influence
the long term results of an ileorectal anastomosis:

1 - Sex of the patient.
2 - Age at onset of Crohn's disease.
3 - Age at operation.
4 - Ileal manifestation.
5 - Pre-existing perianal disease.
6 - Sigmoidoscopical appearance of rectal mucosa.

The present communication reports the results of a retrospective study from the University Medical Centre Leiden, The
Netherlands, and the General Hospital Birmingham, England,
where the importance and influence of the above six mentioned
factors were analysed.

PROCEDURE

In a period of twenty years 105 patients had elective
colectomy and ileorectal anastomosis for Crohn's colitis. In
patients with severe deforming rectal disease, severe perianal lesions or incontinence an ileorectal anastomosis has
never been performed.

The clinical records of the 105 patients were reviewed
and 94 out of 97 patients who were alive at the time this
study was done were interviewed. Those with a functioning

ileorectal anastomosis were examined by sigmoidoscopy whenever possible. Active Crohn's disease in the rectum was classified as mild proctitis when edema of the mucosa was present; as moderate proctitis when bleeding, cobblestone appearance or some ulceration was recorded and as severe proctitis when there was diffuse and deforming disease.

Active disease in the terminal ileum was defined on either the operative or sigmoidoscopic findings or on classical X-ray films taken after the last resection of diseased bowel.

RESULTS

From the 105 patients entering the study 74 [70%] still had a functioning ileorectal anastomosis; 20 [19%] had had an ileostomy; 8 [8%] had died and 3 [3%] were lost to follow-up. The mean follow-up time of the survivors was 7.6 years. Prognosis for males [45] and females [60] was similar with 60% and 69% respectively functioning ileorectal anastomosis.

The age of onset of Crohn's disease, varying between 5 and 60 years, did not seem to influence the outcome of the ileorectal anastomosis.

In half of the patients colectomy and ileorectal anastomosis were performed within less than 4 years, in 2/3 in less than 6 years after onset of Crohn's disease, but the prognosis was not affected.

At the time of colectomy ileal involvement was found in 40 operative specimens; in 49 the small bowel was considered normal and in 16 patients precise information was missing. A success rate of 78% was found both in cases of active ileal Crohn's disease [31 out of 40] and when there was no ileal disease [38 out of 49] at the time of colectomy.

In 29 patients perianal fissures and/or fistulae were recorded; 67 were considered to have a normal perineum, in 9 there were insufficient data. Success rate in this group was 76% [22 out of 29] when perianal disease was present and 72% [48 out of 67] when there was no perianal disease at the time of colectomy.

Pre-operatively, the rectum looked normal on sigmoidoscopy in 30 patients and mild or moderate proctitis was found in 58 patients. In 17 patients the notes were incomplete. Better results were obtained when the rectum was sigmoidoscopically normal at the time of operation with a success rate of 87% [26 out of 30] compared to 69% [40 out of 58] in patients with mild or moderate proctitis. However, this difference did not achieve statistical significance.

On follow-up examination most of the patients with a functioning ileorectal anastomosis for Crohn's colitis were satisfied with the results of the operation. Three patients were dissatisfied and suffering from frequency and urgency of defaecation with sigmoidoscopic evidence of moderate or severe proctitis. Pre-operatively, 2 of these 3 patients were considered to have a normal rectum on sigmoidoscopy.

DISCUSSION

One of the main factor influencing the outcome of colectomy with ileorectal anastomosis for Crohn's colitis both in the medical literature and in the present study seems to be the pre-operative normality of the rectal mucosa. However, it is remarkable that in our series even when mild or moderate proctitis was present pre-operatively a success rate of 69% was achieved. As still quite a proportion of patients with ileorectal anastomosis failed [31 %] and we could not distinguish them from the good responders with the factors studied so far, further studies are necessary.

The measurement of rectal capacity might help in the classification of the patients for advising to perform an ileorectal anastomosis. It has been shown that there is good correlation between the degree of proctitis and the rectal capacity (2).

A last point worth-while consideration might be the risk of cancer in the rectal stump after ileorectal anastomosis for Crohn's colitis. As far as we know there has been no report of cancer in the rectum after following ileorectal anastomosis in Crohn's disease.

CONCLUSIONS

The present retrospective study has shown that the performance of an ileorectal anastomosis should be considered in the treatment of Crohn's disease of the colon even when the rectum appears to be mildly or moderately inflamed, or when perianal disease is not too severe.

The sex, age, length of history of the disease, the prescence of ileal involvement did not have any predictive value in the outcome of the ileorectal anastomosis in this study. Further studies, such as the measurement of pre-operative rectal capacity might be of value in assessing the correct indication of ileorectal anastomosis in Crohn's disease of the colon.

ACKNOWLEDGEMENTS

We would like to thank Mr. J. Alexander-Williams, from the University of Birmingham, who operated on most of the English patients. We are also indebted to Professor Dr. M. Vink, head of the Department of Surgery of the Leiden University Hospital, where most of the Dutch patients were operated.

REFERENCES
1. Buchmann P, Weterman IT, Keighley MRB, Peña AS, Allan RN, Alexander-Williams J. (1980) The prognosis of ileorectal anastomosis in Crohn's disease.Br.J.Surg. in press
2. Buchmann P, Mogg GAG, Alexander-Williams J, Allan RN, Keighley MRB. (1980) Relationship of proctitis and rectal capacity in Crohn's disease. Gut 21:137-140

RECURRENCES AFTER SURGERY IN CROHN'S DISEASE. DOES THE INDI-
CATION FOR SURGERY AND THE CLINICAL PATTERN AT PRESENTATION
DETERMINE THE RELAPSE RATE IN PATIENTS WITH CROHN'S DISEASE?

R.G. FARMER, V. FAZIO and G. WHELAN

To study this question we evaluated 578 patients who
where referred between the years 1966-1969 to the Cleveland
Clinic for management of Crohn's disease. No patient was
originally referred for the management of relapse. The disease status of these patients was determined in 1978-1979
using information obtained from clinical review or, where
this was not possible, telephone contact. The mean age at
operation was 33 years and the mean follow-up, 113 months.
Two assistants who were "blinded" to the hypothesis is being
examined, abstracted data onto coding forms relating to the
clinical pattern at presentation, indication for surgery,
nature of first definitive operation and whether or not recurrences had occured.

There were 398 patients [69%] who had an operation and
180 [31%] who had not. Re-operation was performed for 207
[52%] of those operated. Patients with an ileocolic pattern
at presentation formed the largest subgroup. These 194 patients were more likely to receive a definitive surgical
resection - 166 [86%] vs. 398 [69%] in the total group,
$p < 0.0005$. They also had a higher relapse rate requiring a
second operation - 100 [60%] vs 207 [52%], $p < 0.01$. When analyzed by actuarial methods, patients with ileocolic disease
originally requiring surgery because of internal fistula had
a shorter median interval to relapse than those with other
surgical indication - 64 months vs. 108 months, $p < 0.01$.

This study indicates that over two-thirds of patients
presenting with Crohn's disease will require a surgical procedure. Of those who are operated upon over half will have a
relapse requiring re-operation during the ensuing 10 years.

Operation is more likely to occur if the patient had an ileo-colic pattern at presentation. If the indication for surgery was internal fistula, the median time to relapse is much shorter than for other surgical indications.

Table. Clinical pattern in Crohn's disease. Relationship of location of disease and operation

	Operated no.	%	non-operated no.	%	re-operated no.	%	Total patients no.
Ileo-colic	166	86	28	14	100	60	194
Small in-testine	114	65	61	35	52	46	175
Colon	103	58	73	41	48	47	176
Ano-rectal	15	45	18	54	7	47	33
Total	398	69	180	31	207	52	578

REFERENCES
1. Farmer RG, Hawk WA, Turnbull RB. (1975) Clinical patterns in Crohn's disease. Gastroenterology 68:627-635
2. Farmer RG, Hawk WA, Turnbull RB. (1976) Indications for surgery in Crohn's disease. Gastroenterology 1:245-250
3. Mekhjian HS, Switz DM, Watts HD, Deren JJ, Katon RM, Beman FM, (1979) National cooperative Crohn's disease study: Factors determining recurrence of Crohn's disease after surgery. Gastroenterology 77:907-813

SURGERY IN CROHN'S DISEASE

E.C.G. LEE

INTRODUCTION

Most patients with Crohn's disease can be managed successfully by a judicious combination of medical and surgical treatment, but there are some whose disease progresses inexorably and who develop recurrences rapidly after operation. A particularly difficult problem arises when a stricture develops in a patient who has such widespread disease that it is impossible for it to be excised and for a normal state of nutrition to be maintained. The clinician is faced with a dilemma. On the one hand the patient's condition may gradually deteriorate in spite of the most intensive medical treatment; on the other hand although the blockage should be amenable to operative correction, the diffuseness of the disease is usually seen as a strong contra-indication to surgery. At the best the patient is maintained in a state of chronic malnutrition by periodic hospital admissions for hyperalimentation.

This paper summarises the clinical details of six such patients who were submitted to surgery. It is suggested that operative treatment has an important role to play in their management, and that it can safely be carried out even if active Crohn's disease is left behind.

MATERIALS

All six of the patients suffered with extensive Crohn's disease of the type classified as "discontinuous" in the Cape Town Anatomical Classification (1), and all had been followed for some years in Oxford where they had undergone previous resections. Their average age was 24.3 years when the current surgery was undertaken. All of the patients began having symptoms of Crohn's disease at an early age [average age of

onset-12.1 years]. All of the patients had had previous surgery for their condition. Table 1 summarises the anatomical
extent of the disease and the current problem in each patient.

Table 1. Anatomical extent of the disease and the current
problem in each patient.

No	Patient	Sex	Age	Anatomical Extent of Disease	Current problem
1	EL	F	21	Multiple segments of disease throughout small bowel 2 areas of colonic disease	17 cms - multiple obstructions
2	IB	F	24	Lesions in oesophagus, stomach & throughout remaining 18" of small intestine, ileostomy, diffuse colitis	2 small bowel strictures
3	CD	M	20	Multiple areas small bowel disease, ileostomy, subtotal colectomy	3 intestinal strictures
4	JS	M	34	Previous extensive resections massive recurrence	7 cms of strictures
5	ES	F	24	Proctocolectomy with ileostomy for multiple small bowel disease, duodenal obstruction, 20" of remaining gut with active disease	Complete pre-ileostomy stricture
6	LA	F	23	Gross small & large bowel disease with gross perianal disease	Recurrence causing gangrenous preileostomy intussusception

INDICATIONS FOR SURGERY

The indications for surgery in all the patients was an
increasing intestinal obstruction characterised by weight
loss, abdominal distension, colic and malnutrition. [Cases 1
and 3 [Table 1] suffered from severe hypo-proteinemia]. Patients 5 and 6 developed a more rapid intestinal obstruction
which could be classified as acute, and case 6 required emergency surgery after being transferred from another hospital
to Oxford because of a gangrenous intussusception at the site
of recurrent disease proximal to an ileostomy.

DIAGNOSIS

In all patients a preoperative assessment of the extent of disease and of the point of obstruction was undertaken radiologically by the use of a small bowel barium enema [enteroclysis].

PREOPERATIVE PREPARATION

Except for the case with intussusception, careful preparation was carried out by correcting the fluids, electrolytes if abnormal, anaemia if present, and by the use of preoperative hyperalimentation administered through a central venous line. Prophylactic antibiotics were given consisting of preoperative Flagyl and a broad spectrum antibiotic to cover the operation. The patients received a regimen of intravenous corticosteroids as a cover using the method we have employed for some years (2). All the patients had been on previous corticosteroid medication, and patients 1,3 and 4 had quite marked evidence of hypercorticoidism.

OPERATIVE TECHNIQUE

After the abdomen was opened through the previous incision, adhesions were freed and a careful laparotomy was undertaken. All the cases were found to have extensive Crohn's disease scattered throughout the bowel. If difficulty was experienced in assessing the degree of obstruction, a large oesophageal tube was passed through their mouth by the anaesthesist and was then advanced by the surgeon to test the size of lumen. It was particularly helpful in cases 2 and 3, where it demonstrated areas of nearly complete obstrution.

Three techniques were used to overcome the obstruction:
1. A 'plasty' procedure

If a very narrow segmental obstruction was encountered, this was overcome by a longitudinal incision cut through it along the length of the bowel, which was then sewed up transversely [fig.1 A]. The procedure was used in one stricture in case 2 and one stricture in case 3.

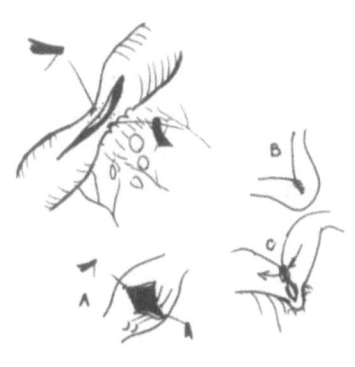

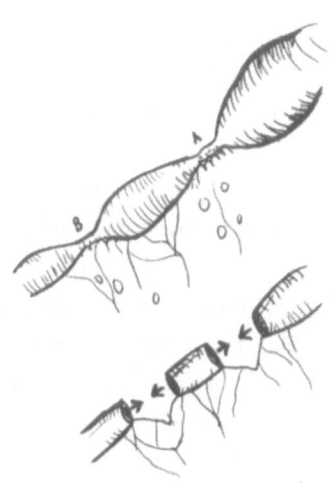

Figure 1. A narrow stricture
is incised along length of
bowel. A]'plasty' procedure.
B] localized by-pass procedure
and C] anastomoses

Figure 2. Multiple stric-
tures at A and B treated
by minimal resections and
anastomosis

2. A localised by-pass

With very active inflammation at the stricture in which
the wall of the bowel was too thick to allow a 'plasty'
procedure, but when the disease appeared too extensive to
resect, small side-to-side anastomoses were made just
proximal and distal to each lesion [Fig. 1 B and C]. This
technique was carried out on some of the strictures in
patients 1,2,3 and 4. Numerous thickened intestinal segments were often found, and it was sometimes difficult to
be sure which lesion was causing the actual blockage. The
use of a small bowel barium enema examination was particularly helpful in localising the obstructions preopera-
tively.

3. Minimal resections

When a segment of bowel was so badly diseased that the

above techniques seemed to be contraindicated, and if the patient had sufficient bowel to warrant a resection, the badly diseased segment was excised and a primary end-to-end anastomosis was carried out in cases 1, 3, 4, 5 and 6. The suture lines were closed with absorbable sutures [catgut or Dexon]. In all the patients extensive inflammation was left behind after the obstructions had been treated. In the majority, it was recognised that active Crohn's inflammation was present at the suture line.

Postoperative course:

No patient suffered a major complication, there were no leaks from suture lines. The length of follow-up of the patients number 1 to 4 is from 12 to 29 months. Patient 1 has recently complained of some abdominal pain and some weight loss and has required a course of corticosteroids to reduce the symptoms. None of the other patients has had an increase of symptoms which could be classified as a major recurrence. None has developed another obstruction. All patients had a marked improvement in general condition which is exemplified by a sustained increase in weight after the operation.

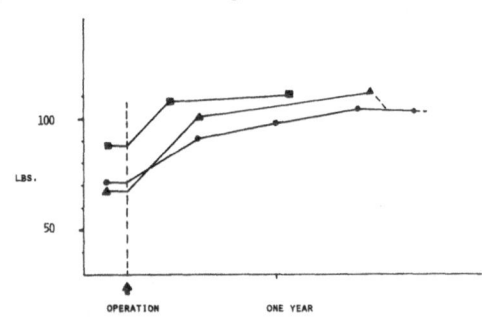

Figure 3. Graph of the pre- and postoperative weights of patients 1,3 and 4 who have been observed for more than one year

DISCUSSION

Many people now consider that Crohn's disease is a diffuse inflammation which affects the intestine throughout its length. Treatment is therefore aimed at reducing the symptoms, diminishing acute inflammation with corticosteroids when a flare up occurs and excising segments of bowel when inflammation becomes severe or when a local complication such as a fistula or stricture develops. Considerable evidence is accumulating to indicate that radical surgery does not reduce the chance of recurrent disease. In Oxford a recent study has shown that the presence or absence of active Crohn's inflammation in the cut ends of the bowel does not influence the incidence or timing of recurrences. What is advocated in this paper is an extension of the conservative view of treatment in which no attempt is made to cure the disease by excision, or even to remove the majority of inflammation. The aim is just to relieve the blockage in patients with extensive disease who have developed an obstruction. Minimal surgery can safely be carried out in such patients even if the intestine is sutured through active Crohn's disease. The marked improvement which followed the operation in all the cases treated so far and the lack of complications is encouraging, but great care must be taken in the preoperative assessment and preparation, in the operative technique and in the postoperative management of patients who are amongst the most difficult problems encountered in gastrointestinal surgery.

CONCLUSION

Minimal surgery for obstruction can safely be carried out in patients with gross diffuse Crohn's disease even though the majority of the disease is left behind.

REFERENCES
1. Lee ECG. (1980) Crohn's disease. A Global Assessment, HM-M Publishers, Aylesbury, England, in press.
2. Allsop JR, Lee ECG. (1978) Factors which influenced postoperative complications in patients with ulcerative colitis or Crohn's disease of the colon on corticosteroids. Gut 19:729-734

H14 Summary of Discussions relating to topics H11 to H13

Terpstra: As Lee has said, recurrence and relapse are
often not correctly defined and are mixed up. We
should define a recurrence as the development of a
new segment of disease, which can be shown patho-
logically, endoscopically or by X-ray, after the
surgeon has removed all obvious evidence of disease. Relapse should be used to describe a flare-up
of symptoms in a patient in whom disease is known
to be left behind after surgery, provided you have
excluded other causes for the symptoms.

O'Morain: Could Farmer correlate the rate of recurrence
with the histological evidence of active inflammation at the cut edges? Secondly, was there any correlation with who did the surgery? Also, did the
rate of recurrence depend on whether the operation
was done as an emergency procedure or as an elective one?

Farmer: All of the operations in question were performed
by only two staff-surgeons, who have worked together for close to 20 years. We have found that it
does not appear to make any difference in terms of
which of these two surgeons performed the operation. The question of whether it is a senior or a
junior surgeon is more difficult, but in our insti-
tution the senior is always present and is in
charge of the operation, so the presumption must be
that the senior surgeon was primarily responsible
for the operation. We have looked at the presence
of microscopic disease at the anastomosis and found
no correlation with recurrence. We are still analy-

sing the data and I cannot tell you whether the recurrence rate depends on whether the operation was performed as an emergency or as an elective procedure.

Lee: We have compared the rate of recurrence in patients who showed evidence of inflammation at the cut edges of resection specimens with the rate in those who did not. There was no difference and therefore I conclude that the surgeon should concentrate on removing only segments of gut that are obviously diseased to the naked eye.

Gilat: What were the indications for performing a proctocolectomy rather than an ileorectal anastomosis in Buchmann's study?

Buchmann: Only the patients with a rectum which appeared normal or only mildly or moderately inflamed were considered suitable for ileorectal anastomosis.

Lee: You have not commented on the high rate of recurrence proximal to the anastomosis after ileorectal anastomosis compared with the low rate after proctocolectomy.

Hellers: I found that the cumulative recurrence rate after ileorectal anastomosis was approximately 55% after 5 years, whereas protocolectomy and ileostomy was approximately 20% after 5 years. Nevertheless, I think that ileorectal anastomosis is still worthwhile in some circumstances. If you have an adolescent who has Crohn's colitis, an ileorectal anastomosis will carry him over a difficult period of life with natural defaecation.

15 General Discussion and Conclusions
on certain topics of the treatment

Reported by B.I. Korelitz

What conclusions can be derived about the therapy of CD based on our cumulative observations on response to specific drugs and to surgical resection?

In the past, the management of regional ileitis and ileocolitis lay essentially in the hands of the surgeon. After a resection, the patient would temporarily disappear from follow-up because he felt well or would infrequently make visits to the man who performed the operation. Should he return to the gastroenterologists at all, there were no medical weapons with which to treat the disease, and evidence of recurrent ileitis led to a referral back to the surgeon. Eventually another resection would be performed. This is well demonstrated by Farmer's contribution.

One of the few observations about the natural course of CD that has withstood the test of time concerns extension of the disease proximally. The inflammatory process tends to remain localized to its original distribution despite increased severity. Though it may extend distally in the colon coincident with clinical exacerbation, it rarely, if ever, extends proximally into the ileum without surgical resection of the bowel. We should accept the recurrence rate at the new terminal ileum after surgical resection as practical evidence that, given enough time, all patients will have a recurrence. This is most likely true following resection with ileostomy as well as with internal anastomosis, even though the recurrence appears earlier in the latter. It is also true whether there are preexisting patches of disease in proximal areas, such as the duodenum or jejunum, or not.

There are now available to us many non-surgical weapons

with which to fight this disease. Some of these are of proven value, such as corticosteroids and sulfasalazine. The efficacy of 6-mercaptopurine and total parenteral nutrition have now been established, but their exact roles require better definition. Experiences with other agents show promise but need more study. These include metronidazole, superoxide dismutase, D-penicillamine and elemental diets. We must use these drugs and non-surgical tools as skillfully as possible, considering choice, dose and timing, in order to smother the disease while awaiting a prevention or more definitive management. Meanwhile, we should continue to be keen observers so as to define the precise role of each form of treatment. The response to each drug or other mode of therapy should provide hints to our colleagues who are performing more basic research.

At the same time it has become apparent that CD surgeons and gastroenterologists are more united in their attitude toward management than ever before. The surgeon remains an essential member of the team. For the most part they agree, however, that new non-surgical options should have their trial short of absolute indications for operative intervention. Even then, the conviction that the least amount of tissue be resected is supported by Lee on minimal surgery in Crohn's disease and by Buchmann on ileorectal anastomosis. All of us seem to agree that margins of resected bowel free of disease does not improve the prognosis and, therefore, the tissue removed should be only that is grossly involved.

CLOSING REMARKS

A.J.CH. HAEX

In this short Afterword to the Proceedings of the Second International Workshop on Crohn's disease I wish to make some general remarks, as counterpart to the Preface in which J.B. Kirsner has dealt with the scientific contents, and to add a few brief comments on the structure of the workshop and the realization of this volume.

Experience has shown that in general the very intensive study of a large number of cases of a particular clinical entity forms the basis for fundamental clinical research in that field. Since it is clear that this holds for Crohn's disease, it will be useful and even necessary to establish a systematic registry of a wide variety of clinical data pertaining to a large number of patients in various phases of the disease in as many countries as possible. This systematic registration will permit the application of modern computer methods to detect interrelationships between the findings. The studies in this field initiated by the OMGE, with which the name of de Dombal in particular is associated, represent pioneering work but as yet concern only clinical data. Our insight into Crohn's disease will be greatly improved by the inclusion of data obtained via the exact scientific disciplines such as immunology, genetics, and cell biology. In the five years which have passed since our first workshop was held in 1975, immunology, cell biology, and genetics have been incorporated into the research done on Crohn's disease. It is to be expected that this trend will continue and that family studies will be given an important place.

In our opinion, an international workshop offers the best situation for the comparison, discussion, and improvement of the methods used and results obtained in different countries. We are already preparing for our next workshop.

A few words on the realization of these Proceedings seem appropriate here. The preparation involved two phases. The first began as early as the organization of the workshop, i.e., the importance assigned to the grouping of the introductions and the planning of the discussions led us to request the experts invited to serve as chairmen of the relevant sections to consult with their participants about the sequence of the presentations and the programming of the discussions and, if necessary, to make changes before and during the workshop. On the last day of the workshop these chairmen gave a short resumé of the results, conclusions, and recommendations of their section, prepared in advance together with the participants. The second phase concerned the editorial work: the chairmen edited the discussions for their own section and the over-all editing was done by the editorial board. The discussions were recorded on tape and typed during the workshop, so that the participants could be given copies for correction on the spot. As was to be expected, it proved necessary to cut the discussions considerably to bring out the essence. The papers of the participants are of course given in full, but minor changes have been made to promote uniformity. Because we considered it of major importance to have the proceedings appear as soon as possible after the workshop, the participants were notified in advance that, in order to save time, proofs would not be sent for correction.

Finally, a few words about the indirect implications of a workshop of this kind. Crohn's disease and the related affections are, because they demand a multidisciplinary approach, extremely informative models with respect to the importance of the evaluation of findings and conclusions at the international level. The old adage 'A good example is the best sermon' applies here too. Unfortunately, clinical research has gained too little acceptance among the practitioners of the exact sciences. Recently, in two articles, C.C. Booth gave a very interesting review of the history of fundamental clinical research and the present status of this research in Britain (1,2). He shows that there as well, the birth of clinical research was far from uncomplicated, even though the proper infrastructure for this research sector had been created by the setting-up of the Medical Research Council at the beginning of this century.

In The Netherlands, this branch of science is still not esteemed to the same degree as the exact sciences, for instance mathematics, physics, and astronomy. Nevertheless, the integration of the exact sciences into the clinical sciences is of the greatest importance. The exact disciplines are indispensable for the analysis — causal, pathogenic, diagnostic, therapeutic, epidemiological, genetic — of the various forms of the course of a disease. I am therefore convinced that meetings like this workshop can be of great importance for governmental bodies responsible for financial and other support for fundamental research, including clinical research. For the proper weighing of priorities in this context, international evaluation with continuity is of primary value. An independent foundation, established with or without government participation [e.g., by pharmaceutical companies, on lines similar to the CIBA Foundation], for the organization of workshops in the field of fundamental clinical research [not to be confused with symposiums] could serve as an important objective instrument in this kind of difficult decision-making. The determination of priorities is even more important in these years of economic recession than it is in times of prosperity, although the decision must be made rationally in any period.

The difficulty that the practitioners of the exact sciences have in accepting clinical research is due to the fact that the clinical sciences are often considered to be only applied sciences. The right reply to this was given by Pasteur: 'Il n'y a pas des sciences appliquées, mais il y a des applications de la science'.

I wish to close by thanking all of the participants of this second workshop on Crohn's disease for their willingness to contribute and for their contributions on many levels, both to the workshop and to this volume.

1. Booth CC. (1979) The development of clinical science in Britain. Brit.Med.J. 1:1469-1473
2. Booth CC. (1980) Clincal science in the 1980s. Lancet ii:904-907

ACKNOWLEDGEMENTS

The second International Workshop on Crohn's disease was held in Noordwijk on June 25-28, 1980. This workshop would not have been possible without the financial support of the following sponsors:

Smith Kline and French B.V., Merck Sharp and Dohme, Gist Brocades farmaca Nederland B.V., Wellcome Nederland B.V., Rhône Poulenc Nederland B.V., Janssen Pharmaceutica Nederland, The University of Leiden and the University Hospital, Leiden, The Netherlands.

We wish to express our thanks for their generous contribution, which permitted clinical investigators and scientists to come together for the advancement of research on Crohn's disease. One of us [ASP] is also indebted to the National Foundation for Ileitis and Colitis, Inc. N.Y., U.S.A.

We should like to express our gratitude to Miss L. Smit and Mr. A.A. Vos of the Department of Gastroenterology, of the University of Leiden, for their invaluable help in organizing the workshop. The help of Mrs. G.H. van der Leeden-Veltman and the members of the Workshop Secretariat is gratefully acknowledged. Hein Verspaget, Walter Mastboom, Niekje Loomans, Jan Paul Giliams, Peter Jongeleen, Tom van Rooyen, Petra Lems-van Kan, Joke van Niewenhuijzen, and Marga Meima gave generously of their time during the running of the workshop and preparation of the book.

De Baak, Noordwijk, provided an excellent atmosphere, for which we thank Mr. Mulder, the manager, and his staff. Holland International, and especially Mr. G.H. de Groot, were responsible for the well-organized transportation arrangements.

Finally, we wish to express our particular indebtness to Miss Gabrielle W. Verhoef and Mr. Izak Biemond, without whom this book could not have been realized in the present form, and to thank Hanna M. Oostvriesland, who provided assistance with the Digital Word Processor.

A.J.Ch. Haex and the Editors

Author Index

Subject Index

540

Addresses of participants

Asquith, P.	The Alastair Fraser and John Squire Metabolic and Clinical Investigation Unit, East Birmingham Hospital, Bordesley Green East, Birmingham B9 5ST, England.
Auer, I.O.	Medische Universitats Klinik, Josef Schneiderstrasse 2, D 8700 Wurzburg, West Germany.
Best, W.R.	University of Illinois Hospital, 1740 West Taylor street, Chicago, Illinois 60612, USA.
Biemond, I.	Department of Gastroenterology, University Hospital, 2333 AA Leiden, The Netherlands.
Bienenstock, J.	c/o E. Davies, Chester Beatty Research Institute, Fullham Road, London SW 36 JB, England.
Binder, V.	Medical-Gastroenterological Department C, Herlev Hospital, University of Copenhagen, Herlev Ringvej, DK-2730 Herlev, Denmark.
Booth, C.C.	Northwick Park Hospital, Clinical Research Centre, Watford Road, Harrow Middlesex HAI 3UJ, England.
Bos, L.P.	Ziekenhuis "De Goddelijke Voorzienigheid", Walstramstraat 23, 6131 BK Sittard, The Netherlands.
Buchmann, P.	Chirurg Klinik und Poliklinik A, Universitatsspital, 8091 Zurich, Switserland.
Burnham, W.R.	University Department of Therapeutics, City Hospital, Nottingham NG5 1PB, England.
Chambers, T.J.	Department of Pathology, St. Bartholomew's Hospital, West Smithfield, London, EC 1A 7BE, England.
Cohen, Z.	Toronto General Hospital, Suite CW1-102, 101 College Street, Toronto Ontario M5G 1L7, Canada.

544

Gebbers, J.-O.	Institut fur Pathologie, Kantonsspital, CH-6004, Luzern, Switserland.
Gilat, T.	Department of Gastroenterology, Ichilov Hospital, Weizmann Street, Tel-Aviv, Israel.
Ginsel, L.A.	Department of Electronmicroscopy, University Hospital, 2333 AA Leiden, The Netherlands.
Gitnick, G.L.	Department of Medicine, University of California, Center for the Health Sciences, 10833 Le Conte Avenue, Los Angeles, California 90024, USA.
Haex, A.J.Ch.	Department of Gastroenterology, University Hospital, 2333 AA Leiden, The Netherlands.
Hees van, P.A.M.	Department of Medicine, Division of Gastroenterology, St. Radboud Hospital, P.O. 9101, 6500 HB Nijmegen, The Netherlands.
Hellers, G.	Department of Surgery, Danderyd Hospital, S-182 03 Danderyd, Sweden.
Hermon-Taylor, J	Department of Surgery, St. George Hospital Medical School, Tooting-London SW17 ORE, England
Hodgson, H.J.F.	Department of Medicine, Royal Postgraduate Medical School, Hammersmith Hospital, London W 12 OHS, England.
Jarnerot, G.	Division of Gastroenterology, Department of Internal Medicine, Region Hospital, 701 85 Orebro, Sweden.
Jeejeebhoy, K.N.	Toronto General Hospital, College Wing 3-302, Toronto Ontario M5G 1L7, Canada.
Jewell, D.P.	John Radcliffe Hospital, Oxford OX 3 9DU, England.
Knapp, W.	Intitute for Immunology, University Vienna, Borchkegasse 8a, 1090 Vienna, Austria.
Korelitz, B.I.	Section of Gastroenterology, Lenox Hill Hospital, 100 East 77th Street, New York, N.Y. 10021, USA.

Kraft, S.C. Department of Medicine, Hospital Box 400, University of Chicago, 950 East 59th Street, Chicago, Illinois 60637, USA.

Krook, A. Department of Clinical Bacteriology, Central County Hospital, S 701 85 Orebro, Sweden.

Kuiper, G Department of Gastroenterology, University Hospital, 2333 AA Leiden, The Netherlands.

Langman, M.J.S. University Department of Therapeutics, City Hospital, Nottingham NG5 1PB, England.

Lee, E.C.G. Department of Surgery, John Radcliffe Hospital, Oxford OX 3 9DU, England.

Lennard-Jones, J.E. The London Hospital, Whitechapel, London E1 1BB, England.

Lloyd-Still, J.D. Northwestern University, Children's Memorial Hospital, 2300 Children Plaza, Chicago, Illinois 60614, USA.

Mayberry, J.F. Department of Gastroenterology, University Hospital of Wales, Heath Park, Cardiff CF 4 4XW, Wales, UK.

McConnell, R.B. Gastro-Enterology Unit, Broadgreen Hospital, Liverpool L14 3LB, England.

MacDermott, R.P. Division of Gastroenterology, Washington University Medical School, 772 Wohl Clinic Building, Box 8124, 660 S Euclid Avenue, St. Louis Missouri 63110, USA.

Meer van der,J.W.M. Department of Cellular Immunology, University Hospital, 2333 AA Leiden, The Netherlands.

Meera Khan, P. Department of Human Genetics, University Medical Centre, 2333 AL Leiden, The Netherlands.

Merwe van de J.P. Department of Microbiology, Erasmus University, P.O. 1738, 3000 DR Rotterdam, The Netherlands.

Meuwissen, S.G.M. Department of Internal Medicine, University Hospital, Free University Amsterdam, De Boelelaan 1117, 1007 MB Amsterdam, The Netherlands.

Meijer, C.J.L.M. Department of Pathology, University Medical Centre, P.O. 9603, 2333 RC Leiden, The Netherlands.

Natarayan, A.T. Department of Radiation Genetics and Chemical Mutagenesis, University Medical Centre, Wassenaarseweg 72, 2333 AL Leiden, The Netherlands.

O'Morain, C. Department of Gastroenterology, Northwick Park Hospital, Clinical Research Centre, Watford Road, Harrow, Middlesex HAI 3UJ, England.

Pajares Garcia,J.M. Department of Medicine, Division of Gastroenterology, Autonoma University, Gran Hospital, Diego de Leon 62, Madrid-6, Spain.

Peña, A.S. Department of Gastroenterology, University Hospital, 2333 AA Leiden, The Netherlands.

Phillpotts, R.J. Department of Surgery, St. George Hospital Medical School, Tooting-London SW17 ORE, England.

Rhodes, J.M. The Royal Free Hospital, Pond street, London NW3 2QG, England.

Riis, P. Department of Gastroenterology, Faculty of Medicine, University of Copenhagen, Herlev Ringvej, DK 2730, Herlev, Denmark.

Rosekrans, P.C.M. Department of Gastroenterology, University Hospital, 2333 AA Leiden, The Netherlands.

Saene van, H.K.F. Laboratory for Microbiology, University Hospital, Oostersingel 59, 9700 HB Groningen, The Netherlands.

Schmitz-Moormann, P. Department of Pathology, Philipps-Universitat, Robert-Koch-Strasse 5, 3550 Marnburg:Lahn, Germany.

Shmerling, D.H. Eleonorenstiftung, Universitats Kinderklinik, Steinwiesstrasse 75, CH-8032 Zurich, Switserland.

Shorter, R.G. Department of Pathology and Medicine, Mayo Clinic, Rochester, M.N. 55901, USA.

Soltis, R.D.   Department of Medicine, Box 308, Mayo, University of Minnesota Medical School, 420 Delawarestreet S.E., Minneapolis, MN 55455, USA.

Sommers, S.C.   Lenox Hill Hospital, 100 East 77th Street, New York, N.Y. 10021, USA.

Stanford, J.L.   Department of Microbiology, School of Pathology, The Middlesex Hospital Medical School, Riding House Street, London WIP 7 LD, England.

Strickland, R.G.   Division of Gastroenterology, Department of Medicine, University of New Mexico, School of Medicine, Albuquerque, New Mexico 87131, USA.

Strober, W.   National Institutes of Health, National Cancer Institute, Building 10, Room 4N 114, Bethesda, Md 20205, USA.

Terpstra, J.L.   Department of Surgery, University Hospital, 2333 AA Leiden, The Netherlands.

Thayer, W.R.   Division of Gastroenterology, Department of Medicine, Brown University, Rhode Island Hospital, 593 Eddy St. A.P.C. Room 421, Providence, Rhode Island 02903, USA.

Thompson, H.   Department of Histology, The General Hospital, Steel House Lane, Birmingham B4 6NH, England.

Tongeren van, J.H.M.   Department of Medicine, Division of Gastroenterology, St. Radboud Hospital, P.O. 9101, 6500 HB Nijmegen, The Netherlands.

Truelove, S.C.   Nuffield Department of Clinical Medicine, The Radcliffe Infirmary, Oxford OX2 6HE, England.

Tijtgat, G.N.   Department of Medicine, Division of Gastroenterology, University of Amsterdam, Eerste Helmersstraat 104, 1054 EG Amsterdam, The Netherlands.

Valkenburg, H.A.   Insitute for Epidemiology, Department of Medicine, Erasmus University, P.O. 1738, 3000 DR Rotterdam, The Netherlands.

Verspaget, H.W.

Department of Gastroenterology, University Hospital 2333 AA Leiden, The Netherlands.

Versteeg, J.

Laboratory of Medical Microbiology, University Medical Centre, 2333 AL Leiden, The Netherlands.

Waaij van der, D.

Laboratory of Medical Microbiology, University Hospital, Oostersingel 59, 9700 HB Groningen, The Netherlands.

Wensinck, F.

Department of Medical Microbiology, Medical Faculty, Erasmus University, P.O. 1783, 3000 DR Rotterdam, The Netherlands.

Weterman, I.T.

Department of Gastroenterology, University Hospital, 2333 AA Leiden, The Netherlands.

White, S.A.

Department of Microbiology, School of Pathology, Middlesex Hospital Medical School, London WIP 7 LD, England.

Yardley, J.A.

Department of Pathology, The Johns Hopkins Hospital, Baltimore MD 21205, USA.